A. C. Yankah · M. H. Yacoub · R. Hetzer

Editors

Cardiac Valve Allografts

Science
and Practice

Foreword
by D. N. Ross

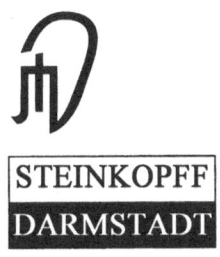
STEINKOPFF
DARMSTADT

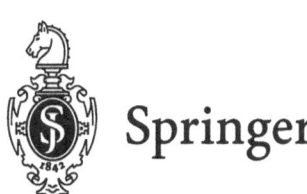
Springer

Editors

Sir Magdi H. Yacoub, FRCS
Professor and Director
Dept. Cardiothoracic Surgery
Harefield Hospital
Royal Brompton Hospital and
National Heart and Lung Institute
London
UK

Roland Hetzer, MD, PhD
Professor, Chairman and Director
Deutsches Herzzentrum Berlin and
Humboldt University
Dept. Cardiothoracic and Vascular Surgery
Augustenburger Platz 1
D-13353 Berlin
Germany

A. Charles Yankah, MD, PhD
Consultant, Assistant Professor
Deutsches Herzzentrum Berlin and
Humboldt University
Dept. Cardiothoracic and Vascular Surgery
Augustenburger Platz 1
D-13353 Berlin
Germany

Die Deutsche Bibliothek – CIP-Einheitsaufnahme

Cardiac valve allografts : science and practice / A. C. Yankah ... ed.
Foreword by D. N. Ross. – Darmstadt : Steinkopff ; New York :
Springer, 1997
   ISBN 978-3-642-63915-9   ISBN 978-3-642-59250-8 (eBook)
   DOI 10.1007/978-3-642-59250-8

© 1997 by Springer-Verlag Berlin Heidelberg
Originally published by Dr. Dietrich Steinkopff Verlag GmbH & Co. K.G. Darmstadt in 1997
Medical Editor: Beate Rühlemann – English Editor: James C. Willis – Production: Heinz J. Schäfer
Cover Design: Erich Kirchner, Heidelberg

Typesetting: Macmillan India Ltd., Bangalore

Printed on acid-free paper

Foreword

Having been associated with the successful launch of the first edition of this book it was clear that it would merit a second edition and this is now provided by Doctor Yankah and my respected colleague Professor Sir Magdi Yacoub.

Although the homograft story goes back a number of years it has progressively gathered strength and new adherents. I for one have never doubled its triumphant progress. Unlike man-made offerings which come and go like the seasons, the homograft was conceived not on this earth but in a celestial design centre with not just several years but millions of years of background and testing. This makes it unlikely to be bettered now or in the future and this message has slowly taken root in the cardiac surgical community.

No particular or spectacular surgical developments have occurred recently apart from technical changes like the free standing root implantation. On the other hand there is a growing awareness that all homologous tissue is subject to the body's antigenic reactions. Consequently for a long-term or permanent valve replacement this reaction must be immunosuppressed or avoided by the use of autogenous tissues. Hence the increasing interest in the pulmonary autograft as a logical development.

This edition quite correctly allocates a good deal of time and space to the problems of immunology and preservation techniques including cryopreservation. The latter is extremely useful for storage and stockpiling but incorporates the not necessarily beneficial effect of preserving antigenicity which in the infant can result in rejection.

The book surveys a wide and increasing spectrum of the work and is right up to date including mitral and tricuspid homografts – aspects of the valve replacement story long overdue.

Xenotransplantation has perhaps not earned its place in this volume but provided the body's acceptance of these tissues can be achieved perhaps by gene manipulation or new immunosuppressives then we should reserve space for this topic in the next edition.

Donald N. Ross

Preface

This book is updating the first edition which was published after an international meeting on the "Use of Cardiac Valve Allografts" in September 1987 in Berlin. The successful meeting commemorated the 25th anniversary of the clinical allograft valve surgery in honour of the two pioneer surgeons Mr. Donald Ross, London, UK and Brian Barratt-Boyes, Auckland, New Zealand. The invited speakers highlighted on the basic immunology of allograft valve surgery, the use of cryopreserved vs. refrigerated (4 °C) valve allograft and orthotopic implantation of pulmonary allografts. Now cardiac valve allograft surgery is being practiced in many centers world-wide for over 34 years. The global acceptance of this operation after some years of unpopularity owning to early valve failures was attributed to factors such as 1. improved preservation techniques (cryopreservation), 2. standardized implantation techniques and 3. defined and established surgical and medical indications for repair or congenital heart valve defects, aortic mycotic infections and complicated endocarditis.

The above mentioned factors have subsequently improved the durability and hemodynamic performance and clinical results as well as patient's survival. The increasing interest in allograft valve surgery has subsequently led to a higher demand for more allograft valves of different sizes than before which is now an issue of great concern to many allograft valve bankers because of the limited supply. The aortic and mitral valves have a highly sophisticated structure best suited to the equally sophisticated function. Recently basic science techniques have allowed valuable insights into both structure and functional aspects of the valves, as well as into factors which could influence durability and thorough understanding of these issues could have a major impact on clinical results.

This book is presenting recently updated knowledge related to harvesting, banking, implantation and also revival of homograft mitral and tricuspid valve surgery, making it a highly authoritative reference source for practising cardiac surgeons and physicians. With the increasing number of surgeons going through the learning curve of allograft valve implantation one will expect reports on varying clinical results. This book will therefore highlight on the views and recommendations from experienced world renowned surgeons on the current controversy on implantation techniques of allograft valves; the subcoronary freehand valve and the root replacement. The readership will be given the option to appreciate the clinical benefits of the pulmonary autograft in aortic position as an alternative valve substitute for immunologically high risk patients. It is hoped that this book will be of value to the practicing cardiologists and cardiac surgeons as well as researchers interested in this field.

We are grateful to Mrs. B. Rühlemann and Mrs. S. Ibkendanz, of the publishers Steinkopff Verlag, for their excellent cooperation in bringing this work to publication in a timely manner. We also wish to thank Mrs. A. Benhennour, our librarian, for her assistance in compiling the bibliographies and Mrs. A. Gaußmann and Mr. H. Hasselbach for their exceptional graphic design work.

Lastly we would like to thank all the contributing authors for their great interests and efforts towards the success of this book.

A. Charles Yankah
Sir Magdi H. Yacoub
Roland Hetzer

Contents

Allograft Aortic Valve and Root Replacement

Alternative Procedures

Autografts

Infectious Aortic Valve and Thoracic Aorta

Aortic and Pulmonary Allografts for Reconstruction of the Right Ventricular Outflow Tract (Orthotopic and Heterotopic Implantation)

Homograft Mitral and Tricuspid Valve Replacement

Contributors

C. Acar, MD
Paris, France

L.C. Armiger, MD
Auckland, New Zealand

D.R. Clarke, MD
Denver, Colorado,
USA

P.E. Dawson
Marietta, GA, USA

W. Daenen, MD, PhD
Leuven, Belgium

X.J. Feng, MD, PhD
Antwerp, Belgium

D.M. Fronk, PhD
Marietta, GA, USA

D.A. Haydock, MD
Auckland, New Zealand

R. Hetzer, MD, PhD
Berlin, Germany

F.M.E. Hoekstra, MD
Rotterdam,
The Netherlands

F.M. Lupinetti, MD
Seattle, Washington,
USA

C.A. Mestres, MD, PhD
Barcelona, Spain

D. Metras, MD
Marseille, France

J.L. Monro, FRCS
Southampton, UK

J.D. Oswalt, MD
Austin, Texas, USA

R. Parker, M.Sc.
London, UK

G. Pettersson, MD
Copenhagen, Denmark

T. Ramos, MD
Santa Cruz, Portugal

J.M. Revuelta, MD, PhD
Santander, Spain

F. Robicsek, MD
Charlotte,
North Carolina, USA

D.N. Ross, FRCS
London, UK

A. Schütz, MD, PhD
München, Germany

E. Simon, MD
Kiel, Germany

K. Turley, MD
San Francisco, CA, USA

P.R. Vogt, MD
Zürich, Switzerland

J. Weipert, MD
München, Germany

T.P. Willems, MD
Rotterdam,
The Netherlands

D. Woloszyn
Harefield, Middx, UK

M.H. Yacoub, FRCS
Harefield, London
UK

A.C. Yankah, MD, PhD
Berlin, Germany

Standards and technical guidelines for heart valve banking

R. Parker

Royal Brompton Hospital London, England

Introduction

The American Association of Tissue Banks (A.A.T.B.) and the European Association of Tissue Banks (E.A.T.B.) have both issued general standards for tissue banking within their continents and several governments and organisations in Europe have formulated their own standards and technical guidelines which can differ from those of the E.A.T.B. The Asia Pacific Association of Surgical Tissue Banks have as yet not issued any standards, but the Australian Government have issued a section in their Code of Good Manufacturing Practice for Therapeutic Goods on Human Tissue, which is more similar to the Standard Operating Procedures issued by some banks. Many non commercial organisations on both sides of the Atlantic have also publicly available guidelines or technical manuals to which they work. There are parts of the A.A.T.B. Standards that are legally required if the bank requests accreditation from the Food and Drug Administration of that country, whereas those of the E.A.T.B. are a voluntary code and have no effect in law. Both sets of standards cover tissue banking in general and are then designed to have specific sections for each tissue, but in the case of E.A.T.B. only the sperm banking specialised section has been completed. The A.A.T.B. document is considerably more complex than the E.A.T.B. one and the aim of this chapter is to give an outline of the topics covered in these standards. The American Standards are subdivided into 12 sections, whilst the European ones have seven, three of the extra sections being needed as tissue banking in America tends to be performed by companies like Cryolife and Lifenet, whereas in Europe tissue banks are usually parts of hospitals or blood transfusion service.

General institutional requirements

It is a requirement in all standards that the purpose of the Tissue Bank is clearly established and documented. In America it is obligatory for the bank to have both a governing body and a medical advisory committee, whereas in the European Standards, the former is not mentioned and the latter is only recommended. The running of the Tissue Bank in America is vested in the Director, who need not be a medically qualified person, while in Europe this power is given to the Medical Director. In America a Medical Director is also required and in Europe the Medical Director can delegate certain responsibilities to a Managing Director. The American Standards lay far more importance to the fact that the staff are suitably qualified, while the European idea relies more on training. Quality Assurance needs independent staff under the American Standards, but only a programme in Europe. It is agreed in both sets of Standards that records must be confidential, accurate, complete, legible and indelible and be kept for a minimum of ten years after the last expiration date of the tissue involved. A tracking system must be used so tissue can be traced from donor to recipient and vice versa. European Standards are more rigorous on environmental safety and facilities and equipment, but these points are covered in greater detail in the technical manuals of A.A.T.B.

Acquisition of tissues

As consent for donation of tissue is covered by federal law in U.S.A. the A.A.T.B. Standards can be explicit on this subject, while the E.A.T.B. Standards have to derogate this to the national legislation of each country. Because of this fact, the E.A.T.B. has produced a fuller set of ethical rules than the A.A.T.B. to provide a minimum level across Europe as some nations have little or no laws on tissue for transplantation. It is agreed on both sides of the Atlantic that no financial inducements should be made to living donors, next of kin or the donor's estate for donation, but that the tissue bank may reimburse parties for costs directly associated with donation. Standards agree that the suitability of a specific individual for tissue donation shall be based upon medical and social history, physical examination, blood tests and autopsy (if performed). It is agreed that donors with a clinical history of viral hepatitis, HIV, active tuberculosis or untreated syphilis should be rejected, together with those who have received pituitary derived human growth hormone or who have died from degenerative neurologic disorders of viral or unknown aetiology. Donors belonging to a high risk category for HIV infection or hepatitis should also be excluded. The acceptability of donors with a history of malignancy must be evaluated by the Medical Director. Both sets of standards agree that the minimum serological tests that must be performed shall include:
  HIV 1 & 2 antibody
  Hepatitis B virus surface antigen
  Hepatitis C virus antibody
  Syphilis.
The A.A.T.B. Standards also require HTLV type 1 antibody. For living donors tissues should be quarantined for 180 days until a repeat test for HIV 1 & 2 and Hepatitis C is performed on donor. Both sets of standards emphasise the importance of restoring the body of cadaveric donors to its original state, out of respect to the deceased and their relatives.

Processing, preservation and storage

Standards dictate that all steps in processing, preservation and storage must be validated to ensure that the procedures render the tissue suitable for its intended clinical use. Pooling of tissues from more than one donor is prohibited because of the risk of cross contamination. The A.A.T.B. Standards are far more explicit in what records must be kept and in the properties of the storage containers. All tissue must be given an expiration date appropriate to its processing, packaging and intended application.

Tissue release

This is one of the sections that only appears in the A.A.T.B. Standards and defines what the Medical Director, or licensed physician designee must review before the tissue can be released for clinical use. This list includes the consent, medical records, autopsy report (if performed), sexual history questionnaire, laboratory tests, the quality assurance review performed by an independent person and that everything was performed according to the Bank's Standard Operating Procedures. The E.A.T.B. Standards do not proscribe in other sections a review procedure either in terms of person responsible or subjects covered.

Labelling

There are two main parts to labelling, the first is what appears on the container holding the heart valve and the second is the package insert. The label on the container must include the name of the tissue, the name and address of tissue bank, the tissue identification number, the expiration date and recommended storage conditions. The American Standards give a far longer list for the package insert than the European ones, but both require statements about serological status of donor, that tissue is for single patient use, indications and contraindications for use and a list of antibiotics and other agents used in the processing of the tissue.

Distribution

All Standards agree that there should be written procedures and documentation for all tissues distributed and that tissues can only be distributed to hospitals, tissue banks, physicians and other qualified medical or research professionals. In addition the American Standards allow distribution to tissue brokers, but the latter agents do not exist in the same form in Europe so do not get mentioned in E.A.T.B. Standards. Tissue Banks must ensure that environmental conditions during transit meet the required parameters and that the packaging ensures integrity and prevents contamination. Tissue Banks must have a policy for authorising or prohibiting the return of unused tissue and a protocol for evaluating that the tissue can still be used clinically if it is accepted back. It is also necessary for tissue banks to have a written procedure for recall of tissue and have suitable tracking procedures to be able to do this. The American Standards have sections on Tissue Dispensing Services and Brokers outlining this responsibilities with regard to the distribution of tissue and stating that they must keep records to the same standard as tissue bank.

Technical guidelines

At the present time the American Association of Tissue Banks are rewriting the technical guidelines for the processing of cardiovascular tissue and the updated version should be finalised during 1996. The European Association of Tissue Banks has completed the technical guidelines for sperm and skeletal tissue banking, but little progress has been made on the section on cardiovascular tissue, so it is likely to be at least 1997 before these are available. Most American Banks already have their own technical guidelines and some like American Red Cross Tissue Services have published theirs. National organisations like the British Association of Tissue Banks, French Blood Transfusion Service and National Blood Service in United Kingdom have set their own standards and produced technical guidelines and these are available from these organisations.

These technical guidelines give further criteria that are specific for cardiac tissue, whereas the main standards are for all tissues. For example they will disqualify heart valve donation from donors who have received significant chest trauma, cardiac massage or have a history of infective endocarditis or rheumatic fever. They set time and temperature limits on each stage of procurement and give additional microbiological testing (such as for mycobacteria) that should be performed. At present most guidelines suggest that heart valves removed under aseptic conditions but not antibiotic sterilised should be used within 48 h if stored at $+4\,^{\circ}$C, antibiotic sterilised valves at $+4\,^{\circ}$C should be used by 21 days and that valves cryopreserved below $-135\,^{\circ}$C can be stored for 5 or 10 years.

References

1. American Association of Tissue Banks Standards for Tissue Banking (1995) Published by A.A.T.B., McLean, VA, U.S.A.
2. Australian Code of Good Manufacturing Practice for Therapeutic Goods – Human Tissue (1995) Published by Commonwealth Department of Human Services And Health, Canberra, Australia
3. British Association of Tissue Banks Standards for Tissue Banking (1995) Published by B.A.T.B., London, United Kingdom
4. European Association of Tissue Banks General Standards for Tissue Banking (1995) Published by E.A.T.B., Vienna, Austria
5. Standards of the American Red Cross Tissue Services (1994) Published by American Red Cross Tissue Services, Costa Mesa, CA, U.S.A.

Author's address:
R. Parker, M.Sc.
Homograft Department
Royal Brompton Hospital
Sydney Street
London SW3 6NP
England

An international survey of allograft banks

R. Parker

Royal Brompton Hospital, London, UK

Introduction

When heart valve allografts were first implanted in 1962, most hospitals procured their own valves by obtaining hearts from donors who had died in local hospitals. In the 1960s the selection criteria was wide and vague, virology testing minimal and follow-up in many centres non-existent. The trend over the years has been to attmept to introduce standards, either voluntary or by legislation (as in U.S.A. and Belgium) which has led to heart valve banking being centralised into fewer centres. For the purposes of this paper the banks have been categorised into four main groups namely Mainland Europe, United Kingdom, North America and Australasia as each area has basically similar procedures.

Number of banks

In 1995, the author knows of 68 heart valve banks world-wide and these are situated in the countries shown in Table 1. It is likely that there are more heart valve banks in China and the former states of USSR than given in the table. The author wrote to all the banks known to him and the results given in this chapter are compiled from the information he received. There was a 76% reply rate to the questionnaire with the non-responders being mostly the small surgeon-run banks. The greatest concentration of heart valve banks in any country is in United Kingdom, where in 1995 nine were active. In the rest of Europe there were another 34. At the present time there is only one active bank on the African continent, but one should open in Ghana in 1996. South America has shown the greatest expansion of heart valve banks over the last few years, with banks open in Argentina and Brazil already and ones likely to begin in Colombia, Venezuela and Chile within 3 years.

Heart valve bank activity

In the 52 banks which responded, 6583 hearts were collected in 1994 with the greatest numbers being by banks in North America, which had one bank obtaining over 2000 hearts in the year. United Kingdom banks processed 127 hearts on average with

Table 1. Location of heart valve banks

Argentina	2	Italy	6
Australia	4	Lithuania	1
Austria	2	Netherlands	1
Belgium	2	New Zealand	1
Brazil	3	Poland	3
Canada	1	Portugal	1
China	1	Russia	5
Czech Republic	2	South Africa	1
France	2	Spain	3
Germany	2	Sweden	3
Hungary	1	Taiwan	1
India	2	United States	7
Iran	1	United Kingdom	9
Ireland	1		

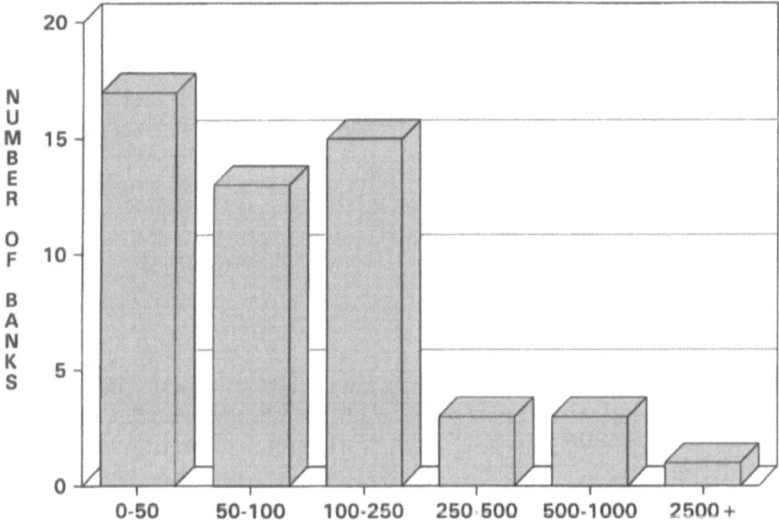

Fig. 1. Annual turnover of allografts.

banks in Mainland Europe and Australasia dissecting half that number normally, and with the banks scattered in the other nations around the world mostly doing less than 40 per year with three in single figures.

The retrieval rate for aortic valves was remarkably consistent in countries throughout the world at an average of 74% whereas pulmonary valve retrieval rates varied from 80% in North America to 49% in Australasia. Figure 1 gives the number of banks and number of aortic and pulmonary valves dissected. The only banks who collect significant numbers of mitral valve allografts are in France and Spain, with these two countries also being the ones who harvested the five tricuspid valves that were banked world-wide in 1994.

Criteria for selection

The general consensus of banks is that the maximum age for heart valve donation should be 55 or 60, with two banks accepting up to 75 years of age in some cases and one bank having a cut off at 40. There is no agreement on the minimum age that is acceptable, with many European banks taking newborn infants, whilst American banks tend to define a minimum weight (often 4.5 Kg) rather than an age.

It is agreed worldwide that the donors of heart valves must be tested for HIV 1 and 2 and Hepatitis B surface antigen (HbsAg) but 60% of banks also test for Hepatitis B core antibody. 94% of banks worldwide test for Hepatitis C and 85% test for mycobacteria with the banks who do not test for the latter being in countries of low tuberculosis incidence. American banks also test for HTLV, but this test is not widely performed in other countries but is likely to be required in Europe within 2 years.

The acceptability of valves taken from donors who have died from brain tumours varies widely between heart valve banks with over 80% of banks in United Kingdom, North America and Australasia accepting them, but only 54% in Mainland Europe and 14% outside the above mentioned areas. Most banks outside North America and United Kingdom will not consider donors who have other malignancies, but U.S.A., Canada and United Kingdom will accept these donors under certain specified conditions.

Timing

Many European banks (see Table 2) rely on beating heart rather than cadaveric donors as their main source for heart valves. These donors can be the recipients of heart transplants or people who have been considered as heart donors, but who do not meet all the criteria. The larger banks in all countries tend to have a higher proportion of cadaveric donors probably to meet the demand of the many hospitals who procure valves from them, whereas the smaller banks which only supply one or two hospitals can obtain sufficient supplies from the beating heart source.

For the cadaveric donors the maximum time between death and removal from the body in bank's criteria varies from 2 to 72 h with the greatest number of banks choosing 24 or 48 h. Once the heart has been removed from the donor (whether beating heart or cadaver) banks mostly consider that the valves should be placed in solution within 12 h, but many banks worldwide stipulate a total time from death to sterilising solution of 24 or 48 h.

Table 2. Percentage of valves from beating heart donors

Mainland Europe	62%
United Kingdom	40%
U.S.A. and Canada	35%
Australasia	29%

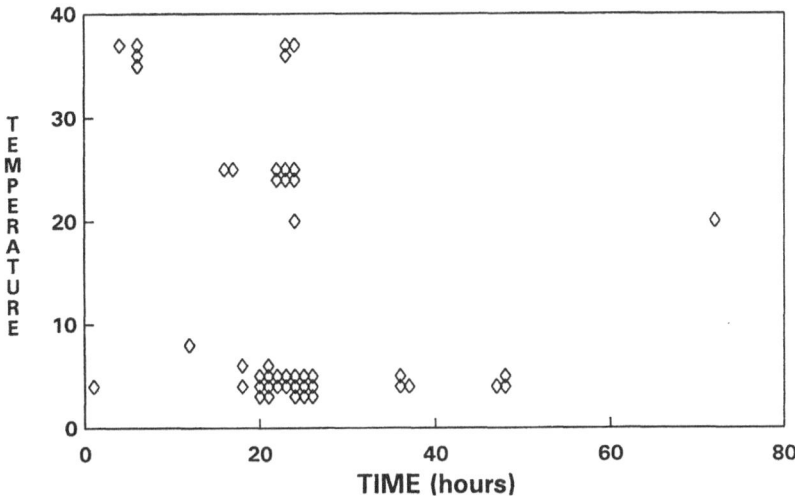

Fig. 2. Antibiotic sterilisation temperature and time.

Method of sterilisation

All banks worldwide now use antibiotic rather than chemical or radiation sterilisaton, but the concentration and composition of antibiotic medium used in heart valve banks varies tremendously, partly depending on whether the heart was removed under sterile or non-sterile conditions, with many banks using separate formulae for valves taken under the two conditions. The majority of banks using cadaveric donors include an antifungal agent (normally nystatin or amphotericin) in their mixture. Figure 2 shows the scatter of antibiotic time and temperature used by banks. Most Mainland Europe and American banks favour 4 °C for the antibiotic phase, whereas United Kingdom banks favour room temperature (20–25 °C) and Australian banks prefer 37 °C.

Preservation

The majority of heart valve banks world-wide store at least a proportion of their valves at cryogenic temperatures, with this being the only method employed in North America and Australia. Some banks store the heart valves removed from heart transplant recipients in nutrient solution without antibiotics for up to 48 h at +4 °C for use as homovital valves, whereas they use low temperature for all other valves. The small number of banks worldwide which store all their valves at +4 °C normally plan on a shelf-life of 6 weeks with one storing for up to 12 weeks, while cryogenically stored valves are given an expiry date 5 years after freezing, but under new guidelines in Europe this is to be extended to 10 years.

Table 3. Processing charge in US$ for heart valves

	Range	Average
U.S.A. and Canada	2225–5700	4804
Mainland Europe	0–3440	1785
United Kingdom	0–2128	1417
Australasia	795–1130	1006

Charges

There is a far greater trade of heart valves between countries in Europe than in other continents, with only one American bank supplying hospitals outside the United States and no Australian banks supplying outside that continent. It also seems that European banks supply to other continents with records of allografts being sent to South America, Asia and Australia from that continent. As money is playing an ever increasing role in medicine it is interesting to note that the processing charges levied by banks for their valves used in other hospitals vary from zero to $5700 with the range and average of charges in the various continents being given in Table 3. In Belgium the price of 85000 Belgian Francs is set by the government and many European countries have legislation outlining that only specific costs may be re-claimed in the price.

Author's address:
R. Parker, M.Sc.
Homograft Department
Royal Brompton Hospital
Sydney Street
London SW3 6NP, UK

Homograft viability, assessment and significance

D. Woloszyn, D. Johnson, M. H. Yacoub

Imperial College, National Heart and Lung Institute, Heart Science Centre, Harefield Hospital, Harefield, Middx., England

Introduction

Human valve allografts have become popular substitutes for diseased valves because in comparison to other valve substitutes (bioprothetic and prosthetic), human cardiac allografts are considered to be superior in haemodynamic performance, relatively resistant to endocarditis, have minimal thromboembolic complications and do not require anticoagulation (1–4). However, the main disadvantages of human cardiac allografts over prosthetic valves are that they have relatively limited availability, they are more difficult to insert and have limited durability (4).

Over recent years, in response to results from different clinical follow up studies, the allograft valve has undergone many changes in methods of procurement, sterilisation and preservation (5–10). The spectrum ranges from chemical treatment (aldehydes, β-propiolactone), irradiation, ethylene oxide to storage in antibiotic, nutrient medium or cryopreservation in the vapour phase of liquid nitrogen (3). This is because these results have shown that heretofore harshly processed valves were not durable (11), suggesting that maintanence of viable valve cusp tissue components may result in optimal valve durability after implantation (1–3, 8–10, 12). In fact since the establishment of the less severe processing techniques used today, there have been significant improvements in the long-term performance of allograft valves (8, 9, 11, 12), although the reasons for this remain obscure and need to be elucidated.

Currently there are three types of human cardiac allograft valves used in heart valve replacement:

Homovital (12): These are harvested under sterile conditions from heart transplant recipients or brain dead multi-organ donors and kept in tissue culture medium and inserted at first available opportunity.

Antibiotic sterilised (*otherwise known as 'fresh homografts'*) (6–7): These are harvested from cadavers or multi-organ donors under aseptic conditions, up to 72 h post mortem. These are then sterilised by exposure to multiple antibiotic, nutrient solution for various brief intervals (usually 24 h) at 37 °C, which can then be stored for up to 6 weeks at 4 °C.

Cryopreserved (8–9): Once homografts have been sterilised they can then be frozen at a controlled rate (-1 °C/min) with 10% dimethylsulphoxide (DMSO) as a cryoprotectant (preventing intracellular and intercellular ice crystal formation) and stored at -140 °C for up to 5 years.

Importance of maintaining viability

Viability is the ability of the system to carry on its physiological function. It is considered reasonable to assume that if a valve is living it should maintain its structure and consequently function for a long time. It has been proposed that the only critical determinants of long-term durability are the quality and stability of the extracellular matrix (ECM) and the collagenous skeleton (14). Nevertheless current research is based on the presumption that high pre-implantation valve *"cellular viability"* is the key to improving long-term performance of homografts (2, 8, 12–13). This is because valve intersticial cells, particularly fibroblasts, possess the capacity to maintain structural and functional integrity through continued synthesis and re-modelling (7, 14, 15) of the amorphous and fibrillar (ECM) (5, 8, 15, 16). However, the viability theory was founded on the "immunological privilege" doctrine, which has now been seriously challenged since valve endothelial cells have been shown to express major histocompatibility complex (MHC) class I and II molecules promoting a potential immunogenic surface (17–20), so it can no longer be assumed that donor cells alive at transplantation will necessarily survive and function indefinitely (21). It has been suggested that donor cells are only likely to persist if there has been a good tissue match (21). Another alternative to the cellular viability rationale is that host endothelial and fibroblast cells can grow into or onto structurally intact leaflet ground substance (10, 22), replacing lost or unviable donor cells, so perhaps donor cell viability itself is not important but preservation of leaflet ground substance is. A homograft with intact ground substance can allow the host cells to repopulate the leaflet; if that is the case presence of viable cells may be important as an index of collagen and the ECM structural integrity (23).

Methods of assessing viability

It is important to assess viability on a quantitative basis (7) in order to determine the overall quality of processing and preservation of allograft valves and subsequently perfect the freezing and storage methods. There are several well established methods for assessing homograft viability. These are listed in Table 1 and discussed below.

1) Measuring the metabolic activity of the cellular components. This can be achieved by:
a) measuring synthesis and release, by endothelial cells, of the vasoactive molecules prostacyclin (PGI_2) (13, 23–26) and nitric oxide (NO) (27) which are thought to be

Table 1. A summary of some of the various methods used for assessing valve allograft viability.

Viability assay	Component tested	References
Protein synthesis	fibroblasts	10, 16, 30–33
Prostacyclin/Nitric oxide release	endothelial cells (ECs)	13, 23–27
Proliferation (in vitro/in vivo)	fibroblasts + ECs	5, 7
Dye exclusion	fibroblasts + ECs	26, 38
Flow cytometry	fibroblasts + ECs	35
Morphological	valve morphology	10, 13, 14
Cell culture	fibroblasts + ECs	26, 36
High performance liquid chromatography	fibroblasts + ECs	37, 38

involved in preventing thrombosis (5). Endothelial cells are also important in that they nourish fibroblasts (24, 28), stimulate collagen production (29), retain proteoglycans in the valve leaflet matrix (13, 25), and reduce calcification (28). In order to distinguish between metabolically responsive and unresponsive cells both the basal and stimulated production of PGI_2/NO is measured. Basal release can occur from dead cells, but if there is a further increase in PGI_2 or NO production in response to stimulation, it is evident that there is intact and actively responsive biochemical machinery (5, 25) (Fig 1).

b) measuring amino acid incorporation into cellular components i.e. protein synthesis. This is an established method for measuring fibroblast viability, using the interchangeable incorporation of the radioactive precursors ^3H proline and ^3H inulin, (10, 16, 30–33). As already discussed, many studies have focused on fibroblast viability, since it is thought to be a pre-requisite for the long-term function of transplanted valves (8, 15, 16). These studies are based on the theory that cells must continually synthesise protein *de novo* in order to remain viable and so is thought to be a reliable assay method. Autoradiography has also been used to distinguish between cell death and impaired protein synthesis of each cell, e.g. one group (15) compared the in vivo uptake of ^3H-methionine, which is predominantly incorporated in non-collagenous proteins, and ^3H-proline which is predominately incorporated into collagen, to look at protein synthesis into aortic valves.

The results of the such experiments can be misleading in that metabolic status is not necessarily associated with the presence of intact viable cells and should not be used as a sole method of assessing status of valves (21).

2) Cellular proliferation, in vitro and in vivo.
This assay gives an indication of the reproductive potential of cells by measuring the incorporation of radioactive nucleic acid precursors, most commonly ^3H-thymidine (8), into newly synthesised DNA. However, this is not give a definitive indication of the reproductive capacity of the cell, as cells may still have the ability to replicate but are not doing so at the time of measurement. Therefore, this may provide an inaccurate measurement giving a low end estimate of viability (5).

3) Dye exclusion (26, 34)
This assay utilizes the difference between live and dead cell membrane permeability. Dyes such as Trypan Blue are unable to penetrate the membrane of viable cells, staining only cells with irreversibly injured cell membranes. The proportion of dead cells can be visualised by light microscopy. This is an insensitive measure of viability (6), as it is based on the absence of an effect. Some cells otherwise incapable of replication, protein synthesis and other essential cellular functions may fail to stain under certain conditions.

4) Flow cytometry (35)
This assay is based on the same principles as dye exclusion. Fluorescein diacetate (FDA) stains viable cells by binding to nucleic acids, acid mucopolysaccharides and polyphosphates. Propidium iodide (PI) enters injured or dead cells forming a complex with nucleic acids. Flourescing cells are counted and the intensity of flourescence measured by FACS analysis. This is a rapid, convenient and sensitive method for assessing cellular viability.

5) Morphology (10, 13, 14)
The morphological integrity of the valve can be examined using immunohistochemistry and scanning or transmission electron microscopy. A major drawback of all these techniques is that they require extensive specimen preparation and highly specialised equipment. It is also difficult to examine large areas thoroughly and it is not always possible to distinguish between the endothelium and underlying structures.

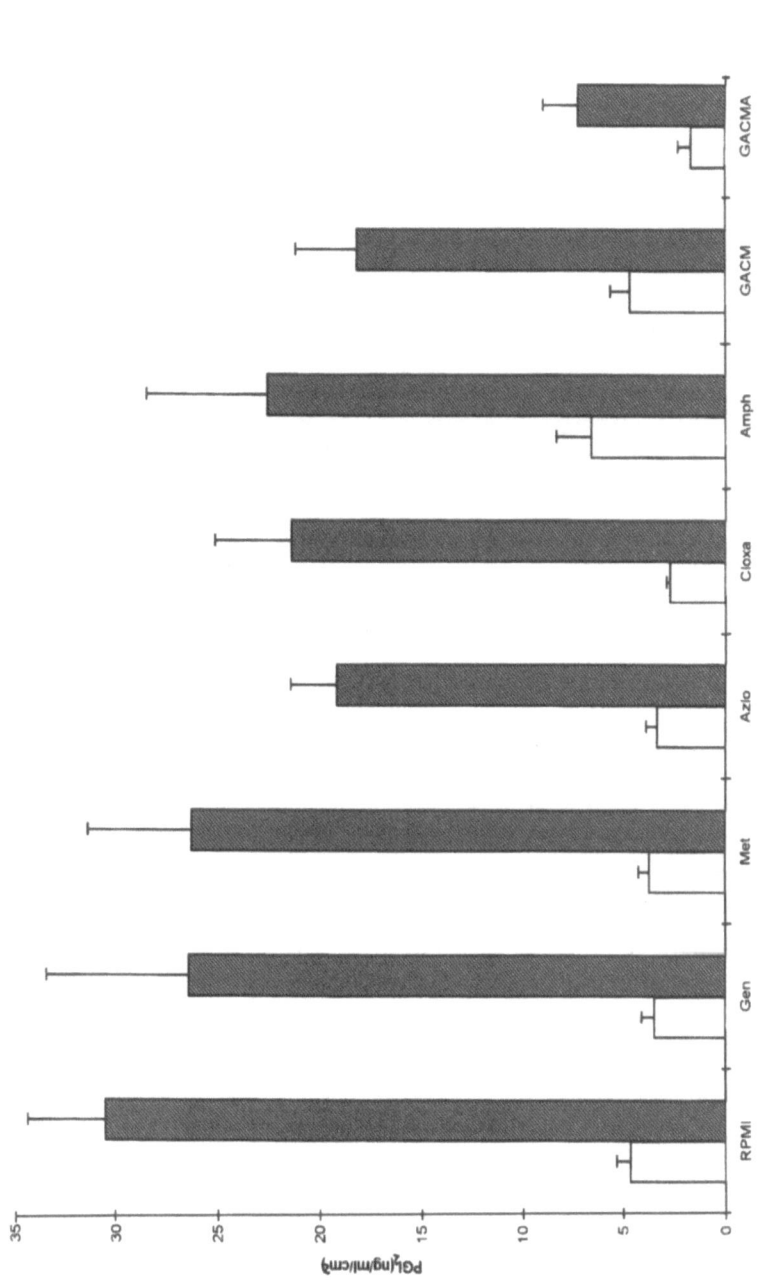

Fig. 1. From X.J. Feng et al. (25). Prostacyclin (PGI$_2$) production from porcine aortic valve cusps after 24 h contact at 4 °C with different antibiotic solutions, RPMI (culture medium RPMI 1640), Gen (gentamycin), Met (Metronidazole), Azlo (Azlocillin), Cloxa (Cloxacillin), Amph (Amphotericin B), GACM (Gentamycin, Azlocillin, Cloxacillin, Metronidazole), GACMA (Gentamycin, Azlocillin, Cloxacillin, Metronidazole, Amphotericin B). The open columns represent the production during the incubation period preceding the stimulation, the hatched columns represent the production in the presence of 10 μM Bradykinin. The stimulated production by the cusps treated with GACMA solution was significantly different from all other groups ($p < 0.05$) ($n \geqslant 6$).

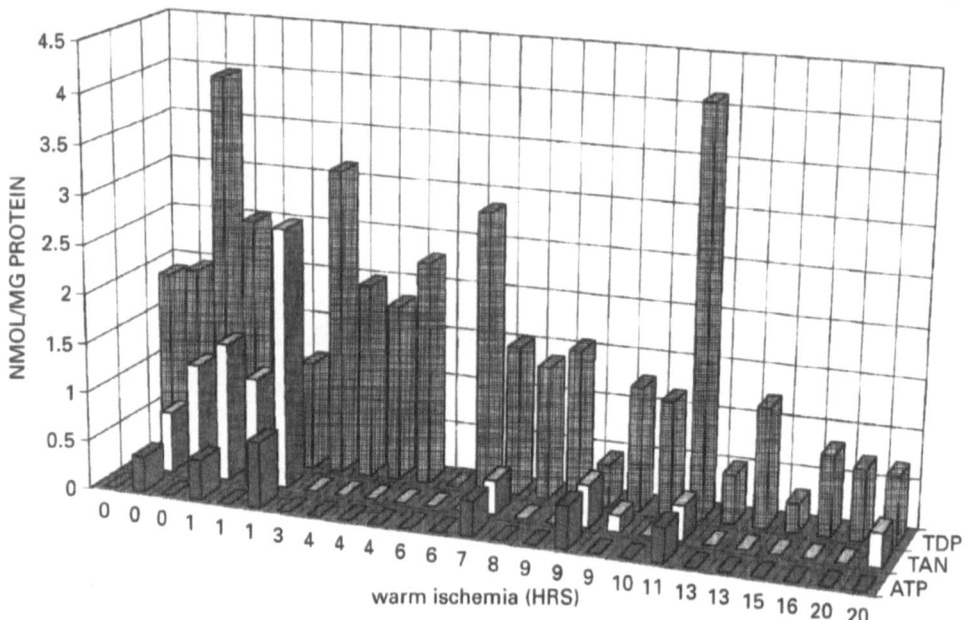

Fig. 2. from R.H. Messier et al. (37). Nucleotides and nucleopurines. Graphic representation of major fluctuating high energy phosphates and catabolites for each valve. This figure powerfully demonstrates the "depletion" of the adenine nucleotide pool in the vast majority of the human valves, with only modest tendency for retention of the higher-energy nucleotides at shorter ischemic intervals (leftward X axis). This pattern plus the obvious "scatter" suggests that there are very significant determinants other than preharvest ischaemia operant in the human clinical transplant situation. X axis represents preharvest ischaemic time to the nearest hour. Key: TAN, $\Sigma[ATP] + [ADP] + [AMP]$; TDP, $\Sigma[adenosine] + [inosine] + [xanthine] + [hypoxanthine]$. Front bars, ATP; middle bars, TAN; rear bars, TDP.

6) Cell culture (26, 36)
The proliferative ability of cells isolated from homografts can be assessed by cell culture. This assessment may be complicated by the variable efficiency of cell attachment and outgrowth. A viable cell may not be capable of proliferation when maintained in culture.

7) High Performance Liquid Chromatography (37, 38) (HPLC)
A metabolically active cell will have relatively large amounts of high energy adenine nucleotides present, these and their catabolites can be quantified using HPLC. This is illustrated in Fig. 2. An advantage of this method is that it assesses the initial metabolic phase of cellular injury caused by allograft processing. However this may not be uniform throughout the valve.

Factors which affect viability

As briefly mentioned in the introduction, all forms of valve processing have the potential to alter the cellular and physical properties of the allograft valve ultimately affecting valve durability. In particular there are several influential factors in contemporary processing techniques, these include pre-implantation ischaemia sterilisation and preservation.

Pre-implantation ischaemia (35, 36, 38–40). This encompasses two types; procurement (warm) ischaemia which is the time between death and valve retrieval, and processing (cold) ischaemia which is the time between retrieval and implantation. Various groups have shown that both types of ischaemia are capable of exerting a deleterious effect on allograft cellular constituents (35, 37). Niwaya et al. (35) found good fibroblast preservation in cryopreserved valves that were harvested within 8.7 h post mortem. Evidence (39) that *"reversible"* cellular injury (i.e. cytoplasmic and mitochondrial oedema, dilation of endoplasmic reticulum) occurs within 1–12 h warm ischaemic time whereas *"irreversible"* cellular injury (i.e. mitochondrial flocculent densities, karyolysis, plasma membrane disruption) is not observed until after 12 h post mortem, slightly extends optimal warm ischaemic time, which according to Fischlein et al. (13) this can be extended even further. In comparing heart beating donor allografts (HBD) that were either cryopreserved or stored in nutrient medium at 4 °C for up to 7 days, they found that processed within 24 h post mortem these allografts exhibited morphologically intact valvular stroma and high endothelial cell viability. Also processing within 48 h led to almost unaltered tissue and cell structure, with a definite increase of endothelial cell loss, which was only further exacerbated by 4 °C storage in nutrient media in excess of 24 h until cryopreservation. However, the proposal that warm ischaemic time can be increased is disputed, Domkowski et al. (37, 38) demonstrated that through reducing harvesting ischaemia to 40 min, valve cells although significantly altered are not "metabolically exhausted" by processing stages. The negative influence of ischaemia is further aggravated by antibiotic treatment, cryopreservation and thawing, resulting in a substantial loss of viability in most commercially prepared cryopreserved aortic heart valves (13, 18, 37).

Sterilisation via antibiotics: Regardless of the ultimate storage technique most valves are sterilised with an antibiotic/antimytotic "cocktail". Examples of some of the antibiotics used in various sterilising mixtures and their effects are listed below.

Amphotericin B

This is a potent antifungal agent that exerts its effect by binding to a sterol present in fungal plasma membranes, ultimately breaking the osmotic barrier (41). However amphotericin also binds to cholesterol of mammalian cell membranes (42) resulting in increased permeability which in turn could potentiate the effect of other antibiotics (24). Amphotericin B alone has been shown to be highly cytotoxic (31) to valve cells particularly at high concentrations, its effect at room temperature was rapid and highly detrimental but at 4 °C this toxic effect was exhibited more slowly. On the other hand it has been demonstrated that low dose amphotericin B e.g. 5 µg/ml can exert adequate fungicidal action without damaging the more sensitive valve endothelial cells (24, 43), in comparison valve fibroblasts are said to be slightly more resistant to the toxic effects of amphotericin B (30). Armiger (30) found a marked or complete loss of cell viability following 24 h exposure to an antibiotic solution containing low concentrations of amphotericin, whereas Lang et al. (33) did not observe significant alteration in proliferation or metabolic status of valve cells following 12–24 h exposure to an antibiotic solution containing high concentrations of amphotericin B (0.5 mg/ml, 20× the dosage used by Armiger) and gentamycin. These discrepancies suggest that factors other than sterilising solution composition and duration of exposure are involved in determining antibiotic effects on cell viability. As discussed above the interval between donor death and valve retrieval is a major influence as injured cells can be expected to be more susceptible to noxious substances than normal ones (21) and this is clearly demonstrated in that valves were collected within 9 h and 30 h after death by Lang et al. and Armiger respectively.

Nystatin

This was a commonly used alternative antifungal agent. It has been shown to have little detrimental effect except at high concentration and long duration of exposure (34). In England nystatin is no longer available in a clinically usable form.

Gentamycin

This inhibits nucleic acid and protein synthesis (24, 33).

Penicillin and streptomycin

These can be directly detrimental to the mechanical strength of the collagen framework (24, 44). Streptomycin binds to the small ribosomal subunit to inhibit protein synthesis (42).

Al Janabi et al. (7) showed that with tissue stored in nutrient, antibiotic medium for up to 8 days, the nucleus still retained DNA synthetic activity, but that protein synthesis decreased rapidly in contrast (31). As the nucleus appears to retain ability to synthesise DNA, it may become functional when the graft is transplanted.

Preservation: The effects of cryopreservation and other preservation techniques on the long-term durability of the allograft valve, particularly the ECM, are unknown. Even though it has been demonstrated that collagen is markedly more resistant to autolysis than cells, processing conditions might adversely influence collagen cross-linking hence ECM integrity. Mitchell et al. (14) found that the collagen network was retained, but due to the lack of interstitial cell viability, the ECM is not continually remodelled and initial autolytic damage to the collagenous skeleton would be cumulative, resulting in potential structural dysfunction.

In usual clinical practise it has been suggested that after cryopreservation the valvular trilaminar appearance was still faintly visible, the density of fibroblasts was equivalent to normal, but that very few endothelial cells remain (5). Fibroblasts and endothelial cells may not necessarily demonstrate a parallel response to preservation techniques (21). However others have found that in the experimental setting, the endothelium is well preserved (45, 46). Mitchell et al. (14) showed that late explants of cryopreserved valves had progressively severe loss of normal layered structure, the elastin rich ventricularis layer of most valves was largely intact, the amorphous extracellular matrix was scant, with nonviable cells and debris and a collagenous skeleton that was largely intact but exceedingly flattened without the normal periodic foldings of collagen bundles (crimping) of a freshly fixed valve.

Thawing: The thawing phase has been observed to have significant effects on cell viability and the mechanical integrity of valves (47). It has been suggested that valves obtained within 12–24 h of donor death usually retain considerable viability, which in all but a minority of cases decreases markedly after antibiotic treatment and further still after cryopreservation, such that most valves were unviable when thawed (28).

Clinical significance of processing techniques

Accumulated evidence indicates that fresh homograft valves continue to function 11–15 years after implantation (48), they retain normal structure (49, 50), and the incidence of late degenerative changes was minimal up to 5 years (51). It has been proposed that cryopreserved valve allografts may exhibit durability superior to that of valves stored at 4 °C in antibiotic solution (2, 8). O'Brien et al. found that 92% of cases that received viable cryopreserved homografts, following an aortic valve replacement (8), were free from valve failure after 10 years. Others have found similar results e.g. freedom from tissue failure for cryopreserved aortic valves was 80% at 10 years in the aortic position in adults as opposed to around 70% at 10 years (1, 2, 9, 11) and 42% after 14 years (11) for fresh valves.

It is important to determine the behaviour of an unprocessed, fully viable homo-graft, ('Homovital') (12). There were good early and medium term results, but this does not eliminate the risk of slow late degeneration. These results suggest that true viability is an advantage, the rate of degeneration was very slow and there was no evidence of accelerated failure caused by rejection or affected by other biochemical or haemodynamic factors (12).

Steps towards achieving high pre-implantation cellular viability

Taking into account all the factors discussed above and their clinical significance we can conclude that if we wish to maintain high pre-implantation viability we must ideally: 1) Reduce the interval between donor death and valve retrieval to the minimum. Practically the most feasible optimal window for valve retreival will be within 12 h post mortem. 2) Harvest the tissue under sterile conditions, whenever possible, to reduce the requirement for exposure to strong antibiotic solutions. However if tissue is retrieved aseptically and requires sterilization, this should be adequate but at the same time have minimal toxicity, which can be achieved by reducing concentration of the antibiotic solution and the duration of exposure. 3) Gently cryopreserve by optimising cryoprotectant (DMSO) concentration/exposure (13, 29) and gradually reducing the temperature by 1 °C every minute until the valve reaches −140 °C.

Conclusion

In order to extend the life span of a homograft, it is important to establish the possible reasons for failure and the criteria for success. To date viability is perceived to be an important issue; this chapter has reviewed the debated importance of maintaining a viable allograft and the various methods available for assessing viability. It seems that viable valves perform better, however a more viable graft may stimulate an immune response (discussed in another chapter). Viability is currently thought to be a desirable property of allograft valves. Discrepancy between results shows that specific methods of valve processing should be closely examined. Subtle differences in methods explain important differences in allograft structure and function. Each group should determine pre-implantation viability status of their own grafts as routinely prepared (21), such that an optimal universal method of allograft processing and storage can be acheived in the future. This could give rise to a large amount of clinical data that would be comparable and possibly help redeem the controversial issues discussed in this chapter. The ultimate goal is to optimise allograft survival.

References

1. Matsuki O, Robles A, Gibbs S, Bodnar E, Ross DN (1988) Long-term performance of 555 aortic homografts in the aortic position: Ann Thorac Surg 46: 187–191
2. O'Brien MF, Stafford EG, Gardner MA, Pohlner PG, McGiffin DC (1987) A comparison of aortic valve replacement with viable cryopreserved and fresh allograft valves, with a note on chromosomal studies: J Thorac Cardiovasc Surg 94: 812–823
3. Ross D, Yacoub MH (1969) Homograft replacement of the aortic valve. A critical review: Prog Cardiovasc Dis 11: 275–293
4. Barratt Boyes BG, Lowe JB, Cole DS Kelly DT (1965) Homograft valve replacement for aortic valve disease: Thorax 20: 495–504
5. Lupinetti FM, Tsai TT, Kneebone JM (1993) Endothelial cell replication in an in vivo model of aortic allografts: Ann Thorac Surg 56: 237–241
6. Yacoub M, Kittle CF (1970) Sterilization of valve homografts by antibiotic solutions: Circulation 41: II29–32
7. al Janabi N, Gonzalez Lavin L, Neirotti R, Ross DN (1972) Viability of fresh aortic valve homografts: a quantitative assessment: Thorax 27: 83–86
8. O'Brien MF, McGiffin DC, Stafford EG, Gardner MA, Pohlner PF, McLachlan GJ, Gall K, Smith S, Murphy E (1991) Allograft aortic valve replacement: long-term comparative clinical analysis of the viable cryopreserved and antibiotic 4 degrees C stored valves: J Card Surg 6: 534–543
9. Kirklin JK, Smith D, Novick W, Naftel DC, Kirklin JW, Pacifico AD, Nanda NC, Helmcke FR, Bourge RC (1993) Long-term function of cryopreserved aortic homografts. A ten-year study: J Thorac Cardiovasc Surg 106: 154–165
10. van der Kamp AW, Visser WJ, van Dongen JM, Nauta J, Galjaard H (1981) Preservation of aortic heart valves with maintenance of cell viability: J Surg Res 30: 47–56
11. Daly RC, Orszulak TA, Schaff HV, McGovern E, Wallace RB (1991) Long-term results of aortic valve replacement with nonviable homografts: Circulation 84: III81–8
12. Yacoub M, Rasmi NR, Sundt TM, Lund O, Boyland E, Radley Smith R, Khaghani A, Mitchell A (1995) Fourteen-year experience with homovital homografts for aortic valve replacement: J Thorac Cardiovasc Surg 110: 186–193. 59: 310–320
13. Fischlein T, Schutz A, Uhlig A, Frey R, Krupa W, Babic R, Thiery J, Reichart B (1994) Integrity and viability of homograft valves: Eur J Cardiothorac Surg 8: 425–430
14. Mitchell RN, Jonas RA, Schoen FJ (1995) Structure-function correlations in cryopreserved allograft cardiac valves: Ann Thorac Surg 60: S108–12
15. van der Kamp AW, Nauta J (1979) Fibroblast function and the maintenance of the aortic-valve matrix: Cardiovasc Res 13: 167–172
16. Livi U, Abdulla AK, Parker R, Olsen EJ, Ross DN (1987) Viability and morphology of aortic and pulmonary homografts. A comparative study: J Thorac Cardiovasc Surg 93: 755–760.
17. Yankah AC, Wottge HU, Muller Hermelink HK, Feller AC, Lange P, Wessel U, Dreyer H, Bernhard A, Muller Ruchholtz W (1987) Transplantation of aortic and Pulmonary Allografts, Enhanced Viability of Endothelial Cells by Cryopreservation, Importance of Histocompatibility. J Cardiac Surg 1: 209–220
18. Hoekstra F, Knoop C, Aghai Z, Jutte N, Mochtar B, Bos E, Weimar W (1995) Stimulation of immune-competent cells in vitro by human cardiac valve-derived endothelial cells: Ann Thorac Surg, 60: S131–3

19. Pober JS, Collins T, Gimbrone MA, Jr, Libby P, Reiss CS (1986) Inducible expression of class II major histocompatibility complex antigens and the immunogenicity of vascular endothelium: Transplantation, 41: 141–146
20. Yacoub MH, Suitters A, Khaghani A, Rose M (1986) Localisation of major histocompatibility complex (HLA ABC and DR) antigens in aortic homografts. Bodner E, Yacoub, M Biologic and Bioprosthetic Valves. Yorke Medical Books
21. Armiger LC (1995) Further comments concerning: biochemical and cellular characterization of cardiac valve tissue after cryopreservation or antibiotic preservation (J Thorac Cardiovasc Surg 1994; 108: 63–7) [letter]: J Thorac Cardiovasc Surg 110: 284
22. Angell WW, Shumway NE, Kosek JC, et al. (1972) A five year study of viable Aortic valve homograft: J Thorac Surg 64: 329
23. Gonzalez Lavin L, Spotnitz AJ, Mackenzie JW, Gu J, Gadi IK, Gullo J, Boyd C, Graf D (1990) Homograft valve durability: host or donor influence? Heart Vessels 5: 102–106
24. Feng XJ, van Hove CE, Mohan R, Andries L, Rampart M, Herman AG, Walter PJ (1992) Improved endothelial viability of heart valves cryopreserved by a new technique: Eur J Cardiothorac Surg 6: 251–255
25. Feng XJ, van Hove CE, Mohan R, Walter PJ, Herman AG (1993) Effects of different antibiotics on the endothelium of the porcine aortic valve: J Heart Valve Dis 2: 694–704
26. Lang SJ, Giordano MS, Cardon Cardo C, Summers BD, Staiano Coico L, Hajjar DP (1994) Biochemical and cellular characterization of cardiac valve tissue after cryopreservation or antibiotic preservation: J Thorac Cardiovasc Surg 108: 63–67
27. Siney L, Lewis MJ (1993) Nitric oxide release from porcine mitral valves: Cardiovasc Res 27: 1657–1661
28. Ferrans VJ, Spray TL, Billingham ME, Roberts WC (1978) Structural changes in glutaraldehyde-treated porcine heterografts used as substitute cardiac valves. Transmission and scanning electron microscopic observations in 12 patients: Am J Cardiol 41: 1159–1184
29. Villanueva AG, Farber HW, Rounds S, Goldstein RH (1991) Stimulation of fibroblast collagen and total protein formation by an endothelial cell-derived factor: Circ Res 69: 134–141.
30. Armiger LC (1995) Viability studies of human valves prepared for use as allografts: Ann Thorac Surg, 60: S118–20
31. al Janabi N, Gibson K, Rose J, Ross DN (1973) Protein synthesis in fresh aortic and pulmonary value allografts as an additional test for viability: Cardiovasc Res 7: 247–250
32. Hu J, Gilmer L, Hopkins R, Wolfinbarger L, Jr (1990) Assessment of cellular viability in cardiovascular tissue as studied with 3Hproline and 3Hinulin: Cardiovasc Res 24: 528–531
33. Hu JF, Gilmer L, Hopkins R, Wolfinbarger L, Jr (1989) Effects of antibiotics on cellular viability in porcine heart valve tissue [published erratum appears in Cardiovasc Res 1990 Feb; 24(2): 168]: Cardiovasc Res 23: 960–964
34. Aguirregoicoa V, Kearney JN, Davies GA, Gowland G (1989) Effects of antifungals on the viability of heart valve cusp derived fibroblasts: Cardiovasc Res 23: 1058–1061
35. Niwaya K, Sakaguchi H, Kawachi K, Kitamura S (1995) Effect of warm ischemia and cryopreservation on cell viability of human allograft valves: Ann Thorac Surg 60: S114–7
36. McGregor CG, Bradley JF, McGee JO, Wheatley DJ (1976) Viability in human heart valves prepared for grafting: Cardiovasc Res 10: 394–397
37. Messier RH, Jr, Domkowski PW, Aly HM, Jones JL, Hilbert SL, Crescenzo DG, Abd Elfattah AS, Wallace RB, Bass BL, Hopkins RA (1995) Adenine nucleotide depletion in cryopreserved human cardiac valves: the "stunned" leaflet interstitial cell population: Cryobiology 32: 199–208
38. Domkowski PW, Messier RH, Jr, Crescenzo DG, Aly HS, Abd Elfattah AS, Hilbert SL, Wallace RB, Hopkins RA (1993) Preimplantation alteration of adenine nucleotides in cryopreserved heart valves: Ann Thorac Surg, 55: 413–419
39. Crescenzo DG, Hilbert SL, Messier RH, Jr, Domkowski PW, Barrick MK, Lange PL, Ferrans VJ, Wallace RB, Hopkins RA (1993) Human cryopreserved homografts: electron microscopic analysis of cellular injury: Ann Thorac Surg 55: 25–30.
40. St. Louis J, Corcoran P, Rajan S, Conte J, Wolfinbarger L, Hu J, Lange PL, Wang YN, Hilbert SL, Analouei A and et al. (1991) Effects of warm ischemia following harvesting of allograft cardiac valves: Eur J Cardiothorac Surg (5) 458–464
41. Kinsky SC (1970) Antibiotic interaction with model membranes: Annu Rev Pharmacol 10: 119–142
42. Craig CR, Stitzel RG (1986) Craig CR, Robert, EC Modern Pharmacology. Little, Brown: Boston, Toronto. (Abstract)
43. Brandsberg JW, French ME (1972) In vitro susceptibility of isolates of Aspergillus fumigatus and

Sporothrix schenckii to amphotericin B: Antimicrob Agents Chemother 2: 402–404

44. Gavin JB, Monro JL (1974) The pathology of pulmonary and aortic valve allografts used as mitral valve replacements in dogs: Pathology 6: 119–127

45. Yankah AC, Wottge HU, Muller Hermelink HK, Feller AC, Lange P, Wessel U, Dreyer H, Bernhard A, Muller Ruchholtz W (1987) Transplantation of aortic and pulmonary allografts, enhanced viability of endothelial cells by cryopreservation, importance of histocompatibility: J Card Surg 2: 209–220

46. Mohan R, Feng XJ, Walter P, Herman A (1994) Cryopreserved heart valve allografts can have a normal endothelium [letter]: J Thorac Cardiovasc Surg 108: 985–988

47. Wolfinbarger L, Jr, Hopkins RA (1989) Biology of Heart Valve Cryopreservation: Hopkins, R. A. p. 21–36. Cardiac Reconstruction with allograft valves. Springer: Berlin, Heidelberg, New York. (Abstract)

48. Jude JR (1970) Fabrication and evaluation of tissue leaflets for aortic and mitral valve replacemant: Ann Surg 171: 939

49. Smith JC (1967) The pathology of human aortic valve homografts: Thorax 22: 114–138

50. Angell WW, Iben AB, Shumway NE (1968) Fresh aortic homografts for multiple valve replacement: Arch Surg 97: 826–830

51. Barratt Boyes BG, Roche AH (1969) A review of aortic valve homografts over a six and one-half year period: Ann Surg 170: 483–492

Authors' address:
M. H. Yacoub
Imperial College
National Heart and Lung Institute
Heart Science Centre
Harefield Hospital
Harefield, Middx., UB9 6JH
England

Human heart cold ischemia and its effect on post-cryopreservation viability of heart valves

P. E. Dawson, K. G. M. Brockbank

CryoLife®, Inc., Marietta, GA, USA

Abstract

The purpose of this study was to determine the effects of varying heart cold ischemia times on post-cryopreservation valve leaflet cellular functions. Cellular viability and function were assessed through measurement of protein synthesis, ribonucleic acid synthesis, and glucose phosphorylation. Cold ischemia times varied from 24 to 113 h before processing and cryopreservation. The results show that valve leaflet cellular functions could be detected for at least 42 h of post-procurement cold ischemia. This information can be used as a guide in further defining the acceptable limits for heart valve donation and processing.

Introduction

Since the inception of heart valve allograft surgery, there have been many questions concerning the best methods for procurement and storage. Early results proved that cellular viability of the tissue is necessary to ensure long-term survival of the graft (1, 5, 9, 12, 15). Practical considerations have dictated that the graft tissue be stored in a readily available format, which has necessitated the evolution of cryopreservation for long-term tissue preservation and storage. This method of valve storage allows for a wide variety of valve types and sizes to be readily available in a stable, sterile, and viable form for transplant. Many questions remain, however, concerning the various effects of pre-cryopreservation variables which a heart faces before the valves are removed and cryopreserved. The clinical need for human heart valves for transplant has produced a great interest in clarifying these issues in order to make as many hearts as possible usable for valve transplants.

To obtain human heart valves for transplant, hearts must be procured, transported, and further processed after donation. As the ischemic period (beginning at the time of cessation of blood flow) lengthens, metabolic alterations occur. Some of the results of this ischemia are accumulation of toxic cell products, ion shifts, cell membrane depolarization, and eventually cell death (2, 13). The simplest approach to slow the rate of tissue deterioration is to reduce the tissue temperature thereby limiting aerobic glycolyis, ATP consumption, and degradative enzyme activity.

Current practice for the handling of hearts for use as valve transplants includes procurement of the heart within 12 h of death. The warm ischemia time period (time of death to organ recovery) is an important factor in the ultimate viability of this tissue.

Crescenzo, et al., have found that minimal irreversible cellular injury occurs in valves exposed to 12 h or less of warm ischemia (7). Indeed, longer ischemia times may provide opportunistic organisms the conditions necessary to proliferate in the tissue as well as increase cellular damage. Following procurement, the heart is rinsed, placed in a cooler at 4 °C, and transported to a tissue preservation facility. During this transport time, whole heart cold ischemia could result in depression of valve cellular functions. The reduction of the temperature to 4 °C aids in slowing the metabolic activity of the tissue and its deterioration.

The purpose of this study was to determine the effects of varying heart cold ischemia times on post-cryopreservation valve leaflet cellular functions. Cellular viability and function were assessed through measurement of protein synthesis, ribonucleic acid synthesis, and glucose phosphorylation. Cold ischemia times were varied from 24 to 113 h before processing for cryopreservation.

Materials and methods

Methods were essentially as discussed previously (5). Thirteen human hearts which were found to be unsuitable for allograft transplantation were selected at the time of procurement or after procurement at arrival to the cryopreservation facility. Hearts were shipped on wet ice and held for varying times from 24 to 113 h at 4 °C before dissection of the valves from each heart. Warm ischemia times were not controlled for and varied from 0 to 12 h. Both the aortic and pulmonic valves were dissected from each heart. The aortic and pulmonic valves were then incubated in an antibiotic solution consisting of DMEM with 12 µg/ml Imipenim at 37 °C for 4 h. Valves were cryopreserved according to methods previously described (11) and stored in liquid nitrogen for 2 to 13 months before thawing and assay. The valves were thawed in a 37 °C water bath, removed from the packaging, and the cryoprotectant was eluted from the tissue in a single step with 5% dextrose in lactated Ringers solution.

Leaflets were removed from the valves after thawing and were labeled with tritiated precursors as follows:

1) ^{3}H-glycine incorporation into trichloroacetic acid precipitated proteins by scintillation counting;
2) ^{3}H-proline incorporation into proteins by scintillation counting and autoradiography;
3) ^{3}H-hypoxanthine incorporation into ribonucleic acids by scintillation counting and autoradiography, and
4) ^{3}H-2-deoxyglucose phosphorylation by scintillation counting.

The leaflet samples used for scintillation counting assays were labeled, washed, dehydrated, weighed, solubilized, homogenized, and labeled products were measured by scintillation counting. All scintillation counting results are expressed as disintegrations per minute (dpm) per milligram of tissue dry weight.

Samples for autoradiography were incubated with ^{3}H-hypoxanthine or ^{3}H-proline at 15 µCi/ml. After incubation, tissue was washed and fixed in buffered formalin. Fixative was removed by soaking the tissue in 15% sucrose in 0.1 M sodium phosphate buffer pH 7.4. The leaflets were then embedded in O.C.T. embedding medium (Miles Laboratory, Elkhart, IN) and frozen in liquid nitrogen prior to cutting in

6-micron sections. Cryosections were processed for autoradiography (Kodak NBT2 emulsion). After staining (hematoxylin-eosin) the number of labeled and unlabeled cells in representative fields were counted to obtain the percent of live cells.

Significance in the differences of the mean values for leaflet function analyses were evaluated by independent t-tests.

Results

Figure 1 shows the results from each of the assays described. The data are grouped into two time periods: 24–42 and 53–113 h. Both aortic and pulmonic valves are grouped together in Fig. 1.

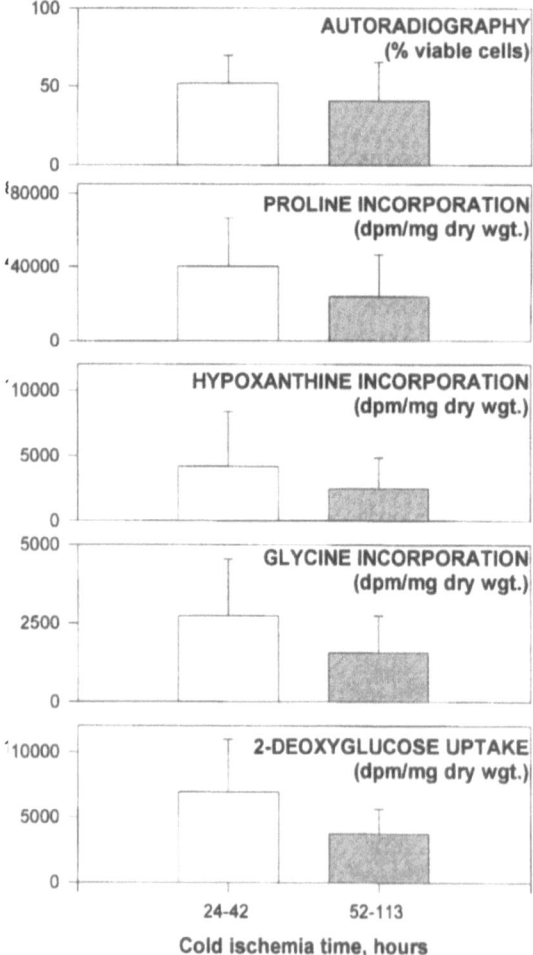

Fig. 1. Average results of functional analyses. Aortic and pulmonic values are grouped together for the two cold ischemic time periods indicated.

Comparisons of valves exposed to 24–42 h ($n = 12$) of cold ischemia with those exposed to 53–113 h ($n = 14$) of cold ischemia demonstrated statistically significant differences by three of the assays used: proline, glycine, and 2-deoxyglucose ($p < 0.1$). The other assays had the same downward trend but were not significant. The warm ischemia time for each group was not statistically different. The mean warm ischemia was 6.25 h for the 24–42 h group and 4.64 h for the 53–113 h group.

Figure 2 shows the data as separated into aortic and pulmonic valves. These are further grouped into cold ischemia times of 24 to 42 and 53 to 113 h. Comparisons of the cellular function of aortic and pulmonic valve leaflets exposed to 24 to 42 h with those exposed to 53 to 113 h of cold ischemia indicate that the pulmonic valves exhibit larger differences in cellular function as ischemia time increases. These observations are true for proline, 2-deoxyglucose, and autoradiography but are not statistically significant due to the smaller numbers of test samples. The results for aortic valves exhibit the same trend.

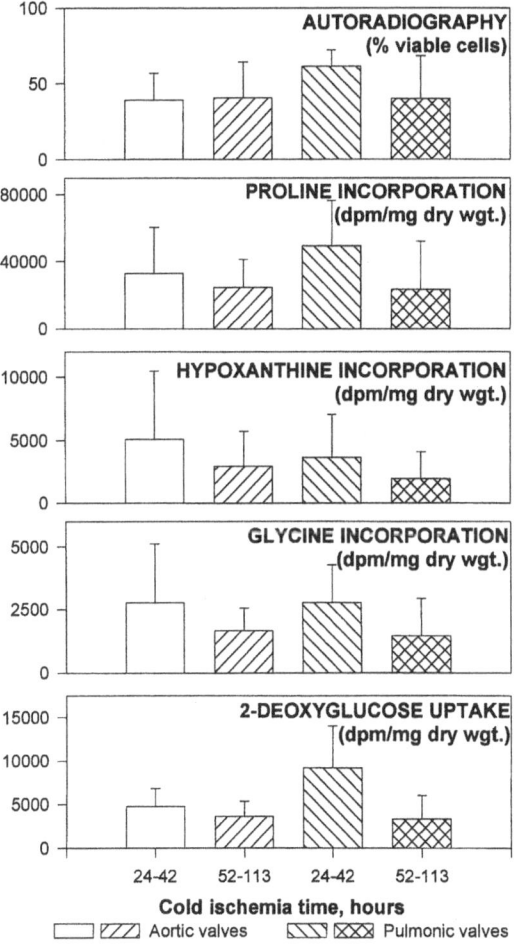

Fig. 2. Average results of functional analyses. Aortic and pulmonic values graphed separately for the two cold ischemic time periods indicated.

Discussion

These results demonstrate that valve leaflet cellular functions could be detected for at least 42 h of post-procurement cold ischemia. An interesting observation concerning this data is seen when the two valve types are examined separately. The pulmonic valves seem to be more sensitive to the test conditions than the aortic valves, although due to the smaller number of samples for this comparison, the differences are not statistically significant. In general, the aortic valves seem less affected by the insults of cold ischemia. On the other hand, our experience shows that aortic valves are more likely to be affected by pathologic/structural defects and degenerative conditions than are pulmonic valves. Pulmonic valves are discarded less frequently than aortic valves for many conditions including calcification and plaque deposition. These observations could explain the higher viability numbers seen with pulmonic valves at the shorter time period. However, during the longer ischemia times, the pulmonic valve viability descends to a level approximately equal to those of the aortic valves at the same time period. Therefore, the difference in viability in the two time frames is larger for the pulmonic than the aortic valves.

Optimal performance of human heart valve allografts after transplantation has been associated with the retention of biochemically functional leaflet cells at the time of implant (1, 5, 9, 12, 15). These cells must have sufficient energy reserves to survive processing and perform their critical roles after transplantation of the valve. Donated human hearts for use as valve allograft sources are subjected to varying warm and cold time periods before they are antibiotic treated and cryopreserved. Cells that are metabolically depressed after tissue procurement and processing may not recover sufficiently to sucessfully endure the added shock of cryopreservation before transplantation into a recipient. We have previously demonstrated that incubation of heart valves at 37 °C ("revitalization") before cryopreservation results in a higher level of tissue metabolic activity after thawing (4, 6). This "revitalization" method was used with these tissues and is used with all CryoLife® processed human tissues for transplant. Adherence to the ischemia limits described above and the use of a warm incubation period prior to cryopreservation provides human heart valve allografts the best opportunity for survival and function at the time of implant. The use of cryopreservation to store these valves long-term has been demonstrated, and stability has been documented for at least 2 years in heart valve leaflets (3). Others have found that 10 years of storage at -196 °C for most biological materials is possible (8). Therefore, if the pre-cryopreservation events which enable the tissues to withstand the initial stresses of cryopreservation can be fully defined, these tissues can then be stored for at least 2 years with the confidence that the recipients are receiving a consistently viable allograft.

The American Association of Tissue Banks currently recommends that "Tissues obtained from living and non-living donors shall be retrieved and preserved within the time interval appropriate for retention of biological functions compatible with intended use of that tissue" (14). The European standards for cryopreserved heart valves permit a maximum combined warm and cold ischemic time of 48 h providing that donor body refrigeration begins within 6 h of death (16). These guidelines are clarified with the results from this study which indicate that valves collected from hearts with a cold ischemic time of 42 h or less, combined with a warm ischemic time of 12 h or less, provide tissue which maintains an acceptable level of viability at the time of implant and allows the procurement and ultimate use of as many heart valves as possible for those patients who need them.

References

1. Angell WW, de Lanerolle P, Shumway NE (1973) Valve replacement: present status of homograft valves. Prog Cardiovasc Dis 15: 589
2. Belzer FO, Southard JH (1986) Organ preservation and transplantation. In: Meryman HT (ed) Transplantation: Approaches to Graft Rejection. Liss, New York, pp 291–303
3. Brockbank KGM, Carpenter JF, Dawson PE (1992) Effects of storage temperature on viable bioprosthetic heart valves. Cryobiology 29: 537–542
4. Brockbank KGM, Dawson PE, Carpenter JF (1993) Heart valve leaflet revitalization. Tissue and Cell Report 1 No. 2: 18–19
5. Brockbank KGM, Dawson PE (1993) Influence of whole heart postprocurement ischemia time upon cryopreserved heart valve viability. Tansplant Proc 25 No. 6: 3188–3189
6. Carpenter JF, Brockbank KGM (1992) US Patent #5,171,660
7. Crescenzo DG, Hilbert SL,Messier RH, Domkowski PW, Barrick MK, Lange PL, Ferrans VJ, Wallace RB, Hopkins RA (1993) Human cryopreserved homografts: Electron microscopic analysis of cellular injury. Ann Thorac Surg 55: 25–31
8. Grout BWW, Morris GJ (1987) Freezing and cellular organization. In: Grout BWW, Morris GJ (eds) The Effects of Temperatures on Biological Systems. Arnold, London, pp 147–173
9. Lockey E, Al-Janabi N, Gonzales-Lavin L, Ross DN (1972) A method of sterilizing and preserving fresh allograft heart valves. Thorax 27: 398–400
10. McGiffin DC, O'Brien MF, Stafford EG, Gardner MA, Pohlner PG (1988) Long-term results of the viable cryopreserved allograft aortic valve: continuing evidence for superior valve durability. J Cardiac Surg 3: 289–296
11. McNally RT, Heacox A, Brockbank KGM, Bank HL (1990) US Patent #4,890,457
12. O'Brien MF (1989) Long-term results of viable cryopreserved allograft aortic valve. In: Clarke DR (ed) Transplantation Techniques and Use of Cryopreserved Allograft Cardiac Valves and Vascular Tissue. Adams, Boston, pp 139–150
13. Ratych RE, Bulkley GB, Williams GM (1986) Ischemia/reperfusion injury in the kidney. In: Meryman HT (ed) Transplantation: Approches to Graft Rejection. Liss, New York, pp 263–289
14. Standards of Tissue Banking: American Association of Tissue Banks (1993) p 11
15. Stark J (1989) Do we really correct congenital heart defects? J Thorac Cardiovasc Surg 97: 1–9
16. Yearly report of the medical director: European Homograft Bank International Association (1991) Brussels

Author's address:
P. E. Dawson
CryoLife®, Inc.
2211 New Market Parkway
Suite 142
Marietta, GA 30067
USA

Effects of storage temperature and fetal calf serum on the endothelium of porcine aortic valves: Functional and microscopic evaluation

X. J. Feng[1], Cor E. J. Van Hove[2], L. Andries[3], P. J. Walter[1], A. G. Herman[2],

Department of Cardiac Surgery[1], Pharmacology[2] and Physiology[3], Faculty of Medicine, University of Antwerp (UIA), Antwerp-Wilrijk, Belgium

Abstract

Endothelial integrity and function may be an important determinant for long-term success of allograft heart valves. To determine the optimal storage temperatures for preserving long-term endothelial function of porcine aortic valves, different storage temperatures and different periods of time were investigated. Fresh valves were either a) stored at 4 °C with or without 10% fetal calf serum (FCS) supplement, for 1, 2, 4, 7, 14, 21, and 28 days. b) cryopreserved for 2, 4, and 8 weeks without FCS in either at -80 °C or at -170 °C. c) cryopreserved in long-term storage (as long as 1 year), with or without FCS, at -170 °C. Viability of endothelial cells was assessed through measurement of the production of prostacyclin (PGI_2) in basal and bradykinin (BK) stimulated conditions, during in vitro incubation of the valve cusps at 37 °C, using a radioimmunoassay for 6-oxo-prostaglandin $F_{1\alpha}$ ($PGF_{1\alpha}$). Endothelial morphological variations in valves stored at 4 °C were evaluated by scanning electron microscopy (SEM), in valves cryopreserved at -80 °C and -170 °C were evaluated by confocal scanning laser microscopy (CSLM). Results: a) With storage at 4 °C, after 4 days the valves produced already significantly less ($p < 0.05$) PGI_2 than fresh preparations in both basal (0.21 ± 0.04 vs 3.56 ± 0.03 ng/ml$\cdot$cm^2) and stimulated conditions (4.17 ± 0.36 vs 24.23 ± 1.83). Morphological changes could not yet be distinguished with SEM at that time. When the storage period was extended, the levels of PGI_2 further diminished; after 14 days, PGI_2 release could no longer be detected. b) In cryopreserved valves, PGI_2 production was similar for as long as 2 weeks of storage either at -80 °C or at -170 °C in basal (2.69 ± 0.63 vs 2.93 ± 0.51) and stimulated (16.43 ± 3.19 vs 16.50 ± 2.57) conditions. After 8 weeks, no PGI_2 release could be detected in valves stored at -80 °C. c) After 6 months storage at -170 °C, the PGI_2 production was significantly ($p < 0.05$) reduced compared with fresh valves; it then remained constant for as long as 1 year. The valves stored with fetal calf serum produced significantly ($p < 0.05$) less PGI_2 than did those without FCS. CLSM showed that large areas of valve cusps retain intact endothelial cells after 1 year stored at -170 °C. For longer cryopreserved banking, we recommend storing heart valves at -170 °C instead of at -80 °C for maintaining viability of endothelial cells. Fetal calf serum would harm endothelial viability during long-term cryopreservation.

Introduction

Since the supply of homograft heart valves is limited and since in most institutions homograft valves are not immediately implanted after procurement, storage of heart valves has therefore become essential.

At present, centers which use many homografts and thus have short delay periods for implantation, continue to store homografts at 4 °C for about 1 week (Yacoub, personal communication). Most other centers prefer to cryopreserve homograft valves (3, 4).

Cryopreservation of valves includes a freezing procedure, a storage process and a thawing protocol. The influence of the freezing program and thawing conditions on the endothelial viability of heart valves has been described previously (8). The effects of both temperature and the duration of the storage will be described in this study.

For cryopreversion of homograft valves, controversies exist about how low the storage temperature should be. Cryopreserved valves are mainly stored at − 80 °C in a solid carbon dioxide refrigerator or at − 196 °C in liquid nitrogen. Yankah (personal communication) has been storing homograft valves at − 80 °C for the last 5–7 years and intends to continue storing these valves for another 5 years. Other centers such as CryoLife Inc. in the USA cryopreserve the valves in liquid nitrogen. The latter is also included in the guidelines "imposed" by EURO TRANSPLANT.

For surgeons, storage in a refrigerator at − 80 °C in the operation room offers practical advantages. It permits inspection of the valves and makes it easier to decide about the size of the homograft valve needed after intraoperative sizing of the aortic root, since preoperative echocardiographic evaluation of the aortic root size often fails to predict the correct size.

On the other hand, Lange and Hopkins (15) indicate that some "physicochemical" changes still continue at − 130 °C, and that even for the optimal preservation of the interstitial matrix, the storage temperature should be below − 130 °C. Since self-repair of the implanted homograft valve by fibroblasts might determine its ultimate durability in the host, and since the endothelium might protect against thrombus formation and might also prevent the loss of subendothelial structures, the pre-implantation viability of all cells comprising the homograft may be critical.

We therefore compared the effect of three different storage temperatures, i.e., + 4 °C, − 80 °C and − 170 °C and various storage periods on the prostacyclin (PGI_2) production in vitro as a viability marker of the endothelial cells of porcine aortic valve cusps. We selected endothelial function for the assessment of homograft cell viability after storage, since an intact endothelium helps in preventing intravascular thrombosis but also can contribute to fibroblast alimentation from the blood stream. Furthermore, the endothelium is the most vulnerable component of the aortic valve cusp, and can therefore be used as a sensitive indicator of overall cell survival. It should be noted that storing the valves in liquid nitrogen vapor-phase temperature (− 190 °C to − 150 °C) is traditionally called storage in liquid nitrogen at − 196 °C. In our study, we cryopreserved valves at − 170 °C which we also used in our clinical homograft valve bank.

Material and methods

The porcine aortic valves were stored for various periods at 4 °C in the nutrient medium, or cryopreserved at − 80 °C and − 170 °C in the cryopreservation freezing medium after a controlled rate freezing process.

Valve preparation

Fresh porcine aortic valves were obtained from a local slaughterhouse. Hearts were removed as aseptically as possible from pigs (weight 100 to 120 Kg, age 180 to 210 days) within 20 min of death. The aortic valve along with 2–3 cm of ascending aorta and 1–1.5 cm of ventricular myocardium was quickly excised from the heart using sterile material in a clean area of the slaughterhouse. The valves were placed carefully in ice cold RPMI 1640 tissue medium and then transported to the laboratory within 40 min. In the laboratory, each valve was longitudinally separated into three tissue pieces. Each tissue piece consisted of the corresponding cusp with 3 cm adjacent aortic wall and some myocardium. A 7/0 proline suture was then passed through the center of the free edge of the cusp for its easy lifting from one solution to another (see below). The distribution of the cusps into control and test groups was either fully randomized or one of the three cusps of a single valve served as control while the other two were used as test material.

Storage procedures

a) Storage at 4 °C

The tissue piece was put into a sterile plastic container containing 100 ml RPMI 1640 tissue culture medium at 4 °C with or without 10% fetal calf serum (FCS) and stored for various periods (1, 2, 4, 7, 14, 21 up to 28 days).

A renewal of the medium was carried out every week till the end of the storage for cusps stored for more than 7 days.

b) Cryopreservation at −80 °C and −170 °C

Freezing conditions and techniques have been previously described (8). Two hemo-freeze bags filled with 100 ml medium were used as the packaging material. As cryoprotective agent dimethylsulphoxide (DMSO) was added at room temperature in a concentration of 10%. The packed valves were kept at 4 °C for 20 min equilibration. The valves were frozen in a freezing chamber with a programmable temperature controller. Temperature was monitored by a temperature probe. A freezing rate at the site of the tissue of −1 °C per min was achieved. Upon termination of the controlled freezing program at −80 °C the valves were immediately removed from the freezing chamber and cryopreserved either in a mechanical freezer at −80 °C or in a liquid nitrogen tank in the vapor phase at −170 °C.

The valves were stored both at −80 °C or −170 °C for 2, 4 and 8 weeks. In addition, longer storage periods of 6 months and 1 year were also studied for valves stored at −170 °C. For long-term storage, cryopreservation solutions with or without 10% FCS supplement were also compared.

Estimation of prostacyclin production

After different storage periods, rapid rate thawing and a gentle cryoprotective agent (DMSO) dilution process were used for all cryopreserved valves (8). Thawing was performed by immersing the frozen valves completely with their internal packaging in a large volume of water at 40 °C and only 2–3 min were required for turning ice to slush. DMSO concentration was decreased from 10% to 7.5%, 5%, 2.5% and finally to 0%. Each step took only 1.5–2 min. For all tested valves, the cusps were dissected free from the valve tissue for estimation of PGI_2 production.

Incubation for assessment of basal and bradykinin (BK) stimulated PGI_2 production have been described earlier (8, 9). Fresh incubation medium, RPMI 1640 supplemented with 1% (g/v) bovine serum albumin and 2% (v/v) 1 M phosphate buffer (pH = 7.4), was kept at 37 °C in the test-tubes each containing 2.5 ml medium. After dissecting the cusp free from the valve tissue, each *cusp* was lifted every 15 min from one test tube to another by a no-touch technique using the 7/0 proline (see above), for 20 periods totalling 300 min. PGI_2 released into the incubation medium of each of these test-tubes was measured by radioimmunoassay of 6-oxo-$PGF_{1\alpha}$, the stable metabolite of PGI_2 (21). To stop the continued PGI_2 production by shed endothelial cells indomethacin (final concentration 10 µg/ml) was immediately added to the medium after the cusp had been removed from the test tube (13). Previous experiments demonstrated that during the incubation period, cusps spontaneously released a bell-shaped PGI_2 production curve. From 270 min on the PGI_2 release, although slightly diminished, was no longer significantly different from the previous incubation period and was therefore called basal production. This period allowed us to study PGI_2 production stimulated by a receptor-mediated mechanism such as bradykinin (final concentration 10 µM) (12) which was added to the incubation medium during the 270–285 min of incubation period.

Calculation of endothelial cell surface area of the cusp

To calculate the amount of PGI_2 produced per square centimeter (cm^2) by the cusp *surface*, the ratio of the weight of the total dried cusp and its measured surface area was used. This was done after the PGI_2 estimation by weighing a circular piece of the cusp, punched out by a circular knife (diameter 0.5 cm) of which the surface area given was known (0.3925 cm^2).

Statistical analysis

A paired Student's *t*-test (5% level of significance) was used to compare the basal and stimulated PGI_2 levels since these observations were made in the same specimens. To compare the PGI_2 release between cusps stored according to different storage treatments analysis of variance (ANOVA) was used.

Scanning electron microscopy (SEM)

The endothelial integrity of valves stored at 4 °C for 2, 4, 7, 14, and 21 days was examined by SEM. The preparation of the tissue specimens and the quantification of the endothelial damage were similar to what has been described previously (9). The valve cusps were fixed using 2.5% glutaraldehyde in 0.1 M cacodylate buffer; specimens were postfixed in 1% osmium tetroxide in 0.1 M cocadylate buffer for 2 h and then rinsed again in cacodylate buffer with 7.5% saccharose. Specimens were dehydrated in an ascending series of ethanol up to 100% and 100% amylacetate followed by critical point-drying in a Balzers apparatus with carbon dioxide as transitional fluid. Each valve cusp was longitudinally divided into two parts. All surfaces were mounted on stubs with double-faced tape, sputter coated with a 15-nm layer of gold and subsequently examined and photographed in a JEOL 1200EX on scanning mode operating at 40 kv. The ventricular and aortic surface of each part was examined. At least 5 random fields, only in the center of each piece were sampled and scored by an independent observer in a rating of $+$, $++$ and $+++$ for each of the variables: i) endothelial coverage, ii) intercellular gaps, iii) membrane damage, iv) basal lamina, v) fibrils exposure.

Confocal scanning laser microscopy (CSLM)

The endothelial viability of valves cryopreserved at $-80\,°C$ and $-170\,°C$ for 1 year was assessed using CSLM. After dissection, the specimens (cusps) were incubated for 15 min in medium containing (0.67 mg/ml) ethidium homodimer 1 (Molecular Probes, USA). The stain penetrates into cells with a damaged cell membrane and will bind to RNA and DNA. Ethidium homodimer 1 can be excited by an argon laser and the emitted light can be visualized by using a GHS filter block of the Biorad 600 confocal microscope. After washing, to remove the unbound stain, specimens were fixed with 4% formaldehyde in Millonig buffer. Small strips from both sides of the valve were cut and stained with Bodipy-phallacidin (Molecular Probes, USA) to reveal the actin filaments in valvular cells. In addition, some specimens were stained with YOPRO (Molecular Probes, USA), which binds to RNA and DNA in damaged cells and which can also be observed with a filter set for fluorescein. Since cells are dead after fixation, this stain will label all nuclei in the valve, which allows the detection of cells with little filamentous actin. Both the YOPRO and the Bodipy-phallacidin staining can be observed with BHS filter block of the confocal microscope. Specimens were mounted as shown in Fig. II.4 and observed with a Biorad MRC-600 confocal scanning laser microscopy. For obtaining dual color images, the A1 and A2 filter blocks were used. Images were printed with a Sony Vidio Printer UP-3000P.

Results

Prostacyclin production

Storage at 4 °C

a) 1 to 21 days period
The prostacyclin production of valves previously stored at 4 °C for various periods of time was compared to fresh valves as control. As shown in Fig. 1, prostacyclin production by fresh valve cusps showed a bell-shaped pattern i.e. rose to a maximum value during the 120–135 min period of incubation and then decreased gradually to a steady basal level at which moment it could still be stimulated via a receptor mediated mechanism (BK) (Fig. 1A). For the stored valves, both the spontaneous release as well as the bradykinin stimulated production diminished as the duration of the storage period increased.

After 1 day of storage (Fig. 1B), the valves retained $93 \pm 4.2\%$ of the basal release (measured in the 15 min period before stimulation) and $74 \pm 3.8\%$ of the stimulated release as compared to fresh cusps. There was no difference in the maximum, basal and stimulated PGI_2 production as compared to control although the bell shaped pattern was delayed for about 40–60 min.

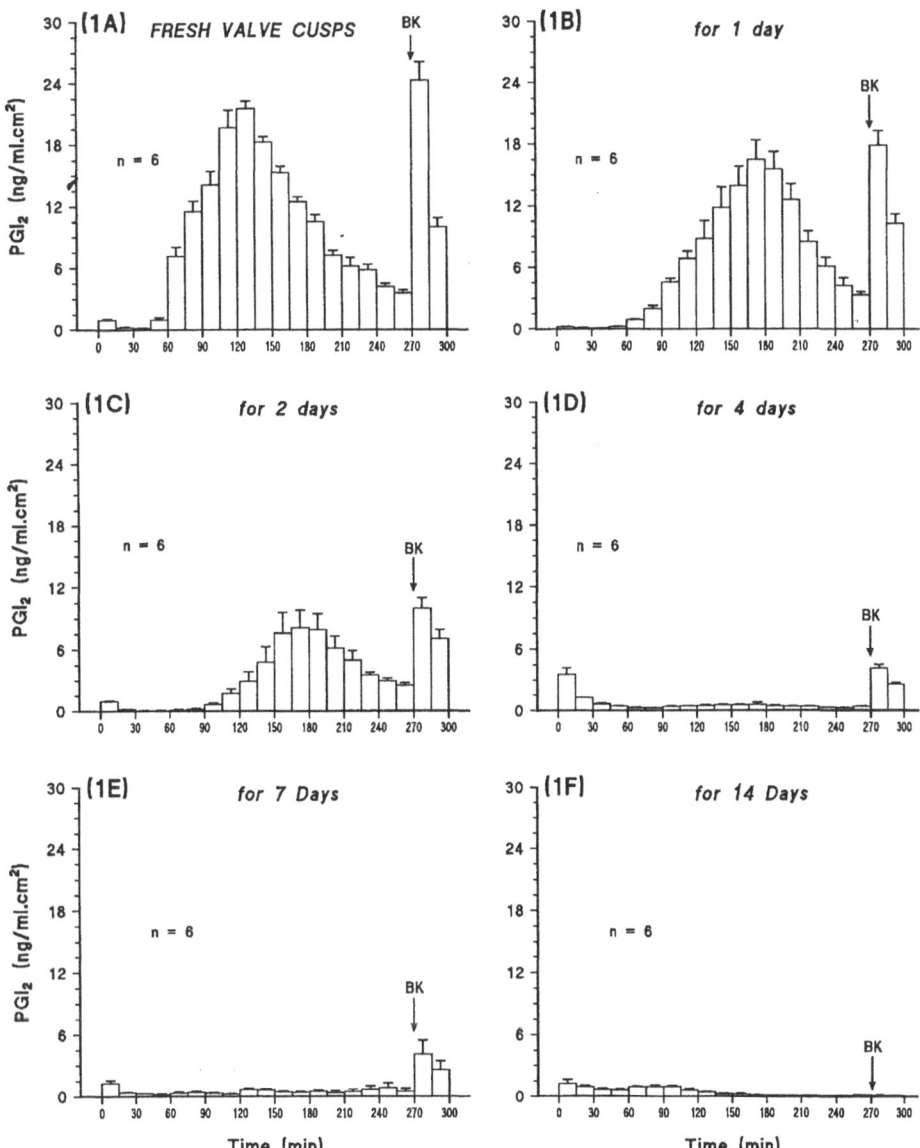

Fig. 1. Prostacyclin (PGI$_2$) production during 300 min of incubation by valve cusps stored for various periods of time (1, 2, 4, 7 and 14 days) at 4 °C compared with fresh valve cusps. The X-axis numbers refer to the time of the consecutive incubation periods. The Y-axis display the PGI$_2$ content in the incubation medium within 15 min of incubation. Bradykinin (BK, 10 μM) was added into the medium as the agonist during the 270–285 min period of incubation. The bell-shaped curve (1A) represents the spontaneous PGI$_2$ production by the cusps. (Reproduction by permission J Thorac Cardiovasc Surg).

After 2 days of storage (Fig. 1C), the basal PGI$_2$ release still maintained its bell shaped pattern although the maximum production was significantly ($p < 0.05$) less as compared to fresh valves. The basal and stimulated PGI$_2$ release was reduced to respectively $63 \pm 2.8\%$ and $41 \pm 1.7\%$ ($p < 0.05$) of the production observed in the fresh valves.

After 4 days of storage (Fig. 1D), the bell-shaped curve was no longer present. The basal release could hardly be detected and after stimulation, the prostacyclin production was reduced to $17 \pm 1.5\%$ of the control.

For as long as 7 days of storage, stimulated production of prostacyclin could still be observed (Fig. 1E). After 14 days of storage, the spontaneous as well as stimulated prostacyclin production was near the detection limit of the radioimmunoassay (Fig. 1F).

b) Influence of fetal calf serum

Valves stored at $4\,^{\circ}$C with or without fetal calf serum added to the storage medium were also compared. Inclusion of fetal calf serum (10%) in the storage medium did not significantly affect the prostacyclin production (Table 1).

c) Renewal of medium

Regular renewal of the storage medium with fresh culture medium resulted in a longer preservation of the bradykinin stimulated PGI_2 production. After 28 days storage in which the storage medium was replaced with fresh medium every 7 days, bradykinin could still significantly increase the PGI_2 production (Table 2), whereas this was no

Table 1. Prostacyclin production by porcine aortic valve cusps after storage at $4\,^{\circ}$C for different periods in RPM1 1640 medium with or without fetal calf serum (FCS) for different periods (in nanograms per milliliter per square centimeter) ($n \geq 6$)

	Without FCS		With FCS	
	Basal	Stimulated	Basal	Stimulated
Control	3.56 ± 0.30	$24.23 \pm 1.83^+$	3.56 ± 0.30	$24.23 \pm 1.83^+$
2 days	2.50 ± 0.25	$9.96 \pm 1.00^+$	3.48 ± 1.49	$10.39 \pm 1.50^+$
4 days	0.42 ± 0.05	$4.17 \pm 0.36^+$	0.41 ± 0.11	$4.01 \pm 0.063^+$
7 days	0.52 ± 0.30	$4.15 \pm 1.34^+$	0.35 ± 0.07	$2.91 \pm 0.55^+$
14 days	0.15 ± 0.008	0.17 ± 0.04	0.13 ± 0.003	0.11 ± 0.07
21 days	0.12 ± 0.03	0.13 ± 0.03	0.07 ± 0.01	0.09 ± 0.01

$^+$ Prostacyclin significantly ($p < 0.05$) increased after stimulation.

Table 2. Prostacyclin production by porcine aortic valve cusps after storage at $4\,^{\circ}$C for different periods in RPM1 1640 medium without or with renewel of the medium (in nanograms per milliliter per square centimeter) ($n \geqslant 6$)

	Without renewal		With renewal[1]	
	Basal	Stimulated	Basal	Stimulated
Control	2.88 ± 0.19	$18.55 \pm 2.07^+$	2.88 ± 0.19	$18.55 \pm 2.07^+$
7 days	0.52 ± 0.30	$4.15 \pm 1.34^+$	–	
14 days	0.15 ± 0.008	0.17 ± 0.04	$0.90 \pm 0.14*$	$2.38 \pm 0.26^{+*}$
21 days	0.12 ± 0.03	0.13 ± 0.03	0.11 ± 0.03	$1.65 \pm 0.36^{+*}$
28 days	–	–	0.08 ± 0.02	$0.43 \pm 0.09^+$

[1] Medium was renewed by fresh medium every 7 days.
$^+$ After stimulation by bradykinin, prostacyclin was significantly ($p < 0.05$) increased compared with basal level.
$*$ Prostacyclin was significantly ($p < 0.05$) higher than the prostacyclin released by the group stored for the same periods without renewal of medium.

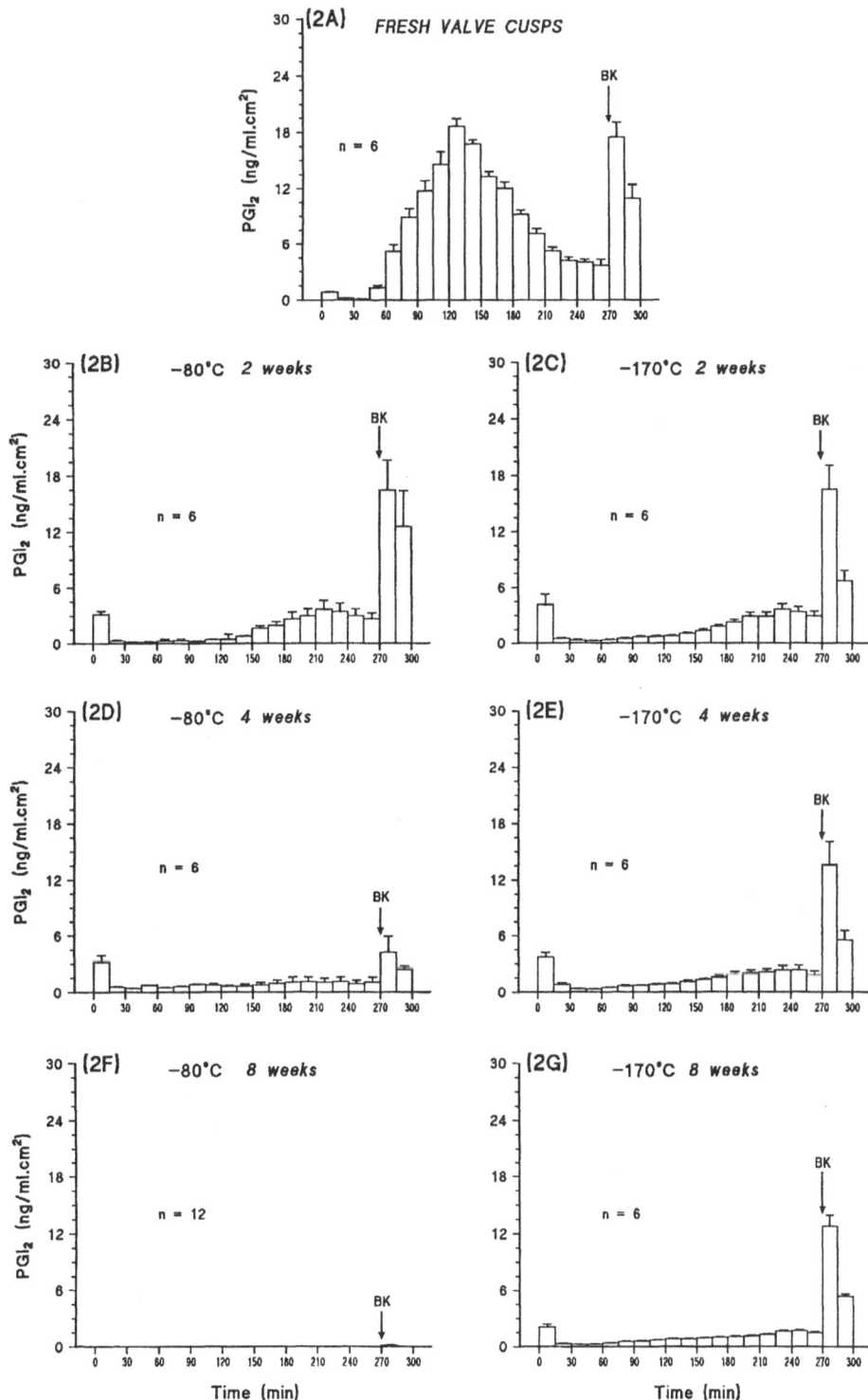

Time (min)

longer possible with the cusps kept at $4\,°C$ for 14 days in the same medium without renewal. The spontaneous release was less affected by the medium renewal and decreased as the duration of the storage increased.

Cryopreservation at $-80\,°C$ and $-170\,°C$

a) Short term storage at $-80\,°C$ and $-170\,°C$ (as long as 8 weeks)

Cryopreservation at either $-80\,°C$ or $-170\,°C$ for as long as 2 weeks showed a comparable PGI_2 production (Figs. 2B and C). Although the spontaneous release of PGI_2 was significantly diminished, the stimulated production was similar to the fresh valves (2A).

Cryopreservation for 4 weeks at $-80\,°C$, significantly reduced the spontaneous as well as stimulated PGI_2 production compared with fresh valves and valves cryopreserved at $-170\,°C$ (Figs. 2D and E).

After 8 weeks of storage at $-80\,°C$, hardly any PGI_2 production (spontaneous and stimulated) could be detected (Fig. 2F). In contrast, valves cryopreserved at $-170\,°C$ for 8 weeks still release PGI_2 (Fig. 2G) and this release was comparable to the production by the valves cryopreserved at $-170\,°C$ for 2 weeks (see Fig. 2C).

b) Long term storage at $-170\,°C$ (6 months to 1 year)

Long-term preservation in liquid nitrogen vapor phase significantly ($p < 0.05$) reduced the basal as well as the stimulated PGI_2 production after 6 months compared

Table 3. Prostacyclin production by porcine aortic valve after storage in liquid nitrogen vapor phase at $-170\,°C$ for as long as one year without or with fetal calf serum (FCS) (in nanograms per milliliter per square centimeter) ($n \geq 6$)

	Without FCS		With FCS	
	Basal	Stimulated	Basal	Stimulated
Control	2.73 ± 0.26	16.55 ± 2.12	2.73 ± 0.26	16.55 ± 2.12
1/2 year	$2.54 \pm 0.33*$	$9.94 \pm 0.77^{+*}$	$1.02 \pm 0.17^{+}$	$6.13 \pm 1.15^{+}$
1 year	1.68 ± 0.24	$9.62 \pm 1.71^{+*}$	$1.24 \pm 0.13^{+}$	$4.73 \pm 0.49^{+}$

After stimulation by bradykinin, PGI_2 could be significantly ($p < 0.05$) increased as compared to basal in all groups.
* Prostacyclin was significantly ($p < 0.05$) higher than the prostacyclin released by the group cryopreserved for the same periods with FCS.
+ Prostacyclin production was significantly less than the control values.

◀───────────────────────────────────

Fig. 2. Prostacyclin (PGI_2) production by valve cusps cryopreserved for different periods of time (2, 4 and 8 weeks) at $-80\,°C$ and $-170\,°C$ compared with fresh valve cusps. The X-axis numbers refer to the time of the consecutive incubation periods. The Y-axis display the PGI_2 content in the incubation medium within 15 min of incubation. Bradykinin (BK, 10 µM) was added into the medium as the agonist during the 270–285 min period of incubation. The bell-shaped curve (1A) represents the spontaneous PGI_2 production by the cusps.

with fresh valve cusps (Fig. 3 and Table 3), but then remained constant as long as 1 year.

When FCS was included in the cryopreservation medium, the PGI_2 production was significantly ($p < 0.05$) reduced at 6 and 12 months of storage compared with the same storage period without FCS.

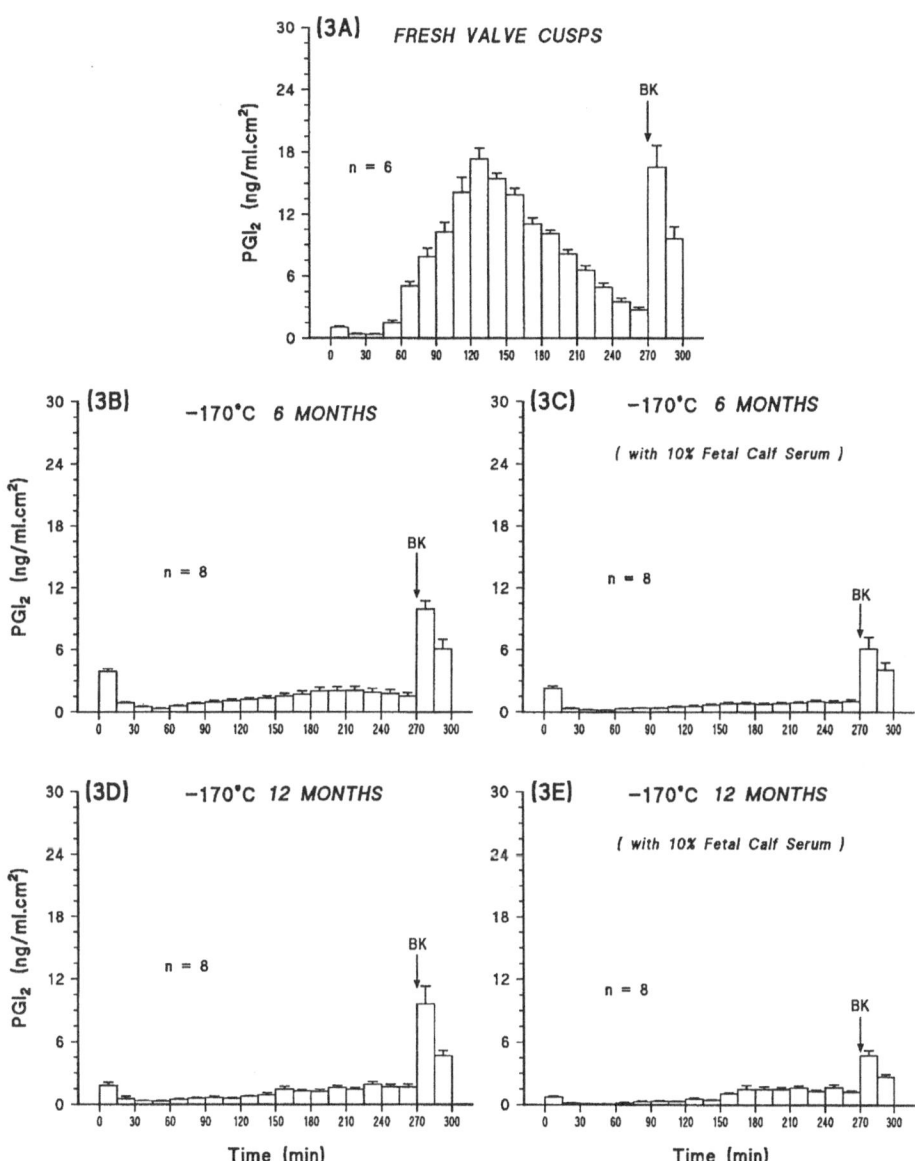

Fig. 3. Prostacyclin (PGI_2) production by valve cusps cryopreserved for as long as 1 year with or without fetal calf serum at $-170\,^\circ$C compared with fresh valve cusps. The X-axis numbers refer to the time of the consecutive incubation periods. The Y-axis display the PGI_2 content in the incubation medium within 15 min of incubation. Bradykinin (BK, 10 μM) was added into the medium as the agonist during the 270–285 min period of incubation. The bell-shaped curve (1A) represents the spontaneous PGI_2 production by the cusps. (Reproduction by permission J Thorac Cardiovasc Surg).

Table 4. Evaluation of scanning microscopy of surface morphologic characteristics of porcine aortic valves after storage at 4 °C for different periods

Scanning electron microscopy of valves surface					
Storange time	Endothelium coverage	Intercellular gaps	Membrane damage	Basal lamina	Fibrils exposure
Fresh	+ + +	0	0	0	0
2 days	+ + +	±	±	0	0
4 days	+ + +	±	±	0	0
7 days	+ +	+	±	±	±
14 days	+	+	+ +	+ +	+
21 days	0	0	+ + +	±	+ + +

+ + +, strongly present; + +, definitely present; +, present to some extent; ±, present or absent; 0, absent.

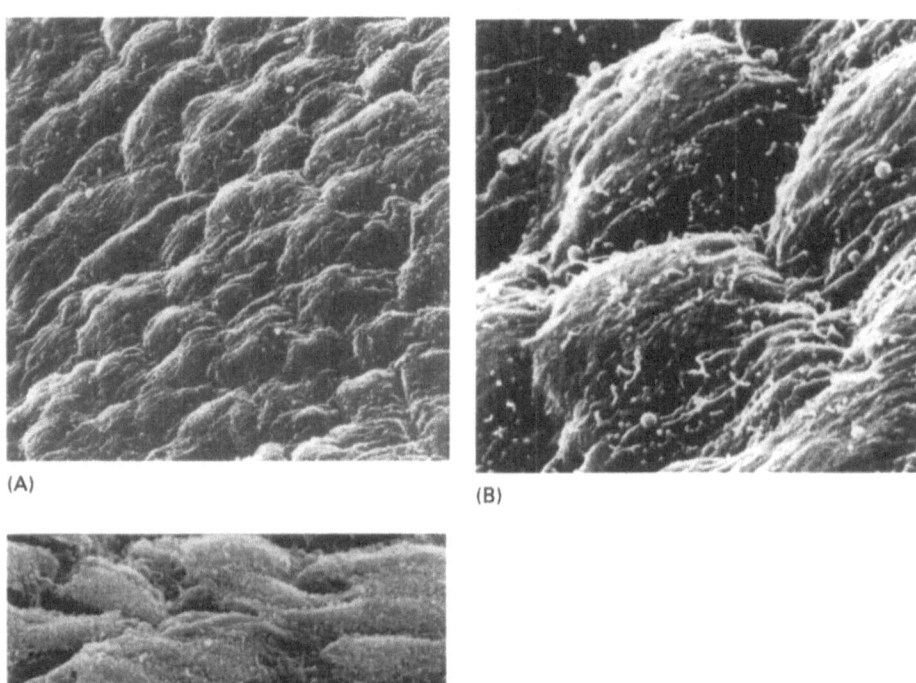

(A)

(B)

(C)

Fig. 4. Scanning electron micrograph of valve cusps stored at 4 °C in RPMI 1640 medium for 7 days. **A and B)** Most of the surface of valve cusp was covered by endothelium which was morphologically normal. **C)** In some areas, the shape of the cells had changed and intercellular gaps and basement membrane could be observed. Magnification: **A)** × 1920, **B)** × 7200, **C)** × 2400 (Reproduction by permission J Thorac Cardiovasc Surg).

Scanning electron microscopy (SEM) of 4 °C stored valves

The results of SEM are shown in Table 4. The morphological alterations of the endothelium appeared later than the biochemical changes, i.e., decrease of PGI_2 production. Up to 4 days of storage at 4 °C, SEM could not clearly distinguish variations of the endothelium. Intact endothelium with numerous microvilli covered the surface of the cusps; almost no subendothelial tissue could be observed and intercellular gaps were occasionally found. Even after 7 days of storage, most areas on the surface of valve cusp were still covered by endothelial cells (Figs. 4A and B). Slight damage was seen in some areas, e.g., the shape of cells had changed and intercellular gaps and retraction fibers revealing underlying basal lamina could be observed (Fig. 4C).

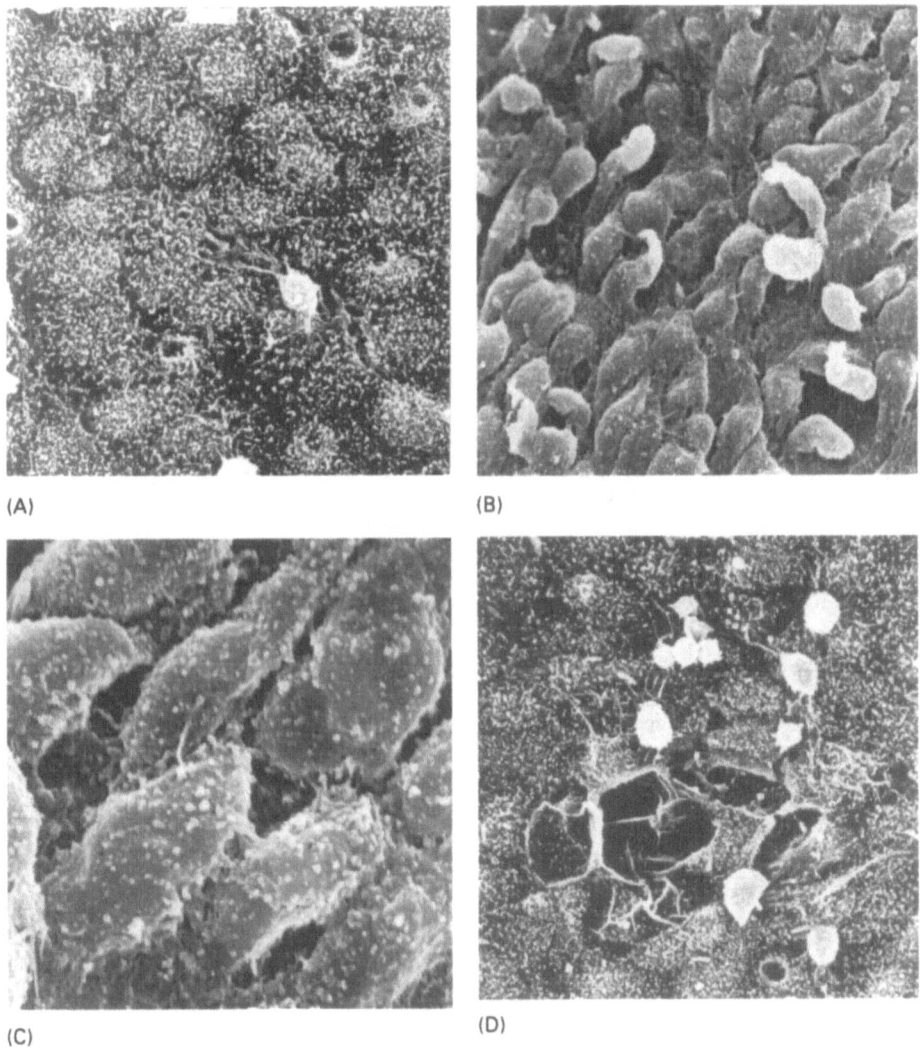

(A)

(B)

(C)

(D)

Fig. 5. Scanning electron micrograph of valve cusps stored at 4 °C in RPMI 1640 medium for 14 days. **A)** Many holes in the membrane of the endothelial cells. **B)** Disordered endothelial cells. **C)** Intercellular gaps and exposure of basement membrane. **D)** Some endothelial cells lost. Magnification: **A)** × 1440; **B)** × 1920; **C)** × 7200; **D)** × 1440 (Reproduction by permission J Thorac Cardiovasc Surg).

The valves stored at 4 °C for 14 days showed a damaged endothelial surface (Table 4). More than 50% of the endothelial cells were destroyed, i.e., displayed numerous holes in their cell membrane (Fig. 5A), had an abnormal arrangement with an abnormal cell shape (Fig. 5C), and large intercellular gaps revealing basement membrane could be detected (Fig. 5D). In some areas, endothelial cells were lost (Fig. 5C).

It was difficult to find morphological intact endothelial cells on the surface of the valves after 21 days of storage at 4 °C. Deendothelialization was common in most areas and only membrane remnants of endothelial cells could be seen (Fig. 6A), less basal lamina was present and underlying collagen fibers were often completely exposed (Fig. 6B and Table 4). A few scattered, remnants and shrivelled endothelial cells could be found in some fields (Fig. 6C).

Confocal scanning laser microscopy (CSLM) on cryopreserved valves

Endothelial cells of fresh valve cusps were intact with some scattered damaged cells (Fig. 7). Most endothelial cells were delineated by a peripheral band of actin filaments.

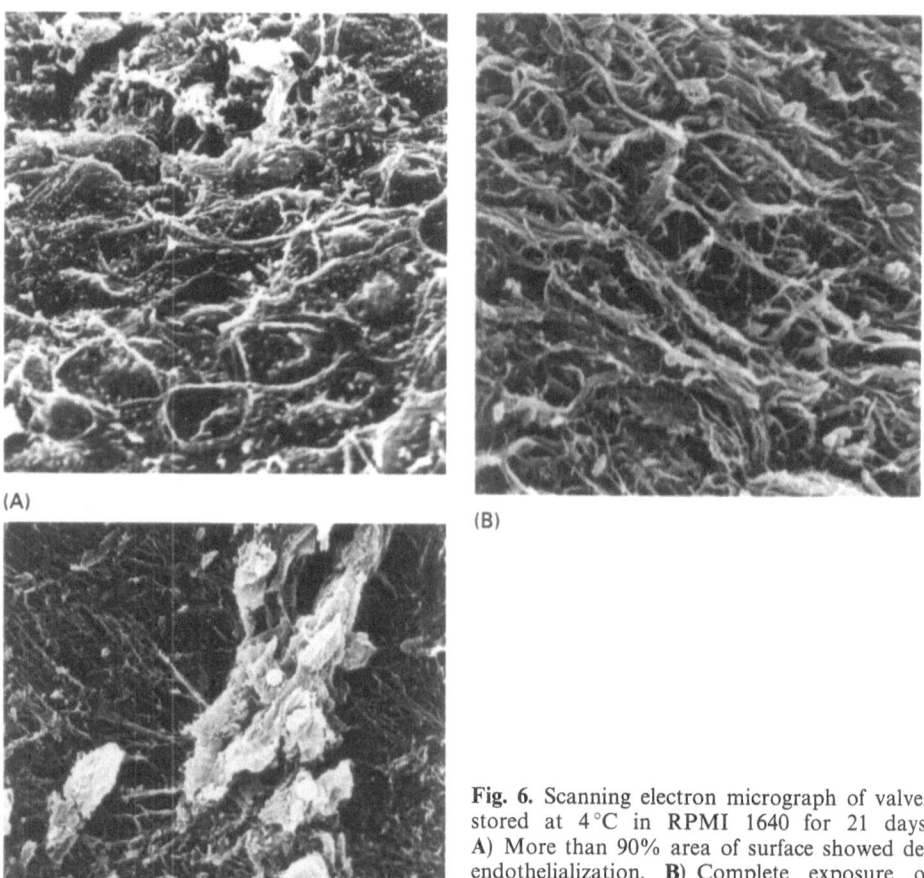

(A)

(B)

(C)

Fig. 6. Scanning electron micrograph of valves stored at 4 °C in RPMI 1640 for 21 days. A) More than 90% area of surface showed de-endothelialization. B) Complete exposure of fibers. C) Some remnant endothelial cells could be found but they are shrivelled. Magnification: A) × 2400; B) × 4800; C) × 1920 (Reproduction by permission J Thorac Cardiovasc Surg).

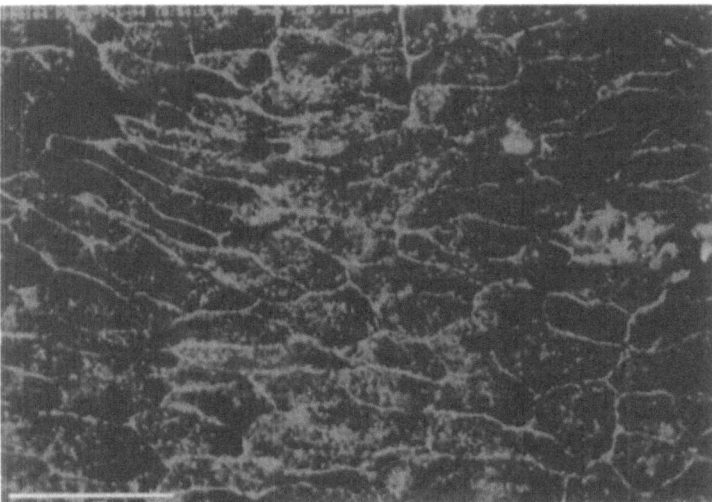

Fig. 7. Confocal Scanning Laser Microscopy images of en face views of endothelium or interstitial tissue. Dual color images were obtained by merging images of the green channel with images of the red channel. The green color represents labeling of actin filaments and the red color corresponds with labeling of nuclei by ethidiumhomodimer I. Fresh valve. Optical section through valvular endothelium along the inflow side of the cusp showing many endothelial cells with peripheral actin bands and small randomly oriented green colored rod-like structures which probably represent actin filament bundles of microvilli. In this field, only two endothelial cells are damaged in this section, as is demonstrated by the two nuclei labeled with ethidiumhomodimer I (red color). (Scale bar: 50 μm.)

The shape of the cells was variable and ranged from polygonal to highly elongated cells. Inside the cells, few actin microfilament bundles (stress filers) were present. Along the inflow side (faces the ventricular cavity which is smooth) of the cusps, many endothelial cells possessed rod-like structures without a specific orientation. These structures might represent the actin filament core of microvilli, which are known to be numerous at this side of the cusp.

In valves of cryopreservation at $-170\,°C$ for 1 year, optical sections through the endothelium demonstrated that large areas showed intact endothelial cells (Fig. 8) with a normal actin filament pattern and occasional scattered damaged cells with nuclei labeled by ethidiumhomodimer I.

Valves stored at $-80\,°C$ for 12 months were characterized by areas with damaged endothelial cells. Moreover, staining of actin filament bundles of the peripheral band was diffuse or interrupted in other cells (Fig. 9). Endothelial nuclei labelled with ethidiumhomodimer I were scattered between viable cells, or grouped together.

Discussion

Depending on the preservation methods used, cells of the homograft valve can be damaged and this will affect valve survival in the recipients after implantation. Therefore, when survival results of implanted valve homografts are evaluated it is necessary to distinguish between viable, nonviable and fresh homograft valves (20).

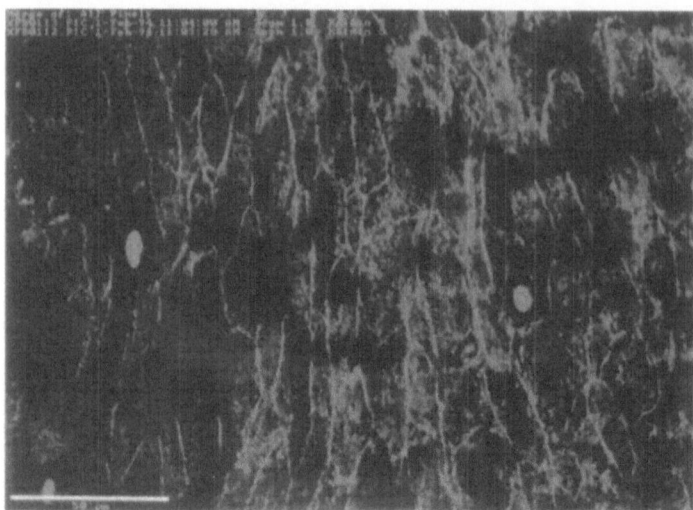

Fig. 8. In valve cryopreserved at −170 °C for 1 year. Optical section through endothelium. Endothelial cells were still outlined by a peripheral actin band. In this field, only three damaged (red stained) cells were found. (Scale bar: 50 μm.)

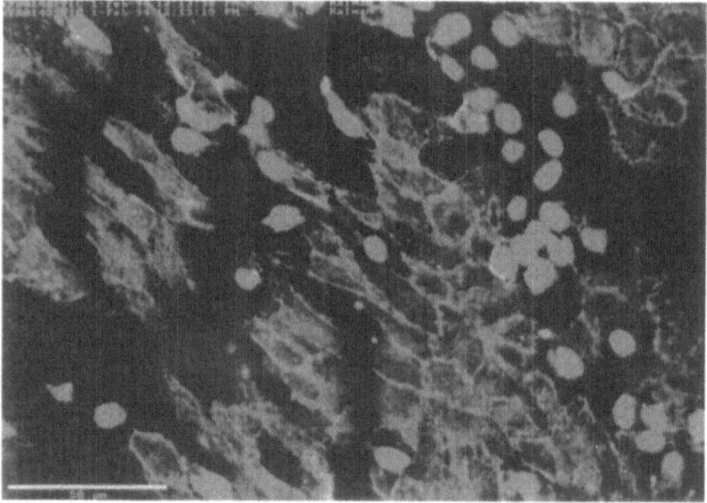

Fig. 9. In valve cryopreserved at −80 °C for 1 year. Optical section through endothelium. In this area, many damaged cells (marked by red nuclei) are present. The peripheral actin band of viable cells is broader and less distinct than in fresh valves. (Scale bar: 50 μm.) (Figs. 7–9 Reproduction by permission J Thorac Cardiovasc Surg).

Comparing three different storage temperatures, i.e., 4°, −80° and −170°C, the main advantage of storage in the unfrozen state at 4 °C is the avoidance of damage by the formation of ice crystals; the disadvantage however, is a limitation of storage duration. The present study demonstrated that after 24 h of storage in a refrigerator at 4°C, endothelial cells of porcine aortic valve cusps retain 93% (basal) and 74% (stimulated) of the PGI_2 production as compared to fresh valves. Up to 48 h of storage, PGI_2 production was reduced to respectively 63% (basal) and 41% (stimulated). After 4 days at 4 °C, the capacity of the endothelial cells to produce PGI_2 had sharply declined. Yankah and associates, using the dye exclusion test technique, identified 76%, 65% and 53% viable endothelial cells after storage at 4 °C for respectively 2, 20 and 30 h (24). Clearly, endothelium loses its viability within a short time at 4 °C.

Additionally, this study on storage at 4 °C also indicated that a functional alteration of endothelial cells (prostacyclin production) occurred earlier than pronounced morphological changes. After 1 week of storage at 4 °C, scanning electron microscopy of the valves still revealed a semi-confluent layer of endothelial cells although their biochemical function had already significantly decreased.

Viability of fibroblasts of heart valves stored at 4 °C has been previously studied. Yankah et al., by the dye exclusion technique, showed that 80% of the fibroblasts were viable after 30 h of storage at 4 °C (24). Mochtar and colleagues stored canine valves at 4 °C and by using the technique of autoradiograph protein synthesis showed that fibroblasts were only viable for 1 week (18). They could not reproduce the results of high viability after storage at 4 °C for more than 1 week, reported by Al-Janabi et al. (1). The observation by Mochtar et al. on fibroblasts viability are similar to our findings on endothelial cells based on their PGI_2 production (Table 2) and both indicate a rapid deterioration of the viability of the cells within 1 week of storage at 4 °C.

The main advantage of cryopreservation is that long-term storage can range from months to years. Preservation periods ranging from 10 years (17) up to 32 000 years (2) have been suggested. Such long periods can only be achieved with the temperature limits below the glass transition point of the freezing solution which is approximately -130 °C (7). In this way changes in frozen tissue structure can be avoided as chemical and physical processes are almost completely inhibited. The results of this study confirmed that a temperature below -130 °C is necessary for long-term preservation of the viability of the endothelial cells of heart valves. Up to 2 weeks, the viability of the endothelial cells was similar whether stored at -80 °C or at -170 °C (Fig. 2). Thus, when valves are intended to be stored for such short periods, we recommend storage at -80 °C since this temperature offers practical advantage over the storage at -170 °C which requires special tank filling with liquid nitrogen.

On the other hand, ice recrystallization has been detected at temperatures as low as -130°C (14, 15) and was accelerated at temperatures higher than -130 °C (14). This could explain that after 4 weeks of storage at -80 °C, the prostacyclin production by the endothelium of cryopreserved valves significantly decreased in our experiments. In contrast, after 8 weeks of storage at -170 °C, PGI_2 production of the cryopreserved valves was not significantly reduced as compared to fresh valves.

In this study, confocal scanning laser microscopy confirmed that numerous endothelial cells of the valve were still viable after more than 1 year of cryopreservation at -170 °C. This result was identical with the results of prostacyclin production by the cusps after 1 year of cryopreservation at -170 °C.

Fetal calf serum is commonly added to tissue culture medium as protein supplement (16) since it is considered to induce RNA and DNA synthesis (23). For this reason, FCS is widely utilized in the cryopreservation media for a variety of tissues and cells including human (6, 10, 19, 22). It was also used to enhance viability of preserved aortic homograft valves (11, 24). On the other hand, FCS is a potent heterologous antigen (4). In a previous study, we have indicated that fetal calf serum was not required for cryopreservation of porcine aortic valves (8). In this study, we demonstrated the negative influence of FCS, i.e., the loss of endothelial function during long-term cryopreservation. The results showed a lower PGI_2 release after bradykinin stimulation in valves stored at $-170°$ for 6 months when fetal calf serum was used as a supplement in the medium (Table 3). Although we cannot explain this observation, we can state that contrary to what has been usually recommended, the addition of fetal calf serum to the cryopreservation medium is not advisable for maintaining the functional integrity of the endothelial layer.

From our results we can conclude:

A) Endothelial viability of aortic valve cusps is retained until 4 days of storage at $4°C$ but is remarkably decreased there after. Morphologic alterations appeared later. Viability of the entire valve storage at $4°C$ should be assessed by measuring viability of endothelial cells because implanting a homograft valve, even with a morphologically apparently normal endothelial structure but with reduced or absent function, might mean that the collagen-laying self-repair function of the underlying fibroblasts could also be disturbed.

B) There was no difference in PGI_2 production after 14 days of cryopreservation at either $-80°C$ or $-170°C$. Although $-80°C$ is a more convenient technique for storage, liquid nitrogen vapor phase storage at temperatures below $-130°C$ is required for long-term preservation of endothelial function.

C) Fetal calf serum is not only unnecessary for short-term storage, but might be deleterious to the functional integrity of the endothelial cells.

Acknowledgment

The authors wish to thank Dr. Ai H. Lin for her important help with the radioimmunoassay of 6-oxo-PGF$_{1\alpha}$ and the laboratory personnel from the division of Electron Microscopy of University Instelling Antwerp for their invaluable help with the SEM.

References

1. Al-Janabi N, Gibson K, Rose J, Ross DN (1973) Protein synthesis in fresh aortic and pulmonary valve allografts as an additional test for viability. Cardiovasc Res 7: 247–250
2. Ashwood-Smith MJ, Farrant J (1980) Low temperature preservation in medicine and biology. Tunbridge Wells, Kent: Pitman, p 22
3. Barratt-Boyes BG, Roche AHG, Subramanyan R, Pemberton JR, Whitlock RML (1987) Long term follow-up of patients with the antibiotic sterilized aortic homograft valve inserted free hand in the aortic position. Circulation 75(4): 768–777
4. Bodnar E, Matsuki O, Parker R, Ross DN (1989) Viable and nonviable aortic homografts in the subcoronary position: a comparative study. Ann Thorac Surg 47: 799–805
5. Bodnar E, Olsen EG, Florio R, Guerreiro D, Ross DN (1988) Heterologous antogenicity induced in human aortic homografts during preservation. Eur J Cardiothorac Surg 2(1): 43–47
6. Dong JF, Detta A, Hitchcock ER (1993) Susceptibility of human foetal brain tissue to cool- and freeze-storage. Brain Res 621(2): 242–248
7. Dowell LG, Rinfret AP (1960) Low temperature forms of ice as studied by X-ray diffraction. Nature 188: 1144–1148
8. Feng XJ, van Hove CE, Mohan R, Andries L, Rampart M, Herman AG, Walter PJ (1992) Improved endothelial viability of heart valves cryopreserved by a new technique. Eur J Cardiothorac Surg 6: 251–255
9. Feng XJ, van Hove CE, Mohan R, Walter PJ, Herman AG (1993) Effects of different antibiotics on the endothelium of the porcine aortic valve. J Heart Valve Dis 2(6): 694–704
10. Fisher RL, Hasal SJ, Sanuik JT, Scott KS, Gandolfi AJ, Brendel K (1993) Cold- and cryopreservation of human liver and kidney slices. Cryobiology 30(3): 250–261
11. Gonzalez-Lavin L, Bianchi J, Graf D, Amini S, Gordon CI (1987) Homograft valve calcification: Evidence for an immunological influence. In: Yankah AC, Hetzer R, Miller DC, Ross DN et al. (eds) Cardiac Valve Allografts 1962–1987. New York: Springer-Verlag, pp 69–74

12. Hong SL (1980) Effect of bradykinin and thrombin on prostacyclin synthesis in endothelial cells from calf and pig aorta and human umbilical vein. Thromb Res 18: 787–792
13. Jaffe EA (1987) Cell biology of endothelial cells. Human Pathology 18: 234–239
14. Karow AM, Pegg DE (1981) Organ preservation for transplantation. New York: Marcel Dekker, p 118
15. Lange PL, Hopkins RA (1989) Allograft valve banking: Techniques and technology. In: Hopkins RA (ed) Cardiac Reconstruction with Allograft Valves. Springer-Verlag, New York, pp 37–64
16. Leibfried-Rutledge ML, Critser ES, First NL (1986) Effects of fetal calf serum and bovine serum albumin on in vitro maturation and fertilization of bovine and hamster cumulus-oocyte complexes. Biol Reprod 35(4): 850–857
17. Luyet BJ (1960) On various phase transitions occurring in aqueous solutions at low temperature. Ann NY Acad Sci 85: 549–552
18. Mochtar B, Van Der Kamp AWM, Roza-De Jongh EJR, Nauta J (1984) Cell survival in canine aortic heart valves stored in nutrient medium. Cardiovasc Res 18: 497–501
19. Muller-Schweinitzer E, Hasse J, Swoboda L (1993) Cryopreservation of human bronchi. J Asthma 30(6): 451–457
20. O'Brien MF, Stafford G, Gardner M, et al. (1987) The viable cryopreserved allograft aortic valve. J Cardiac Surg 2(suppl 1): 153–167
21. Salmon JA (1978) A radioimmunoassay for 6-Keto-prostaglandin $F_{1\alpha}$. Prostaglandins 15(3): 383–397
22. Settmacher U, Jahn S, Grunow R, Mehl M, von Baehr R (1989) Cryopreservation of newly formed human and mouse hybridoma cells. Allerg Immunol 35(3): 195–201
23. Supino R, Casazza AM, Di Marco A (1977) Effect of daunorubicin and adriamycin on nucleic acid synthesis of serum stimulated mouse embryo fibroblasts. Tumori 63(1): 31–42
24. Yankah AC, Hetzer R (1987) Procurement and viability of cardiac valve allografts. In: Yankah AC, Hetzer R, Miller DC, Ross DN et al. (eds) Cardiac Valve Allografts 1962–1987. New York: Springer-Verlag, pp. 23–26

Author's address:
Dr. X. J. Feng, MD, PhD
Department of Pharmacology
University of Antwerp (UIA)
Universiteitsplein 1, B-2610 Wilrijk
Belgium

Pre-implantation viability of cryopreserved valves prepared by the Green Lane Technique

L. C. Armiger, B. G. Barratt-Boyes

Department of Pathology, University of Auckland School of Medicine, and Green Lane Hospital, Auckland, New Zealand

Abstract

Objective: The importance of a viable donor cell population to the durability and clinical performance of the allografted heart valve is still disputed. The aim of our investigations has been to establish the pre-implantation viability status of the cryopreserved valves currently prepared for use as allografts at Green Lane Hospital and to correlate this with the cellular status of explanted cryopreserved grafts recovered at re-operation.

Methods: Viability was assessed primarily by an autoradiographic assay for the incorporation of glucosamine into proteoglycan matrix and results were compared with cell culture assays and cell ultrastructure. Twenty-six valves were obtained at autopsy and assayed sequentially 1) at collection; 2) after disinfection in antibiotic solution; 3) after thawing following cryopreservation and storage. A second group of 45 similarly disinfected and cryopreserved banked valves considered unsuitable for clinical use was assayed after thawing.

Results: Most of the banked valves showed only sparse radiolabelling confined to the hinge area of the leaflet. By electron microscopy, the unlabelled cells showed severe damage to plasma membranes and cytoplasm. In the autopsy series, valves obtained 24–48 h after donor death were non-viable at collection. Those obtained within 24 h of donor death showed variable extents of radiolabelling, but this declined markedly after 24 h of exposure to antibiotics and progressively still further after 48 h of antibiotic treatment and cryopreservation. Whereas 85% of all valves collected were viable initially, only 15–20% remained viable following disinfection and storage.

Conclusions: The majority, though not all, of the cryopreserved valves prepared at Green Lane Hospital are currently non-viable when implanted. The first 25 explanted cryopreserved valves examined histologically all show some focal fibroblastic growth which may presumably be either donor or recipient in origin. The disinfection and cryopreservation procedures in use at present have additive adverse effects on the cell viability of hypoxically-injured cadaver-derived valves.

Cryopreserved human heart valves have come to be widely regarded as the closest possible approach to the "fresh" untreated valves used initially as allografts: these performed better than later grafts which were freeze-dried or wet-stored relatively long-term (1, 5) and their superior durability was attributed by Angell (1) to the presence of a viable donor cell population. Few centres, however, have attempted to define the pre-implantation viability status of their cryopreserved valves and to correlate this with the cellular status and tissue architecture of the grafts when recovered at autopsy or re-operation (9).

Moreover, little attention has hitherto been paid to the potential additive effects of autolysis, antibiotic treatment, and cryoprotectant on donor cell viability, or to the possibility that such factors may result in phenotypic alteration of any cells surviving the valve preparation phase. These considerations can be expected to be significantly influenced by local differences in the collection and processing procedures employed from institution to institution, which thus may be largely responsible for the persistent difference of opinion in relation to the importance of using "viable" valve grafts.

In Auckland, therefore, we have been attempting to resolve some of these issues for our own locally-produced cadaver-derived cryopreserved valves and the present paper outlines our studies to date.

Materials and methods

To allow viability to be quantitated and related to leaflet histology, and to assess cellular synthetic activity rather than mitotic potential, we have used an autoradiographic assay for the incorporation of glucosamine into the proteoglycan matrix material of the valve leaflet. The method had been used previously for blood vessels (8) and its applicability to valve tissue was first tested by comparing the effects of wet-storage and cryopreservation on the viability of canine aortic valve leaflets procured immediately after sacrifice of the animals. Details of the technique have been published previously (4). Briefly, 1–2 mm radial blocks of leaflet and supporting tissues are incubated for 24 h at 37 °C in medium 199 containing 50 μCi [^{3}H]-glucosamine/3 ml. Following a 2-h cold chase the blocks are fixed in buffered 10% formalin containing 0.5% cetylpyridinium chloride and processed for histology. Autoradiographs are prepared from three levels of each block and grain counts/unit area are determined for ventricularis, spongiosa, and fibrosa in ten leaflet transects of each autoradiograph.

This assay has been used in two major studies:

1) Twenty-six valves (19 pulmonary, 7 aortic) obtained at post-mortem examination have been assayed sequentially after each phase of our routine valve preparation procedure, i.e. initially when procured, then following each 24 and 48 h in antibiotic solution (2, 11) (cefoxitin 240, lincomycin 120, polymyxin B 100, vancomycin 50, amphotericin 25 mcg/ml in Hanks' solution), and finally after thawing following cryopreservation (3) and storage for 4–81 days. Most of these valves have also been cultured for viable cells and all have been examined by electron microscopy (4).

2) Forty-five banked cryopreserved valves (25 pulmonary, 20 aortic) classed as unsuitable for clinical use have been thawed and assayed and examined by electron microscopy. These valves were all disinfected and cryopreserved by the same methodology as used for the post-mortem series (11, 3) but were stored for a wider range of time intervals and had a considerably longer mean storage duration.

Both studies included material covering a wide range of potential variables other than storage times. They were approved by the University of Auckland Human Subjects Ethics Committee.

Concurrently, 25 explanted cryopreserved valves have been examined histologically.

Results

The preliminary assessment of the autoradiographic technique in the freshly pro-cured dog aortic valves revealed a striking difference between normal and cryopreser-ved leaflets (Fig. 1). There was a very marked loss of viability following processing and this occurred preferentially from both surface layers and from the thinner co-apting regions of the leaflet.

The sequential study of the human post-mortem material showed that most of this loss resulted from the antibiotic treatment phase of the procedure (Figs. 2, 3). It also showed, however, that most valves collected 24 or more hours after death of the donor were non-viable initially (Fig. 3). In the viable group procured within 24 h of donor death the intensity of radiolabelling at collection varied considerably from valve to valve and did not appear to be consistently correlated with duration of autolysis.

Grain counts were particularly high in residual endothelium, which was generally lost during subsequent processing. The cryopreservation procedure itself was not totally without effect on residual viability following decontamination (Fig. 3). Results obtained by cell culture and autoradiography were closely similar (Fig. 4) when autoradiographs were scored simply as positive or negative.

Very few of the banked valves retained significant viability after thawing. When present, radiolabel was usually confined to the hinge area of the leaflet (Fig. 5).

By electron microscopy, unlabelled cells in both series of experiments typically showed nuclei that were relatively little changed from the normal but very severely damaged cytoplasm (Fig. 6).

The histology of the explanted cryopreserved valves showed variable focal growths of fibrous tissue in one or more leaflets of all these grafts. The foci were sometimes relatively diffuse but often dysplastic (Fig. 7). In no instance was a normal leaflet histology observed and considerable extents of leaflet in each valve remained acellular or populated only by host macrophages and/or insudations of blood cells.

Discussion

Recently, definitive evidence of early post-operative recipient immune response to cryopreserved valves has been obtained (6,10). This strengthens the possibility that the donor fibroblasts of viable cryopreserved valves may survive implantation only if there is a fortuitously good tissue match and that the good clinical performance of cryopreserved valves in general may more often be due to better preservation of the acellular ground substance of the leaflets than to a persistent cell population. It is of more interest than ever, therefore, that the viability status of these valves at implanta-tion should be known.

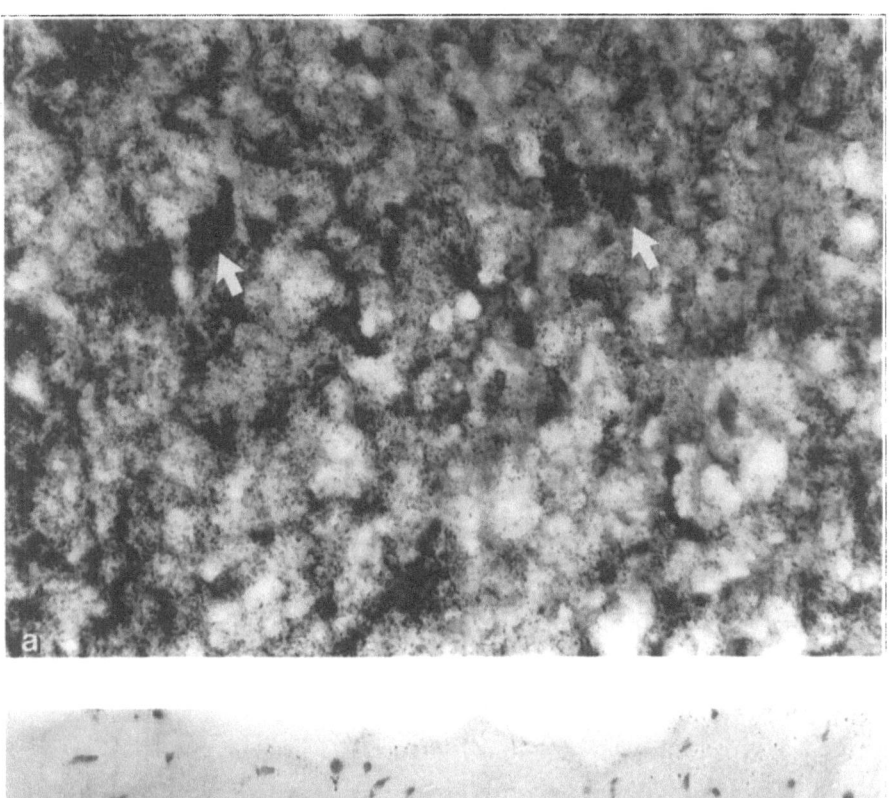

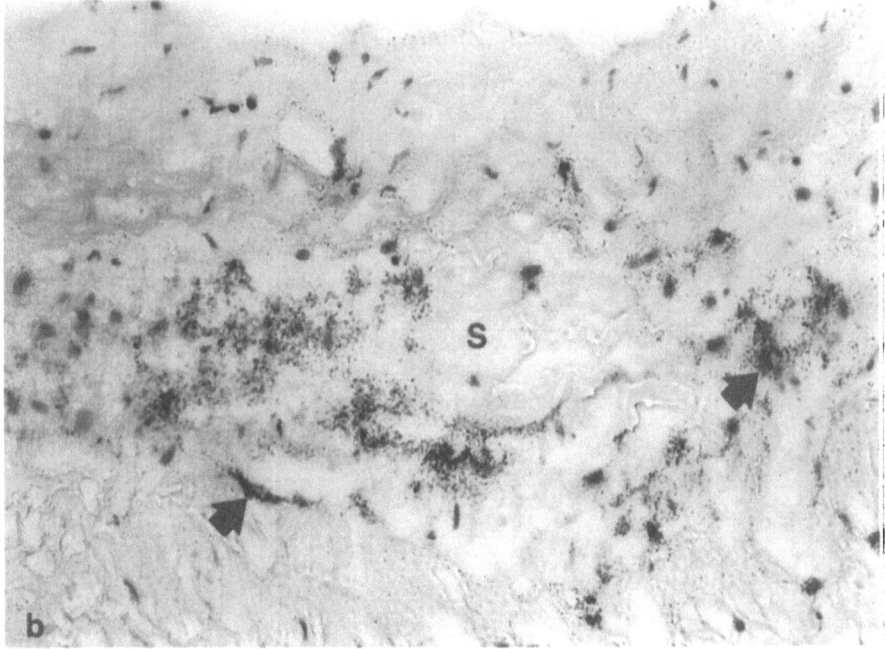

Fig. 1. Autoradiographs from the same dog aortic valve: a) control leaflet assayed immediately after procurement, showing widespread radiolabel which is particularly dense around cells (arrows); b) cryopreserved leaflet assayed after thawing, showing sparse, discontinuous radiolabel (arrows) in the spongiosa layer (S) only. LM × 550.

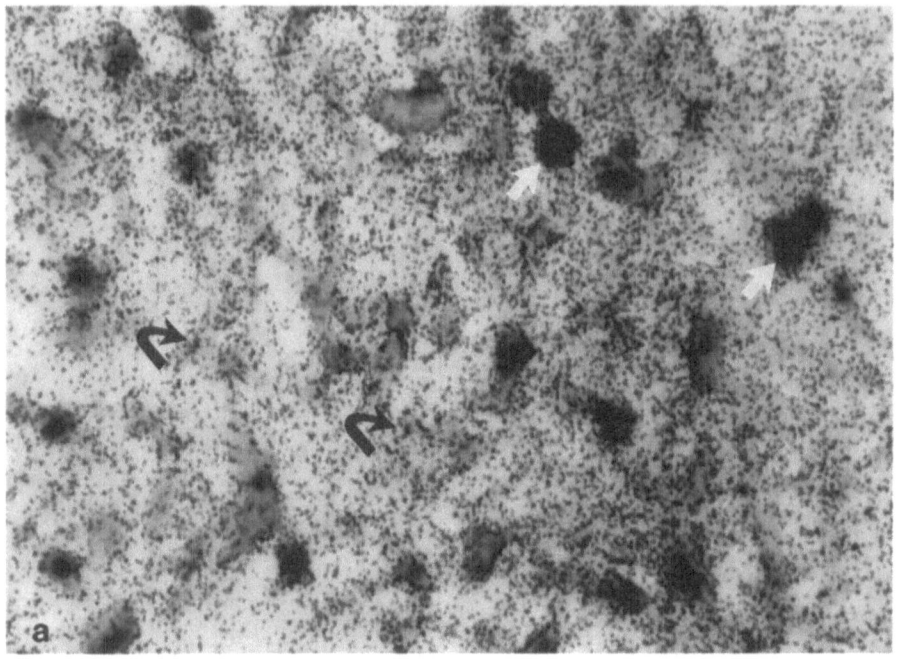

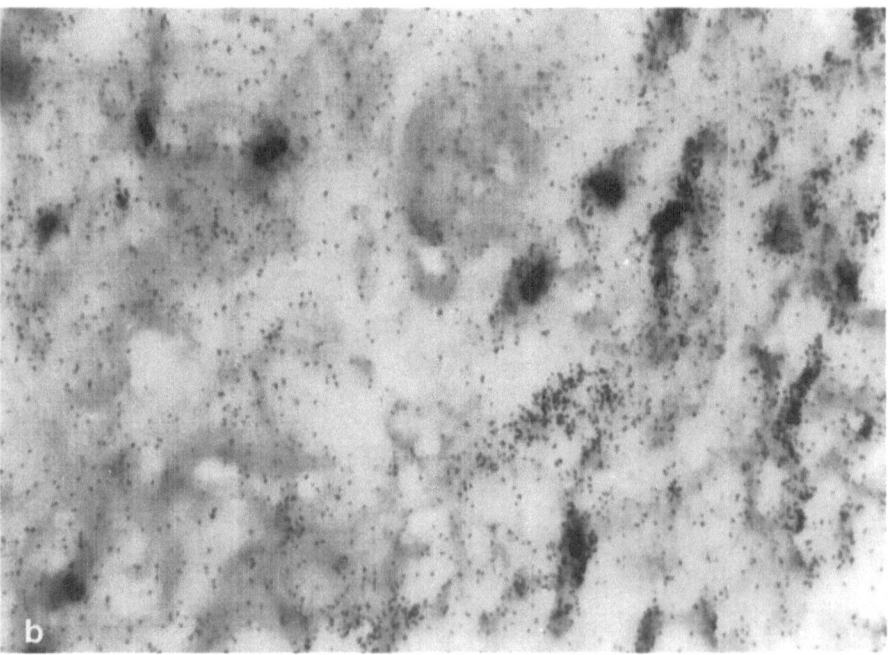

Fig. 2. Sequential autoradiographs from the same human aortic valve, showing progressive loss of viability during graft preparation procedure: a) good radiolabelling of cells (arrows) and matrix (curved arrows) in leaflet spongiosa at valve procurement 12 h after death of donor; b) diminished cell labelling after 24 h of antibiotic treatment; c) loss of cell labelling after 48 h of antibiotic treatment; d) minimal labelling of matrix only, following cryopreservation and thawing. LM × 1100.

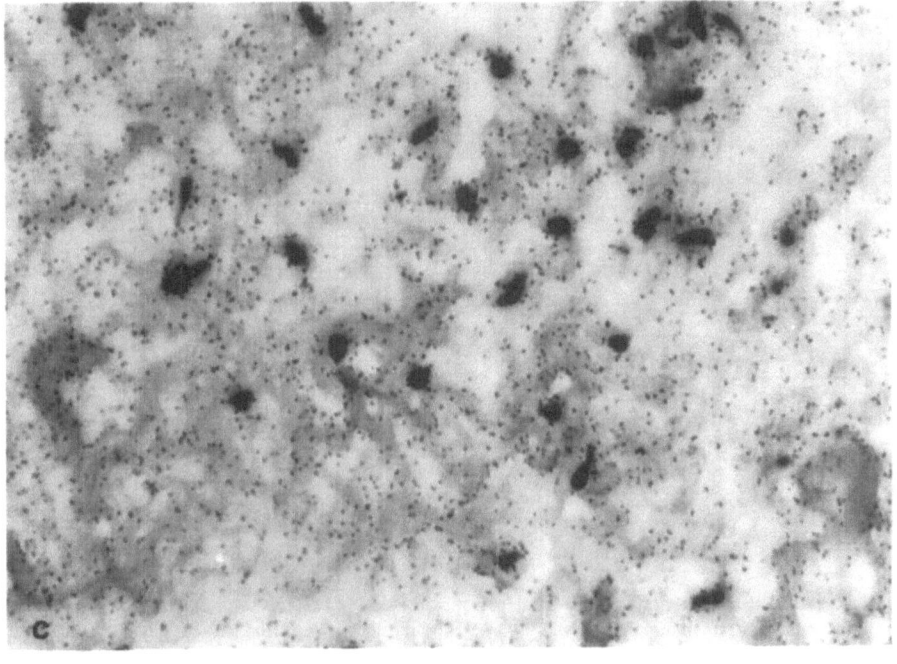

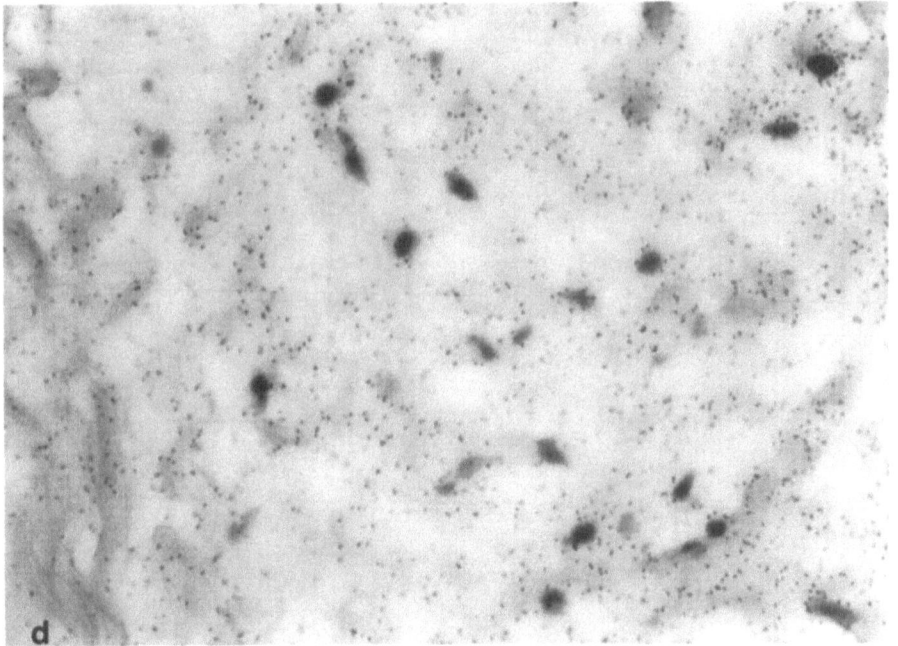

Fig. 2. c and d.

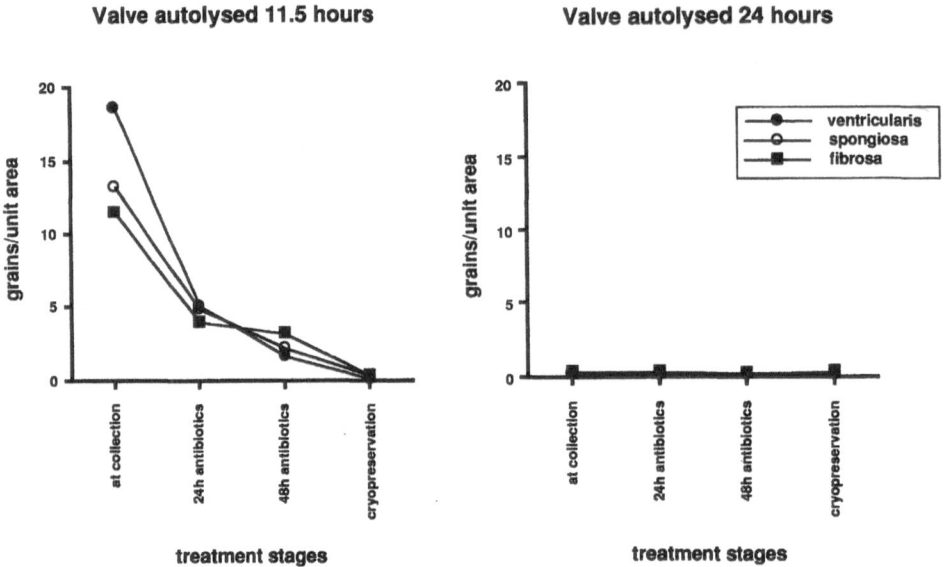

Fig. 3. Graphs showing: (left) in a valve procured 11.5 h *post mortem*, the progressive loss of radiolabel (viability) from all three tissue layers of the leaflet during the graft preparation procedure; (right) in a valve procured 24 h *post mortem*, the virtual absence of labelling throughout the tissue at all stages.

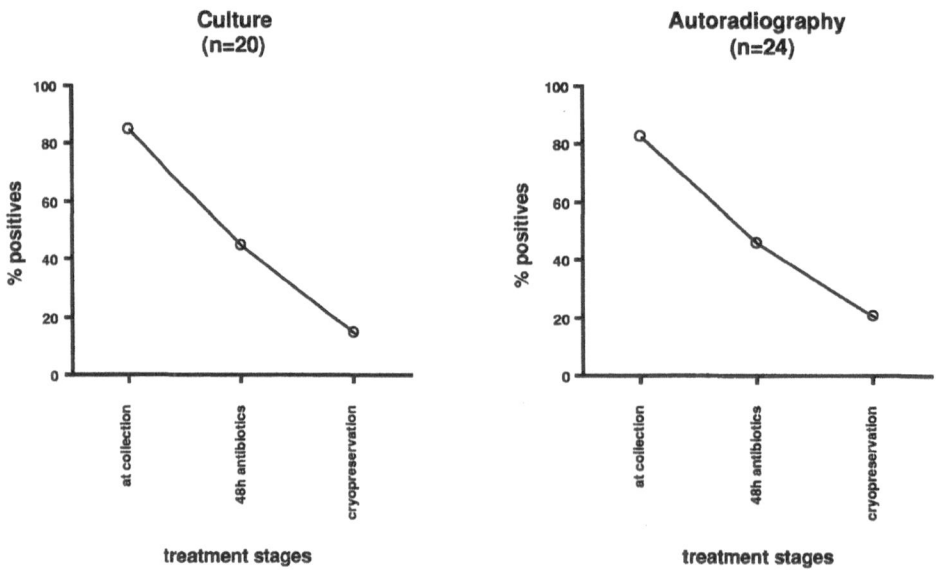

Fig. 4. Graphs illustrating the closely similar incidence of valve viability (following collection, antibiotic treatment, and cryopreservation) obtained by culture and autoradiographic assay.

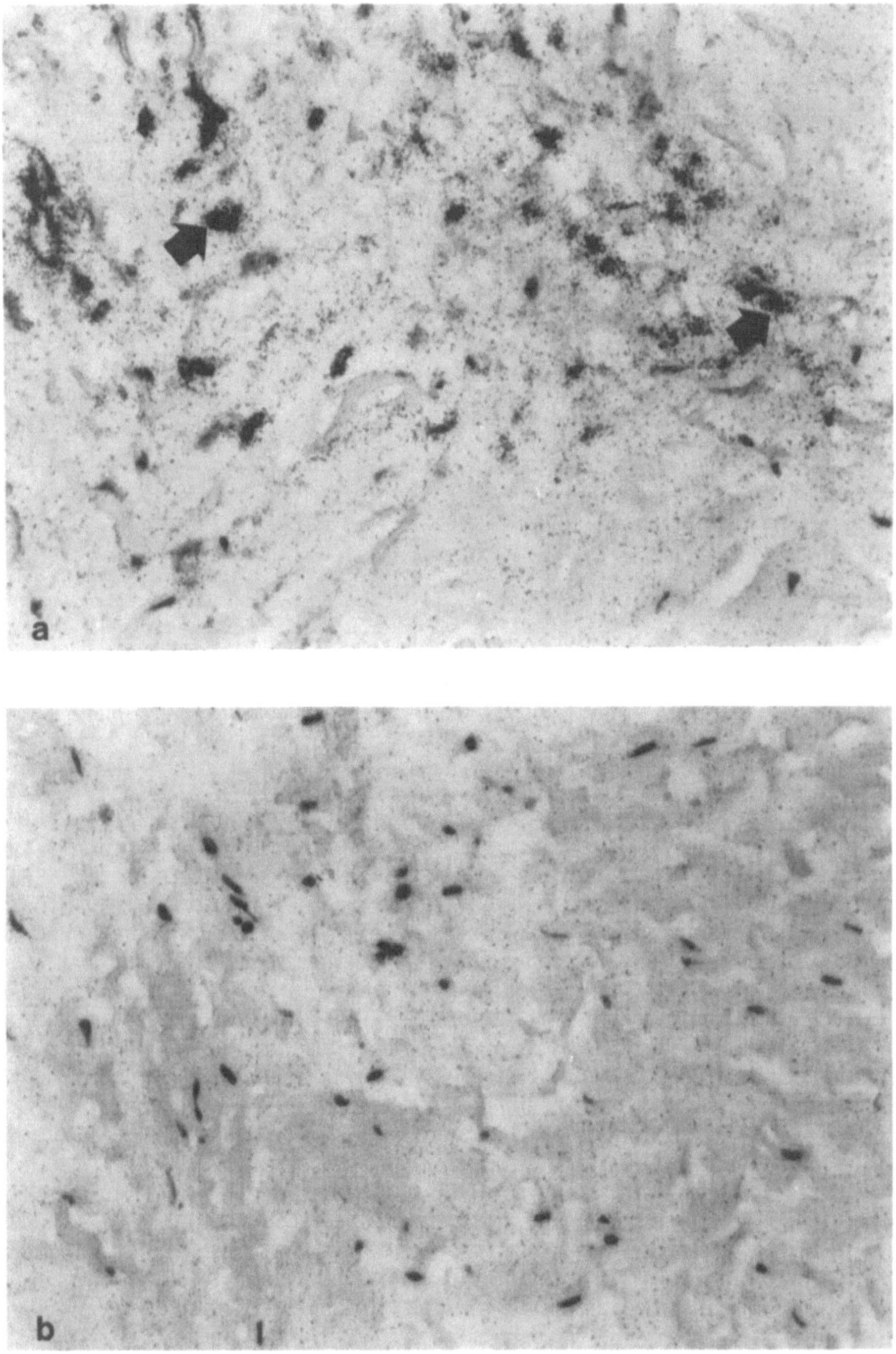

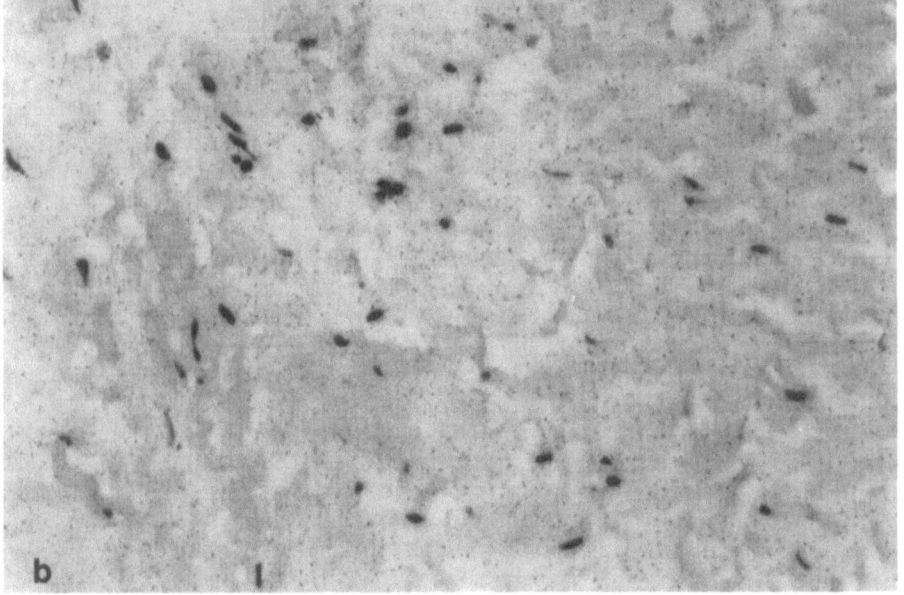

Fig. 5. Autoradiograph showing variable persistence of viability in one leaflet of a banked cryopreserved pulmonary valve: a) cell-associated radiolabel (arrows) in the spongiosa of the hinge (proximal) region; b) unlabelled cells with pyknotic nuclei in the belly (mid-region). LM × 550.

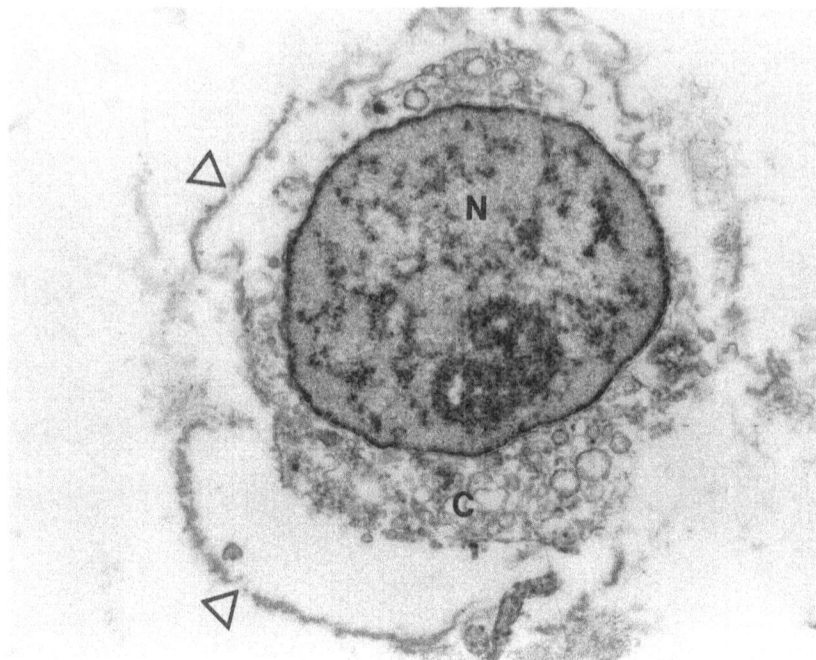

Fig. 6. A typical cell from a banked cryopreserved pulmonary valve collected 15 h *post mortem*. The nucleus (N) remains intact but the cytoplasm (C) and cell membrane (arrowheads) are markedly degenerate. EM × 23 650.

Our studies have shown that the cryopreserved valves produced in Auckland are in fact predominantly non-viable when inserted. Most of those obtained 24–48 h after death of the donor are already non-viable at collection. Although most collected within 24 h of donor death are viable initially, viability is progressively lost during processing and becomes insignificant in all except a relatively small percentage. The maximum drop in viability is seen in the first 24 h of disinfection with antibiotic solution and it is possible that the antifungal agent Amphotericin B is responsible for most of the cell injury, which specifically affects the cytoplasm and cell membrane (7, 10). Exposure to cryoprotectant appears to have a small additive effect on loss of viability in these previously hypoxic and antibiotic-treated cell populations. The exceptionally low incidence of viability in the banked valves we examined suggests that long-term storage in liquid nitrogen may also have some adverse effect, but this rather surprising possibility requires more intensive investigation.

The autoradiographic method we have developed distinguishes as viable only those cells still capable of synthesising matrix material and thus contributing to the coherence of the leaflet tissue. Unlike cell culture assays, it has revealed important differences in both numbers and distribution of these cells, which vary considerably from valve to valve even at procurement and are lost preferentially from the thinner and more superficial parts of the valve leaflet.

In addition to continuing normal production of ground substance, a donor cell population should maintain a normal or near-normal cell distribution and tissue architecture in order to be of long-term benefit to the valve graft. Convincing evidence that this can occur has yet to be obtained. The focal fibroblastic growth observed in our own explanted valves must be presumed to be of either donor or recipient origin,

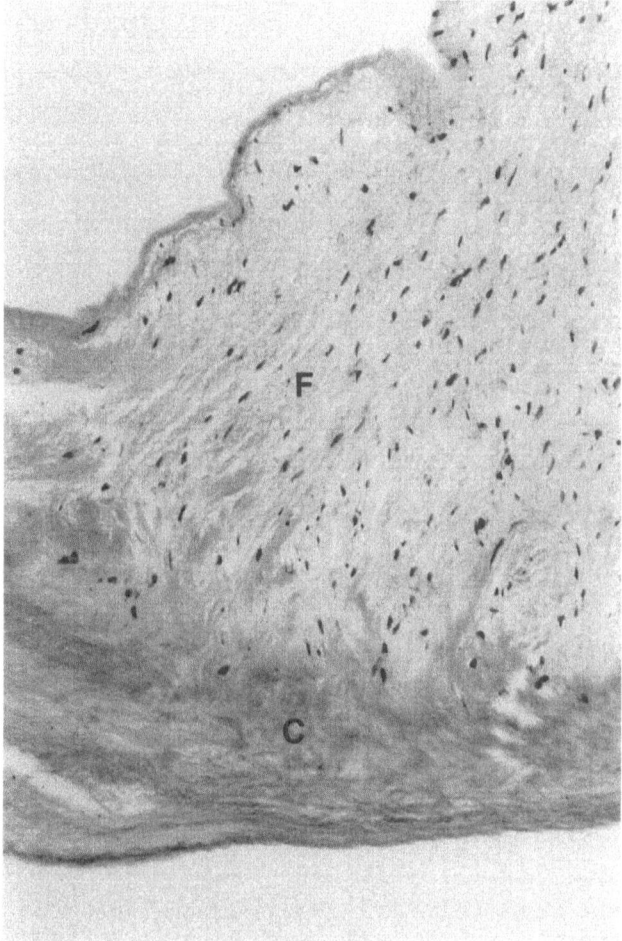

Fig. 7. A large, dysplastic focus of fibrous tissue (F) adjoining typical acellular collagenous graft tissue (C) in one leaflet of an explanted cryopreserved aortic valve. LM × 275.

but regardless of its origin it clearly did not contribute to the persistence of a normal leaflet histology. It should be remembered, however, that failed valves are recovered at re-operation and that the more successful grafts still in place may be showing a different picture.

Acknowledgements

These studies were supported by the Health Research Council of New Zealand, the Auckland Medical Research Foundation, and the New Zealand Lotteries Board.

Marianne Strickett of the Heart Valve Laboratory, Green Lane Hospital, and Tessa Collecutt, Anne Gordon, and Louise Allison of the Department of Pathology provided valuable technical assistance.

References

1. Angell WW, de Lanerolle P, Shumway NE (1973) Valve replacement: present status of homograft valves. Progr Cardiovasc Dis 15: 589–622
2. Armiger LC, Gavin JB, Barratt-Boyes BG (1983) Histological assessment of orthotropic aortic valve leaflet allografts: its role in selecting graft pre-treatment. Pathology 15: 67–73
3. Armiger LC, Thomson RW, Strickett MG, Barratt-Boyes BG (1985) Morphology of heart valves preserved by liquid nitrogen freezing. Thorax 40: 778–786
4. Armiger LC (1995) Viability studies of human valves prepared for use as allografts. Ann Thorac Surg 60: S118–121
5. Barratt-Boyes BG (1971) Long-term follow-up of aortic valvar grafts. Br Heart J 33(Suppl): 60–65
6. Fischlein T, Schutz A, Haushofer M, Frey R, Uhlig A, Detter C, Reichart B (1995) Immunological reaction and viability of cryopreserved homografts. Ann Thorac Surg 60: S122–126
7. Hu J-F, Gilmer L, Hopkins R, Wolfinbarger L (1989) Effects of antibiotics on cellular viability in porcine heart valve tissue. Cardiovasc Res 23: 960–964
8. Merrilees MJ, Scott L (1982) Organ culture of rat carotid artery: maintenance of morphological characteristics and of pattern of matrix synthesis. In Vitro 18: 900–910
9. O'Brien MF, Stafford EG, Gardner MAH, Pohlner P, McGiffin DC, Johnston N, Tesar P, Brosnan A, Duffy P (1988) Cryopreserved viable allograft aortic valves. In: Yankah AC, Hetzer R, Miller DC, Ross DN, Somerville J, Yacoub MH (eds) Cardiac valve allografts 1962–1987. Steinkopff, Darmstadt; Springer, New York, pp 311–321
10. O'Brien MF, Stafford EG, Gardner MAH, Pohlner PG, Tesar PJ, Cochrane AD, Mau TK, Gall KL, Smith SE (1995) Allograft aortic valve replacement: Long-term follow-up. Ann Thorac Surg 60: S565–570
11. Strickett MG, Barratt-Boyes BG, MacCulloch D (1983) Disinfection of human heart valve allografts with antibiotics in low concentrations. Pathology 15: 457–462

Author's address:
Dr. L. C. Armiger
Department of Pathology
School of Medicine
University of Auckland
Private Bag 92019
Auckland 1
New Zealand

The anatomic and physiological properties of the semilunar valves

A. C. Yankah

German Heart Institute Berlin, Berlin, Germany

Introduction

Since its introduction in clinical surgery in 1962 (2, 26) and in 1966, (27) respectively, implantation of aortic valve allografts in the systemic and pulmonary circulations has become a standard procedure in patients with congenital and acquired heart valve diseases. Currently, the pulmonary autograft and allograft valves, following their clinical use in 1967 and 1983 by Ross as valve substitutes in the systemic and pulmonary circulation, respectively, have been receiving much more attention and interest among cardiac surgeons (10, 12, 13, 18, 28).

Improvement in long-term durability of these grafts has been the subjects of interest with regard to better understanding of their anatomic, physiological properties and implantation techniques. Recent descriptions of the anatomy of the aortic valve and root have documented the importance and impact of the early descriptions on the reconstructive aortic root surgery of today. The shape of the aortic valve leaflet was first described by Philistion in the 4th century BC as semilunar (21, 30) while Eras Tistratos in the 3rd century suggested a sigmoid shape to describe the aortic valve leaflet (19, 20). Leonardo da Vinci demonstrated in 1513 in his drawing from autopsy specimens the geometry of the orifice of an opened and closed aortic valve as triangular and formation of three adjacent hemispheres, respectively (19, 20). Valsalva described the aortic sinuses in 1740 and suggested that the coronary artery filling takes place in the sinuses during the diastole (34). Recently, investigators have studied the aortic valve function by cineangiography and found that the aortic root alters its radius during the cardiac cycle and the semilunar valve leaflets initially opens during the early systole with stellate and triangular and completes with circular orifice (5, 32, 33) (Fig. 1). Gross and Kugel as well as others (38) described the aortic valve as a crown-like structure (Fig. 2). Mercer and colleagues in their studies on aortic valve leaflet described it as a parabolic structure which enables it to support the blood volume and pressure (22).

Surgical anatomy of the aortic valve

A completely dissected aortic and pulmonary valve is a crown-like structure and consists of three anatomic units: 1) a fibrous annulus, 2) three semilunar leaflets, and 3) commissures anchored within the expansible sinuses of Valsalva forming the prongs of the crown (Fig. 3). A good knowledge of the surgical anatomy of the aortic

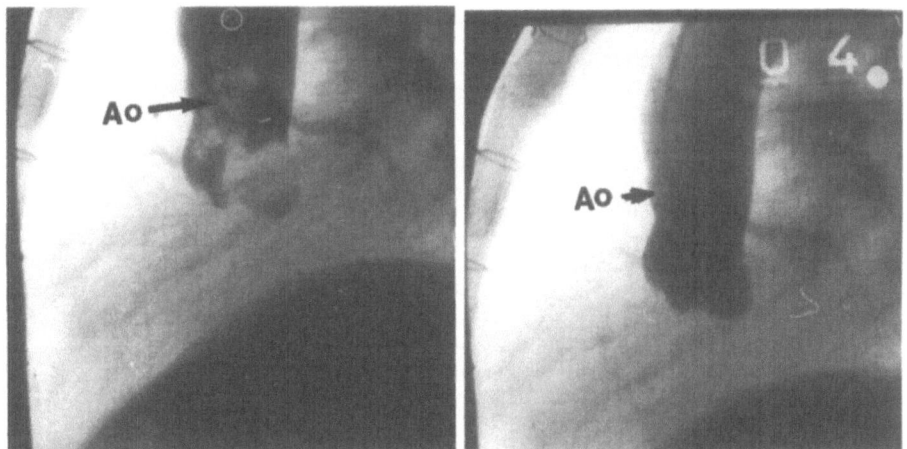

Fig. 1. Supraaortic angiogram of an implanted allograft aortic valve in subcoronary position demonstrating a) the aortic valve opening during systole with a circular orifice, b) competent valve closure during diastole.

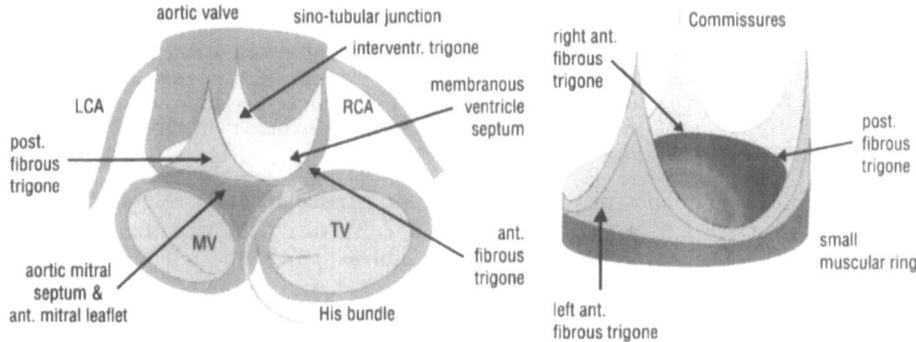

Fig. 2. Illustrations of a) aortic and b) pulmonary valves as crown-like structures.

root is a prerequisite for a valve and root replacement particularly for reconstructive procedures.

Semilunar leaflets

The three leaflets are anchored within the sinus walls and run nearly parallel to each other with the free margin in circumferential direction with the lowest point of attachment in the fibrous annulus, each forming a pocket. At the center of each free edge is a small, tough, fibrous structure, corpus or nodulus Arantii. From each side of the nodulus towards the lowest site of attachment of the leaflet is a thin, occasionally fenestrated portion. The free margins of the three leaflets make surface-to-surface contact during diastolic valve closure to achieve valve competence (Fig. 3).

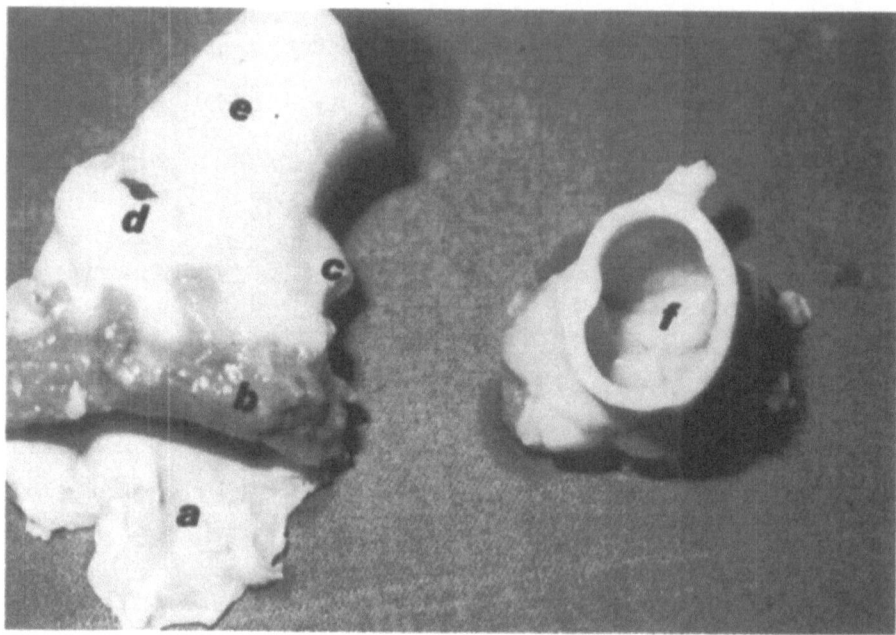

Fig. 3. Dissected aortic root: a) anterior mitral valve leaflet b) myocardial segment of the aortic annulus c) sinus of Valsalva with left coronary artery, d) sinus of Valsalva with the right coronary artery, e) sino-tubular junction with a short segment of the ascending aorta, f) view of the aortic root from above showing coapted trileaflet valve, the commissures and the right coronary ostium.

The surgical anatomies of the leaflets are designated by their relationship to the coronary artery origins within the sinuses of Valsalva: 1) the right coronary leaflet (RCL) which is also described as anteromedial leaflet, 2) the left coronary leaflet (LCL) which is also described as anterolateral leaflet, and 3) the non-coronary leaflet (NCL) which is also described as the posterior leaflet. The RCL lies a little lower than the LCL and the NCL while the RCL and the LCL originate in the myocardium (Fig. 1).

Physical properties

The physical properties of the aortic and the pulmonary valves may be influenced by many factors such as hypertension, immune response, pharmacological and chemical agents and warm ischemia. Elastin, collagen and proteoglycan are major extracellular matrix components (ECM), which provide structural strength to the valve and arterial wall as well as expansibility to the arterial wall. Collagen is very sensitive to pH changes because of its crosslinking polypeptide structure, and therefore vulnerable to the above factors. Elastin in contrast is more resistant. The vascular smooth muscle cells synthesize the majority of the ECM in the adult arterial wall and can modulate ECM production depending on the external stimuli (6, 16). While remodeling of the ECM is a physiologic response hypertension and immune response can cause pathologic remodeling process with increased synthesis and deposition of type I collagen and elastin (6, 16, 37). In tensile strength of the aortic valve and wall there is a difference between female and male aortic walls. Tensile strength is defined as the maximum response of a tissue to stress loading over the shortest period of time before tissue ruptures. There is a reduction in tensile strength of male aortic walls beyond 35 years to 20% of control values at 70 years of age (15). While in the females there is a minimal reduction in tensile strength of 20% until age 75 years. The largest expansibility of the sinuses is near the commissures and the lowest is at the sinus bottoms, which might constitute a stress-reducing mechanism. Aortic valve leaflets however show no differences in tensile strength with age and sex.

Distensibility of the aortic root

The expansibility of the aortic root is the percent difference change in diameter during the cardiac cycle, i.e., systole and diastole. This can be measured by echocadiography or by supraaortic angiography. The distensibility measurements of the aortic root provides information on the dynamic changes of the anatomic units of the aortic root after subcoronary freehand aortic valve and root replacement using allografts or xenografts (Fig. 5). Distensibility of the aortic annulus after subcoronary freehand aortic valve replacement using single multiple interrupted sutures in patients below 50 years of age was 3.2–5.8% and 2.5–4.5% in patients above 50 years of age (37).

Functions of the endothelium

The endothelium of the aortic and pulmonary valves is multifunctional. It coordinates the permeability, thus transportation of substances from the blood to the valve tissue and vice versa. The transport system is closely related to metabolic activities and cellular interactions of the endothelium. It contributes to the maintenance of the hemostasis by synthesizing highly active anti-platelet-aggregating prostacyclin (PGI2) from the endoperoxides (23). The endothelial cells synthesize type IV collagen and release it into the extracellular matrix (17).

Role in the immune system

The semilunar valves are by virtue of possessing endothelial cells, antigenic. The endothelial cells can express MHC Class I and II antigens, Factor VIII antigens as well as adhesion molecules H/Y, ICAM-1 and ELAM-1 (31, 35, 36). Expression of Class II antigens by dendritic cells in the valve strome has also been demonstrated (35). The endothelium also possesses receptors for the component C3a of the complement system (9, 24). On the basis of these properties the semilunar valves when used as allografts for valve replacement should be histocompatible. Alternatively, the potential immunological structures should be eliminated otherwise immunosuppressive treatment of the recipient might be considered.

Histological structure of the aortic valve

The leaflet has ventricular and aortic endothelial layers, between which are 1) loose circumferential connective tissue with a few elastic fibers, 2) radial collagen and elastic fibers, and 3) coarse circumferential collagen bundles. There are basic structural differences between the aortic wall and the valve leaflets. The leaflet contains a few collagens and abundant elastin at the base and its attachment to the sinus, while at the free margins more collagens and a few elastin are found. In the aortic wall the collagen and the elastin are uniformly distributed. The sinus walls consist of mainly circumferentially arranged smooth muscular tissue embedded in a network of arbitrarily oriented elastic fibers. These structures are anchored into the fibrocartilaginous aortic ring. Chromosomal analysis of the valve cells can be employed to identify male or female valve. This study is therefore useful in allograft valve surgery to identify cell origin in donor valve or persistence of donor cells in the event of explant (25).

Aortic annulus

The aortic annulus is a fibro-cartilaginous structure, which is the site of attachment of the lowest segments of the valve leaflets. The dimensions of the annulus determine the size of the valve, which in adults ranges from 17–25 mm in diameter at a mean of 22 mm. In males the dimensions of the aortic annulus are greater than in females. The average aortic annulus diameter in males is 24 mm as compared to 22 mm in females (Table 1).

Subannular structures

The fibrous trigones: They are fibrous structures between the commissures of two valve leaflets at the point of annular attachment and the membranous or the muscular

Table 1. Annular dimensions of aortic and pulmonary allograft valved conduits in adults

Diagnosis of heart donors	Aortic annulus (mm)	Sino tubular ridge (mm)	Pulmonary annulus (mm)
Noncardiac diseases n = 171	22.1 17–25 (range)	19.3 15–22 (range)	25.2 16–29 (range)
Ischemic heart diseases n = 114	23.5 23–27 (range)	20.4 21–24 (range)	28.8 23–31 (range)
Dilating cardiomyopathy n = 285	26.0 23.29 (range)	23.5 21–26 (range)	29.7 25–33 (range)

septum (Fig. 2). In a surgical anatomy the fibrous trigones are designated 1) the right anterior (RAT), 2) the left anterior (LAT) or posterior intervalvular trigone, and 3) the interventricular trigone (IVT). The RAT is the most prominent, through which passes the main conduction bundle of His from atrial to ventricular side. The mitral-aortic septum (MAS) is mobile fibrous structure which lies between the RAT and the LAT and is closer to NCL and is in continuity with the anterior mitral valve leaflet forming a curtain between the aortic and the mitral valves, which is also described as the aortic-mitral fibrous continuity (1) (Fig. 3). It moves back and forth during the cardiac cycle and is the shortest distance between the base of the NCL and the LCL and the annulus.

Sinuses of Valsalva

The aortic sinuses are thinner, onion-shaped vascular walls of bulbus aortae which lies between the sino-tubular junction of the ascending aorta and the aortic annulus. The right and the left aortic sinuses give origin to the right and the left coronary arteries, respectively, and are in surgical anatomy designated as the right coronary (RCS), the left coronary (LCS), and the non-coronary (NCS) sinuses. The RCS has its origin in the myocardium and lies lower than the LCS and the NCS (Figs. 1, 3).

Pulmonary valve

Surgical anatomy

The pulmonary valve has all the characteristics of the aortic valve with exception of its anatomic position. It is a crown-like structure with 1) three semilunar leaflets, while the commissures are anchored into the sinus walls, and 2) a small fibrous annulus (Fig. 2b). The PV lies superior and sinistral to the aortic valve. The adventitia is confluent with the epicardium of the right ventricle. There are two anterior leaflets and one posterior leaflet. Its posterior sinus is closed to the right aortic sinus (RAS). The sinuses do not give origin to coronary arteries and the annulus dimensions are greater than that of the aortic annulus, ranging from 16 to 29 mm in diameter with a mean of 25 mm in adults (Table 1). The average female PV annulus diameter is 23 mm as compared to 25 mm in male.

Relationship of the left anterior descending coronary artery to the pulmonary root

An absolute knowledge of the surgical anatomy of the pulmonary root and its relationship to the first septal branches of the left anterior descending (LAD) branch of the left coronary artery is a *sine qua non* for the transplantation of the pulmonary autograft in the aortic position. The first septal artery branches of the left anterior descending coronary artery lie 2–6 mm from the posterior leaflet of the PV and occasionally with atypical courses. There are three major types of branching of the first septal arteries of the LAD classified as types I, II and III. Type I (30%) is about 3 mm above, type II (25%) is about 3 mm at the level of and type III (45%) is more than 3 mm away and below the posterior sinus of the PV. Types I and II first septal branches of LAD might be vulnerable during harvesting of pulmonary autograft and implantation of homograft to the posterior and lateral myocardium of the right ventricular outflow tract. The surgical anatomy of the pulmonary root and its relationship to the left main coronary artery and LAD has been described in detail by Geens et al. (11).

Opening mechanism of the semilunar valves

The mechanism of opening of the semilunar valves is governed by the law of La Place and it occurs because of the distensible nature of the aortic and pulmonary root structures (the annulus and the incorporated commissures in the sinuses). The aortic valve (AV) and the pulmonary valve (PV) are passive structures. In each cardiac cycle when the ventricular pressure equals the aortic and the pulmonary pressure the sinuses expand and the intercommissural distances increase (7). An expansion of the sinuses and the annulus by 5% would result in a radial movement (vector force) of the commissures (the prongs of the crown-like structures) outwardly and create a tangential tension on the leaflets which pulls the leaflets open to produce a stellate orifice and completes with a circular orifice (Fig. 1). Further opening of the leaflet is determined by the annulus dilatation in response to increase in pressure gradient between the right ventricle/pulmonary artery and left ventricle/aorta and forward flow velocity in every cardiac cycle. Expansion of the annulus by more than 10% results in a change of configuration of the valve orifice from stellate to triangular to, lastly, circular in order to accomplish a complete opening. If the leaflets are attached to a non-distensible structure, the AV can open only when the leaflets are forced apart by the systolic forward flow velocity of the blood from the ventricle. This mode of opening would result in an initial circular orifice. The leaflets are therefore subjected to an additional flexion at the center being the greatest (5, 33).

Mechanism of valve closure

A complete competence of AV and PV at diastolic valve closure is obtained when the diameters of annulus and the sinus as well as the commissural perimeters are reduced to their physiological diastolic dimensions at every cardiac cycle. The free margins of the leaflets and the noduli Arantii will come surface-to-surface in contact (Figs. 1, 3).

An increase in leaflets stress or a change in the geometry of the crown-like valve structure (annulus, leaflets and commissures) and the sinotubular junction such as dilatation, stenosis, undersized allograft or geometric distorsion of the annulus might prevent the leaflets from coming in apposition (3, 8).

Comments

The pulmonary (PV) and the aortic valve (AV) are crown-like structures, each of which consists of three anatomic units: 1) the fibrous annulus, 2) three semilunar valve leaflets, and 3) the commissures. The three commissures are anchored within the expansible sinuses and are distally stabilized at the sino-tubular junction. The pulmonary valve lies superior and sinistral to the aortic valve and its posterior conus is closed to the right aortic sinus. The first septal artery branches of the left anterior descending coronary artery lie 3–6 mm from the posterior leaflet of the PV and occasionally with atypical courses. The average annulus dimension is 25 mm in diameter which is greater than that of the aortic annulus (23 mm). The histological structure consists of two ventricular and pulmonic single layers of endothelial cells which are encoded with MHC Class I and II surface antigens (35, 36). Between the two endothelial layers are elastic and collagen fibers; the former diminish with age. The normal function of the PV is primarily dictated by its shape, geometry, and the physical properties of the anatomic units. There are basic structural differences between the pulmonary arterial wall (PAW) and PV leaflets. At the base and the attachment site to the sinuses, the leaflets contain a high proportion of elastin and a low proportion of collagens while the reverse is true of their free margins. The PAW contains uniformly distributed elastin and collagens. Elastin, collagen as well as proteoglycans are major extracellular matrix components (EMC) which provide structural strength and elasticity to the pulmonary arterial wall and sinuses.

In patients with high pressure VSD, a viable pulmonary valve and arterial wall can withstand three times the normal right ventricular pressure load (13, 14). From anatomic and histologic view points, viable autograft and allograft have the ability to remodel their structures under acute and chronic pressure conditions by increasing the synthesis of elastin and collagens. However, in allografts this can contribute to pathologic processes, such as structural deterioration and calcification. A non-viable PV and PAW might have a limited or no capacity to remodel their structures in response to systemic pressure. As increased elastin and collagen production is a physiologic response to remodel the pulmonary root under systemic high pressure, it might be more accelerated in viable allografts in which immune response and high pressure are the two major contributing factors. In contrast to aortic root in pulmonary circulation the low pressure and the low oxygen saturation might be the other contributing factors for accelerated degeneration. A change in the geometry of the AV and PV (annulus diameter, leaflet radius, and commissures perimeter) either by dilatation of the annulus, sinuses and the sino-tubular junction in association with dilatation of the ascending aorta as well as ring distorsion might therefore effect the function of the valves, thus preventing the leaflet coapaptation.

Surgical implications: To prevent geometric distorsion of the aortic or pulmonary root autograft or allografts root replacement might be a preferred implantation technique. While viable pulmonary autograft might adapt to pressure change in the systemic circulation the pulmonary allograft might therefore not prevent acute or subacute dilatation of allograft pulmonary root in systemic high pressure, particularly in hypertensive patients; root replacement by intraaortic cylinder might be preferable. Subcoronary freehand implantation technique needs proper fixation of the allograft annulus into a normal undistorted host annulus, and proper position of the commissural post at the sino-tubular junction for stabilization of the anatomic units without geometric distorsion during the cardiac cycles.

References

1. Anderson RH, Becker AE, Losekot TG, Gerlis LM (1975) Anatomically corrected malposition of great arteries. Br Heart J 37: 993

2. Barratt-Boyes BG, Christie GW, Raudkivi PJ (1992) The stentless bioprosthesis: surgical challenges and implications for long-term durability. Eur J Cardio-thorac Surg 6 (suppl. I): S39–S43

3. Barratt-Boyes BG (1964) Homograft aortic valve replacement in aortic incompetence and stenosis. Thorax 19: 131–150

4. Bellhouse BJ, Bellhouse F, Abbot JA, Talbot L (1973) Mechanism of valvular incompetence in aortic sinus dilatation. Cardiovasc Res 7: 490–494

5. Brewer RJ, Deck JD, Capati B, Nolan S (1976) The dynamic aortic root. Its role in aortic valve function. J Thorac Cardiovasc Surg 72: 413–417

6. Campbell JH, Tachas G, Black MJ, Cockerill G, Campbell GR (1991) Molecular biology of vascular hypertrophy. Basic Res Cardiol 86: (Suppl. 1): 3–8

7. Christie GW (1992) Anatomy of aortic heart valve leaflets: the influence of glutaraldehyde fixation on function. Eur J Cardio-thorac Surg 6 (Suppl. I) S25–S33

8. David TE (1995) An anatomic and physiologic approach to acquired heart disease. Eur J Cardio-thorac Surg 9: 175–180

9. Denny JB, Johnson AR (1979) Uptake of 125-J-labelled C3a by cultured human endothelial cells. Immunology 36: 169–177

10. Elkins RC (1994) Pulmonary autograft – the optimal substitute for the aortic valve? N Engl J Med 330: 59–60

11. Geens M, Gonzalez-Lavin L, Dawbarn C, Ross DN (1971) The surgical anatomy of the pulmonary artery root in relation to the pulmonary valve autograft and surgery of the right ventricular outflow tract. J Thoracic Cardiovasc Surg 62: 262–267

12. Gerosa G, McKay R, Davies J, Ross DN (1991) Comparison of the aortic homograft and the pulmonary autograft for aortic valve and root replacement in children. J Thorac & Cardiovasc Surg 102: 51–61

13. Gerosa G, McKay R, Ross DN (1991) Replacement of the aortic valve or root with a pulmonary autograft in children. Ann Thorac Surg 51: 424–9

14. Gorczynski A, Trenkner M, Anisimowicz L et al. (1982) Biomechanics of the pulmonary autograft valve in the aortic position. Thorax 37: 535–9

15. Harris PD, Kovalik ATW, Marks JA, Malm JR (1968) Factors modifying aortic homograft structure and function. Surgery 63: 45–52

16. Jacob MP, Moura AM, Tixier JM et al. (1987) Smooth muscle-mediated connective tissue remodeling in pulmonary hypertension. Science 237: 423–429

17. Jaffee EA, Minick CR, Adelman B, Becker CB, Nachman RL (1976) Synthesis of basement membrane collagen by cultured human endothelial cells. J Exp Med 44: 209

18. Kay PH, Livi U, Parker R, Ross DN (1988) The pulmonary allograft for the right ventricular outflow tract reconstruction. In: Cardiac valve allografts 1962–1987. (AC Yankah et al. eds.), Steinkopff Verlag, Darmstadt, Springer-Verlag, New York, pp 189–193

19. Keele KD (1952) Leonardo da Vinci. On movement of the heart and blood. Harvey and Bluth Ltd., London, pp 81

20. Leonardo da Vinci (1977) Anatomical drawings from the Royal collections. The Royal Academy of Arts, London, pp 35A

21. Leboucq G (1944) Une anatomie antique du coeur humain. Philision de Locroi et le timee' de Plation. Rev Grecques 57: 7

22. Mercer JL, Benedicity M, Bahnson HT (1973) The geometry and construction of the aortic leaflet. J Thorac Cardiovasc Surg 65: 511–518

23. Moncada S, Gryzlewski RJ, Bunting S, Vane JR (1976) An enzyme isolated from arteries transforms prostaglandin endoperoxides to an unstable substance that inhibits platelet aggregation. Nature 261: 663–665

24. Müller-Hermelink HK, Yankah AC (1988) Immunohistopathology of cardiac valve allograft explants. In: Cardiac valve allografts 1962–1987 (AC Yankah et al. eds.), Steinkopff Verlag, Darmstadt, Springer-Verlag, New York, pp 89–94

25. O'Brien M, Stafford EG, Gardner MAH et al. (1987) A comparison of aortic valve replacement with viable cryopreserved and fresh allograft valves, with a note on chromosomal studies. J Thorac Cardiovasc Surg 94: 812–823

26. Ross DN (1962) Homograft replacement of the aortic value. Lancet 2: 487–492

27. Ross DN, Somerville J (1966) Correction of pulmonary atresia with a homograft aortic valve. Lancet 2: 1446–1477

28. Ross DN (1967) Replacement of the aortic and mitral valves with a pulmonary autograft. Lancet 2: 956–8

29. Rowlatt UF, Rimoldi HJ, Lev M (1963) The quantitative anatomy of the normal child's heart. Pediatr Clin North Am 10: 499–588
30. Sarton G (1952) A history of science. I Ancient science through the golden age of Greece. Harvard University Press, Cambridge, Massachusetts
31. Simon A, Zavazava N, Sievers HH, Müller-Ruchholtz W (1993) In vitro cultivation and immunogenicity of human cardiac valve endothelium. J Card Surg 8: 656–665
32. Stein PD (1971) Roentgenographic method for measurement of the cross sectional area of the aortic valve. Am Heart J 81: 622
33. Thubrikar M, Boster LP, Nolan SP (1979) The mechanism of opening of the aortic valve. J Thorac Cardiovasc Surg 77: 863–870
34. Valsalva AM (1740) Arteria magnae sinus. In: Opera (Morgagni JB ed.), Venice, 1: 129
35. Yacoub MH (1988) Applications and limitations of histocompatibility in clinical cardiac valve allograft surgery. In: Cardiac valve allografts 1962–1987 (AC Yankah et al. eds.), Steinkopff Verlag, Darmstadt, Springer-Verlag, New York, pp 95–106
36. Yankah AC, Wottge HU, Müller-Hermelink HK et al. (1987) Transplantation of aortic and pulmonary allografts, enhanced viability of endothelial cells by cryopreservation. Importance of histocompatibility. J Card Surg I (Nr. 3 Suppl.): 209–220
37. Yankah AC, Wottge HU, Müller-Ruchholtz W (1995) Increased elastin in medial smooth muscle induced by humoral response as a trigger mechanism for early degeneration of allograft conduit. Cardiovasc Surg 3 (Suppl): 95
38. Zimmerman J (1969) The functional and surgical anatomy of the aortic valve. Israel J Med Sci 5: 862–866

Author's address:
A. Charles Yankah, MD, PhD
Consultant, Assistant Professor
Duetsches Herzzentrum Berlin and Humboldt University
Dept. Cardiothoracic and Vascular Surgery
Augustenburger Platz 1
D-13353 Berlin
Germany

Antigenicity of human cardiac valve allografts in vitro

F. M. E. Hoekstra[1], C. Knoop[1], E. Bos[3], N. Jutte[1], C. Wassenaar[2], W. Weimar[1]

Departments of Internal Medicine I[1], Heart Valve[2] Bank and Thorax Center[3], University Hospital Rotterdam, The Netherlands

Abstract

Fresh and cryopreserved human valves are used to reconstruct ventricular outflow tracts. Valve donor and recipient are not matched for blood group or human leukocyte antigens (HLA) and immunosuppressive therapy is not routinely given to valve recipients. Therefore, immunologic activity of the valve acceptor against allogeneic tissue may play a role in valve destruction. In this study, we examined the immunogenicity of human donor valves in vitro. Pieces of fresh and cryopreserved leaflets derived from the same valve allograft, and endothelial cells derived from fresh valve leaflets, were tested as stimulator in a lymphocyte proliferation assay. Lymphocytes mismatched or matched for HLA-DR with the valve donors were used as responders. The proliferation was expressed as Stimulation Index (SI). The SI was significantly higher with fresh valve pieces as stimulator (median SI: 9; range 4–117) compared to cryopreserved valves ($p = 0.002$, Wilcoxon), although the latter were still able to induce lymphoproliferation (median SI: 2; range 1–9). The SI was significantly lower when lymphocytes were matched for HLA-DR with the valve donor (median SI: 1, range 1–5) compared to the HLA-DR mismatched group (median SI: 5; range 2–117, $p = 0.006$, Wilcoxon). Endothelial cells derived from six different valves, incubated with lymphocytes mismatched for HLA-A, B and DR, induced a median SI of 8 (range: 3–15). These results indicate that both fresh and cryopreserved human valves are able to evoke a proliferative response of immune competent cells in vitro. Also, both matching for HLA-DR between valve donor and responder lymphocytes and the cryopreservation procedure are associated with a significantly decreased lymphoproliferative response. Finally, the endothelial cells present on fresh valves probably play a prominent role in the immune response against human valve allografts.

Introduction

The durability of human valve allografts is dependent on many factors, such as surgical technical procedures (for example sizing) and preservation methods. Clinical follow-up studies concerning patients receiving fresh or cryopreserved valve allografts, show better long-term graft survival for patients with cryopreserved valves (9). Nevertheless, cryopreserved valves can show severe degeneration in the long-term, although this does not necessarily lead to valve dysfunction (10). On the other hand, in some series the shortterm allograft failure rate is high, especially in young recipients (1). Immunological causes for valve degeneration could also be contemplated as valve donor and acceptor are not matched for blood group or human leukocyte antigens (HLA). Immunological studies after human valve allograft transplantation are infrequently found in the literature. In contrast, animal studies show a benificial effect on graft survival when valves are transplanted between histocompatible compared to histoincompatible rat strains (11). Lymphocytes have been observed in explanted clinical allografts (12), but their origin and role in valve destruction are not well understood. The aim of the present study is to evaluate the capacity of human valves to stimulate immune competent cells in vitro, and to assess the effect of cryopreservation and HLA-DR matching on this response. Because endothelial cells form the first barrier between donor and acceptor, these cells were isolated from fresh valve leaflets and their stimulatory capacity was also measured in a lymphocyte proliferation assay.

Material and methods

Human aortic and pulmonary valves were obtained from the Heart Valve Bank Rotterdam, The Netherlands, from heart-beating and nonheart-beating donors and prepared under sterile conditions according to Standard Operation Procedures (7). After sterilization of the valves in a low concentration antibiotic bath, containing flucytosine 0.03 mg/mL; vancomycin, 0.012 mg/mL; amikacin 0.012 mg/mL; ciprofloxacin 0.003 mg/mL and metronidazole, 0.012 mg/ml in medium 199 (Gibco, Paisley, Scotland), at 4 °C for 24 h. Thereafter, two fresh leaflets were prepared from the allograft and one was cut into pieces with a 2-millimeter diameter biopsy punch (Stiefel Laboratories, Inc., Coral Gables, Fl.). The fresh valve pieces were each placed in a well of a 96-well culture plate (Costar Corp., Cambridge, Mass.), with culture medium, consisting of RPMI 1640 Dutch Modification solution (Gibco) supplemented with 10% heat-inactivated human serum, L-glutamine 4 mmol/l, penicillin 100 IU/mL, and streptomycin 100 µg/ml. The third leaflet, remaining attached to the aortic or pulmonary root, was cryopreserved (-1 °C per minute) in medium 199 (Gibco) with 10% dimethylsulfoxide (DMSO). The cryopreserved valves were thawed according to the Standard Thawing Protocol of the Heart Valve Bank and washed with medium 199 (Gibco), containing penicillin 100 IU/mL and streptomycin 100 µg/ml. The cryopreserved leaflets were further treated as described before for the fresh leaflets. The second fresh leaflet was used to isolate endothelial cells, according to the method of Johnson and Fass (5). The fresh leaflet was gently rinsed in medium 199 after the antibiotic bath, then placed for 5 min in a 1 mg/mL collagenase solution (Collagenase A, Boehringer, Mannheim, Germany) in Hanks Balanced Salt Solution (Gibco) at 37 °C. The specimen was rinsed gently in Hanks balanced salt solution without calcium and magnesium (Gibco) and thereafter placed in 1 mL endothelial cell culture medium (RPMI 1640 to medium 199 1:1, Gibco, 30% heat-inactivated serum with 50 µg Endothelial Cell Growth Supplement (Collaborative Research Inc, Bedford, MA) and 50 µg/mL Heparin (Sigma, Sl Louis, MO). After 1 min of gently shaking by hand, the valve leaflet was taken out of the tube and the culture medium containing the endothelial cells was put into a well of a 24-well Primaria-coated dish (Becton Dickinson, Mountain View, CA). At confluence, the endothelial cells were trypsinized in trypsin ethylenediamine tetraacetic acid (0.05%/0.02%). In total, six endothelial cell cultures were obtained from six valve leaflets from six different allografts. The purity of the cell lines was assessed by double staining with fluorescein isothiocyanate-labelled Ulex Europaeus lectin (E-Y Laboratories Inc, San Mateo, CA) and the monoclonal antibody EN4 (Sanbio, Uden, The Netherlands) in combination with anti-mouse kappa-PE (Becton Dickinson), and the samples were subsequently analyzed on a FACScan flow cytometer (Becton Dickinson).

As responder cells, two sets of lymphocytes were used; one set consisted of lymphocytes mismatched for HLA-A, B and DR antigens with the valve, and the second set consisted of lymphocytes matched for HLA-DR only. These peripheral blood mononuclear cells were isolated on Ficoll-paque (Pharmacia, Uppsala, Sweden). The 2-millimeter diameter pieces and endothelial cells were irradiated (30 Gy) and incubated with $0.5 \ 10^5$ lymphocytes in a total volume of 200 μl culture medium at 37 °C in a humidified atmosphere of 5% CO_2 in air. After 7 days the valve pieces were removed and tritiated thymidin (0.5 μCi per well) was added. After further incubation for 8 h 37 °C, the lymphocytes were harvested on glass fiber filters. The Beta Plate Counter (LKB, Sweden) was used to measure the tritiated thymidin incorporation. The test was performed with 10 valve pieces per valve leaflet. As positive controls, irradiated (60 Gy) third party Epstein-Barr virus infected B-lymphoblastoid cell-lines were used, and irradiated (30 Gy) autologous lymphocytes served as negative controls. The results were expressed as Stimulation Index (SI): The counts per minute incorporated by stimulated lymphocytes are divided by the counts per minute incorporated by negative controls.

Results

Both fresh and cryopreserved valve pieces induced significant proliferation of HLA-DR mismatched lymphocytes. Expressed as counts per minute (cpm), incorporation of tritiated thymidin ranged from 588 to 5999 cpm (median: 998 cpm) for fresh valve pieces ($n = 12$), and from 67 to 1690 cpm (median: 309) for cryopreserved valve pieces. Cpm incorporated by negative controls ranged from 40 to 342 (median: 67 cpm). Expressed as Stimulation Index, fresh valve pieces induced a higher SI: 9 (median, range 4–117) than cryopreserved valve pieces derived from the same valve (median SI: 2, range 1–9), $p = 0.002$, Wilcoxon, Fig. 1.

Fresh leaflets ($n = 3$) and cryopreserved leaflets ($n = 4$) incubated with HLA-DR matched lymphocytes induced significantly less lymphoproliferation compared to the HLA-DR mismatched lymphocytes incubated with valve pieces derived from the same valve leaflets. The median SI for HLA-DR mismatched lymphocytes was 4 (median, range 2–117) while the median SI was 2 (range 1–5) for HLA-DR matched lymphocytes ($p = 0.006$, Wilcoxon) (Fig. 2).

Endothelial cell cultures could be obtained in 14 out of 15 fresh valve leaflets, whereas cryopreserved leaflets did not contain viable endothelial cells in any of the five cryopreserved leaflets tested. Indeed, histological examination of cryopreserved valves in our institution does not show the presence of endothelial cells on most of the valves examined. In the proliferation assay, endothelial cell cultures ($n = 6$) induced a median SI of 8 (range 3–11), whereas fresh valve pieces derived from the same valve ($n = 3$) induced a median SI of 10 (range 5–35). Cryopreserved valve pieces derived from the same valves as the endothelial cells ($n = 4$) induced a lower median SI

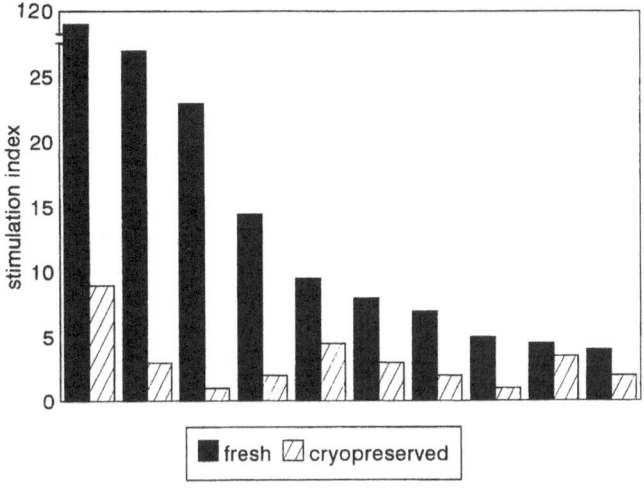

Fig. 1. Median Stimulation Index induced by fresh versus cryopreserved human valve pieces. Lymphocytes mismatched for HLA-A, B and DR were used as responder cells.

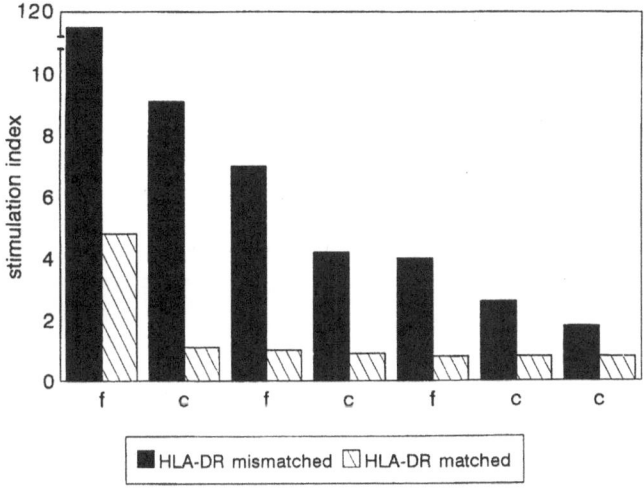

Fig. 2. Median Stimulation Index induced by human valve pieces with HLA-DR matched versus HLA-DR mismatched lymphocytes. F = fresh valve pieces, C = cryopreserved valve pieces.

(median SI: 2; range 1–9), possibly representing the loss of endothelial cells caused by the cryopreservation procedure.

Discussion

Earlier animal studies showed that valve allografts are able to stimulate the immune system (4, 7) that at least in one study this response is donor-specific (13), and that matching for major histocompatibility complex antigens (MHC) can improve graft survival (2, 8, 11). In the present study, we showed that fresh and cryopreserved human cardiac valves are able to evoke a proliferative response of immune-competent cells in vitro, and that both cryopreservation and HLA-DR matching is associated with less lymphoproliferation.

Manipulation of valve allografts could alter the antigenic properties of valve allografts as was earlier shown in animal studies (2). In the present study, we illustrate this phenomenon in the clinical situation by the reduced proliferative response of lymphocytes to cryopreserved human valve pieces. This reduced immune response in vitro could be the result of reduction or even the absence of endothelial cells. These cells are capable of triggering immune responses by expressing HLA class II. Nevertheless, after the cryopreservation procedure we are still able to detect immune responses against donor valves and we can still detect an effect of HLA class II matching. This can be explained by the presence of other class II bearing cells, different from endothelium, e.g., dendritic cells or even fibroblasts in the donor valve. Although valve allograft dysfunction does not necessarily result in cardiac failure, clinical follow up studies show that a significant number of valve replacements is necessary, especially in young recipients (1). Our results may have clinical importance, because valve allografts are allocated to recipients without matching for HLA-antigens. In patients with a high risk of valve allograft failure (young children, in case of second replacements) both cryopreservation and HLA-DR matching of valve donor and recipient conceivably could improve the graft survival. Cross-matching between valve donor and recipient could help to select sensitized patients. Another option remains the use of immunosuppressive agents, although one has to balance their potential benefits with their adherent side-effects.

Acknowledgements

We thank Corina van Tricht and Zohara Aghai for preparation of the valves.

References

1. Clarke DR, Campbell DN, Hayward AR, Bishop DA (1993) Degeneration of aortic valve allografts in young recipients. J Thorac Cardiovasc Surg 105: 934–42
2. Douglas Calhoun A, Baur GM, Porter JM, Houghton WH, Templeton JW (1977) Fresh and cryopreserved venous allografts in genetically characterized dogs. J Surg Res 22: 687–96
3. El Khatib H, Thompson SA, Lupinetti FM (1990) Effect of storage at 4 °C in a nutrient medium on antigenic properties of rat aortic valve allografts. Ann Thorac Surg 49: 792–6
4. Gonzalez-Lavin L, Bianchi J, Graf D, Amini S, Gordon CI (1988) Degenerative changes in fresh aortic root homografts in a canine model: evidence of an immunologic influence. Transplant Proc 20: 815–9
5. Johnson CM, Fass DN (1983) Porcine cardiac valvular endothelial cells in culture, a relative deficiency of fibronectin synthesis in vitro. Lab Invest 49: 589–98
6. Khatib H, Lupinetti FM (1990) Antigenicity of fresh and cryopreserved rat valve allografts. Transplantation 49: 756–67
7. Lange PL, Hopkins RA (1989) Allograft valve banking: techniques and technology. In: Hopkins RA (ed) Cardiac Reconstructions with Allograft Valves. New York: Springer-Verlag
8. Lupinetti FM, Cobb S, Kioschos HC, Thompson SA, Walters KS, Moore KC (1992) Effect of immunological differences on rat aortic valve calcification. J Cardiac Surg 7: 65–70
9. O'Brien MF, Stafford EG, Gardner MAH, Polner PG, Mc Giffin DC, Kirklin JAW (1987) A comparison of aortic valve replacement with viable cryopreserved and fresh allograft valves, with a note on chromosomal studies. J Thorac Cardiovasc Surg 94: 812–23

10. Schoen FJ, Mitchell RN, Jonas RA (1995) Pathological considerations in cryopreserved allograft heart valves. J Heart Valve Dis 4: 72–76
11. Thiede A, Timm C, Bernhard A, Muller-Ruchholz W (1978) Studies on the antigenicity of vital allogeneic valve leaflet transplants in immunologically controlled strain combinations. Transplantation 26: 391–5
12. Yankah AC, Muller-Hermelink HK, Muller-Ruchholz W, Bernhard A (1992) Antigenitat allogener herzklappen. Z Herz Thorax GefaBchir 6: 41–7
13. Zhao X, Green M, Frazer IH, Hogan P, O'Brien MF (1994) Donor-specific immune response after aortic valve allografting in the rat. Ann Thorac Surg 57: 1158–63

Authors' address:
F. M. E. Hoekstra, MD
Department of Internal Medicine I, room Bd 293
University Hospital Rotterdam-Dijkzigt
Dr Molewaterplein 40
3015 GD Rotterdam
The Netherlands

Immunology of homograft valves

A. Schütz

Klinikum Bogenhausen, München

Introduction

The clinical use of cryopreserved homograft valves has become a well-accepted method for aortic valve replacement. Cryopreserved allografts have shown a superior long-term performance compared with grafts stored at 4 °C (14). In contrast to these fresh-wet-stored valves, it seems that cryopreserved grafts keep their viability undamaged, allowing storage at −196 °C for years of these rare and precious prostheses (12).

Despite encouraging data that suggest markedly improved results with the use of cryopreserved allograft valves, there are numerous areas of controversy and mystery. The role of the endothelium in the presumably viable allografts is clearly not understood. It can be argued that it protects the physicochemical balance of the matrix, but it can be counterargued that the endothelium is antigenic and incites host rejection (9). So far, immunological reactions during the early postoperative course following homograft replacement have not been examined, and we are additionally faced with the questions concerning the need for ABO-compatibility. Since the cytoimmunological monitoring (CIM) represents a well established procedure for the diagnosis of acute rejection after allograft transplantation, this noninvasive method was chosen for controlling potential immunological reactions (7, 18).

How long and intensive the endothelium remains viable and therefore capable of inducing host rejection is not yet clarified. Endothelial cell (EC) viability of cryopreserved homografts was investigated by measurement of secreted prostacyclin (PGI_2), which is a reliable marker for endothelial activity (19), and by application of a cell proliferation assay.

Material and methods

Preservation and replacement of the valves

The aortic valves harvested from the hearts of transplanted patients, e.g., from so-called heart-beating donors (3), were dissected, exactly measured and classified according to a detailed quality score. We preserved the valve in culture medium consisting of 90% medium 199 and 10% Dimethylsulfoxide (DMSO) and froze them linearly up to −40 °C. Afterwards, the grafts were stored in vapor liquid nitrogen (−196 °C) which makes unlimited preservation possible. Thawing was performed by immersing the graft in a 40 °C waterbath for 10 min, with subsequent rinsing and gradual dilution of the dimethyl sulfoxide in 4° buffered M199. Before cryopreservation and implantation, samples were taken for microbiological investigations to screen for possible graft contamination. For graft implantation a suitable valve of optimal size, if possible ABO-compatible, was thawed. Our implantation method corresponded in a partly modified way to the technique according to Ross, in the subcoronary position (15).

Cytoimmunological monitoring

The laboratory method has already been described in detail (7, 18). Cytoimmunological monitoring of peripheral blood was performed daily. Three millimeters of heparinized venous blood was drawn. The blood was layered over a Ficoll-Hypaque gradient ($d = 1.077$) and a mononuclear cell concentrate was obtained at the interphase following centrifugation. Cytocentrifuge preparations were made of the mononuclear cell concentrate and were stained according to the Pappenheim method. Then 3×100 cells were counted, and activation indices were determined by forming the ratio between the number of lymphoblasts and the total number of lymphoid cells. These results were computed in percentages:

$$AI = \frac{Lymphoblasts}{Lymphoid\ cells} \times 100$$

An AI > 1 was rated as an immunological reaction. During the first 21 days following allograft implantation CIM was performed daily in 16 patients, and also in eight patients with procine bioprosthesis as a control.

Echocardiography

All patients underwent transthoracal and transesophageal echocardiography as well as Doppler examinations before[1], during and after the operation.

Statistical analysis

Continuous data were expressed as the mean ± standard deviation. All significances were determined by the Mann-Whitney U-Test. The value of $p < 0.05$ was considered statistically significant.

Light and electron microscopy

Homograft valves were fixed in 4% buffered formalin for light microscopy examinations. Paraffin sections were stained with hematoxylin and eosin and elastic van Gieson.

For scanning electron microscopy, the valves were rinsed in Hank's balanced salt solution and fixed in 2% glutaraldehye -0.05 mol/L cacodylate buffer (pH 7.) at 4°. Tissues were dehydrated with acetone to the critical point of carbon dioxide, coated

---

[1] Sonos 1200, Siemens, Munich, Germany

Table 1. Score system for the description of the homograft valve endothelium by scanning electron microscopy

	Score (SEM)
1.	Completely confluent endothelium
2.	Partially confluent endothelium
3.	Loosely netted endothelium
4.	Islands of endothelium
5.	No endothelium

with gold palladium, and examined with a JEOL JSM 5200 (JEOL Ltd., Tokyo, Japan). In order to define the integrity of the endothelium and the quality of the surface area a special score system (from 1 to 5) was introduced (Table 1).

Prostaglandin I₂ release and cell proliferation

Homograft valve leaflets ($n = 16$) were incubated in 3 ml of nutrient medium (M199) at $37\,^{\circ}\text{C}$ and 5% CO_2 for 24 h. Prostaglandin (PG) I_2 release was measured in the incubation medium as the stable metabolite 6-keto-$PGF_{1\alpha}$ by means of an enzyme immunoassay (Advanced Magnetics Inc., Cambridge, Mass.). The reaction was terminated by the addition of stop solution, and the absorbance was established at 405 nm. The absorbance was correlated with the concentration level using a standard curve. In addition, the PGI_1 secretion of the same leaflets was stimulated with 25 µmol/L arachidonic acid.

To investigate EC viability of the valve leaflets, we used a nonradioactive cell proliferation and cytotoxicity assay (EZ4U-Elisa-kit; Biomedica, Vienna, Austria). This process requires functional ribosomes, which turn tetrazolium salt into intensely colored (orange-red) formazan derivates. After incubation of valve leaflets ($n = 8$), the absorbance was measured by a spectrophotometer (Shimadzu UV-1202, Duisburg, Germany) set at 450 nm, with 620 nm as a reference.

Results

Sixteen patients received cryopreserved aortic allografts in the orthotopic position, whereby nine ABO-compatible and seven ABO-incompatible aortic valves were inserted. In total 336 CIM examinations were obtained.

All patients ($n = 16$) showed an increase of the AI due to a T-cell activation, as a sign of immunological reaction occurring. The comparison of ABO-compatible with ABO-incompatible grafts revealed that the AI maximum in the compatible group was 1.4 ± 0.9 with a mean duration of 1.5 ± 0.9 days, while the immunological activation in ABO-incompatible allograft recipients lasted 3.3 ± 1.4 days and the AI of this group was characterized by a higher elevation ($\bar{x} = 2.3 \pm 1.9$) as well (Figs. 1 and 2). This difference between ABO-compatible and ABO-incompatible allografts was significant ($p < 0.05$). After implantation of porcine bioprostheses in eight patients, the CIM results ($n = 98$) did not show a relevant elevation of the activation index in contrast to allograft valve recipients ($p < 0.01$) (Fig. 1). The average AI detected in the blood of these patients was 0.1 ± 0.01 during the first 2 postoperative weeks.

Common to all immunological events of the allograft valves was a reversible course without any immunosuppressive treatment, presenting a moderate elevation of the AI (2.5–5) between 2 and 5 days in ABO-incompatible recipients (0.5–2.5) and for a short time in ABO-compatible recipients (Figs. 3 and 4). The onset of the immunological reaction did not vary in either group and started on the 5th day on average.

The transthoracic and transesophageal echocardiographic studies carried out 3 months postoperatively demonstrated regular function and morphology of cryo-preserved allogeneic heart valves in 14 cases. The transvalvular pressure gradient ranged from 6.9 mmHg to 16.7 mmHg as a maximum with a mean of $\bar{\chi} = 11.4 \pm 3.1$. In two patients a hemodynamically irrelevant valve insufficiency was found.

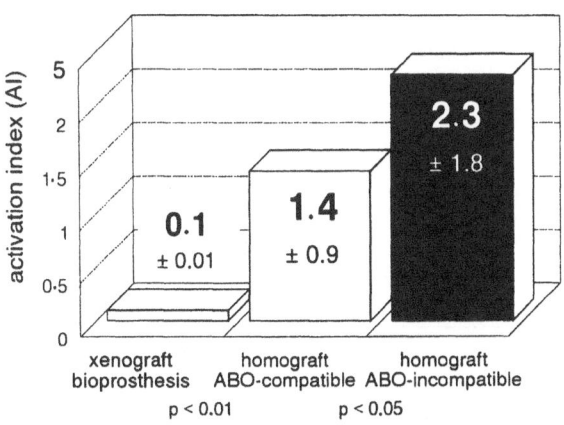

Fig. 1. Intensity of the immunological reaction after allograft valve replacement as determined by the activation index in the CIM routine test.

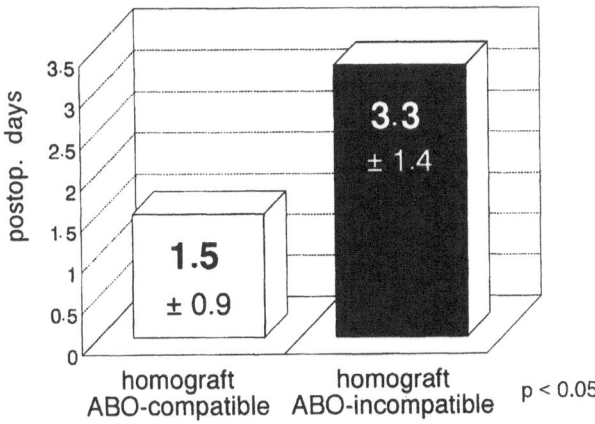

Fig. 2. Duration of the immunological reaction after allograft valve replacement, measured by the activation index.

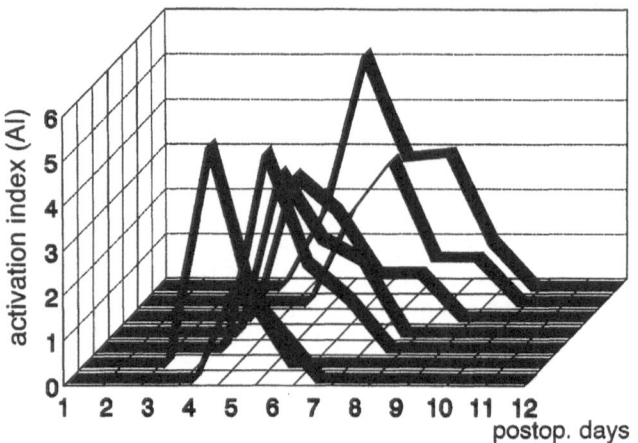

Fig. 3. CIM kinetics after ABO-incompatible allograft replacement.

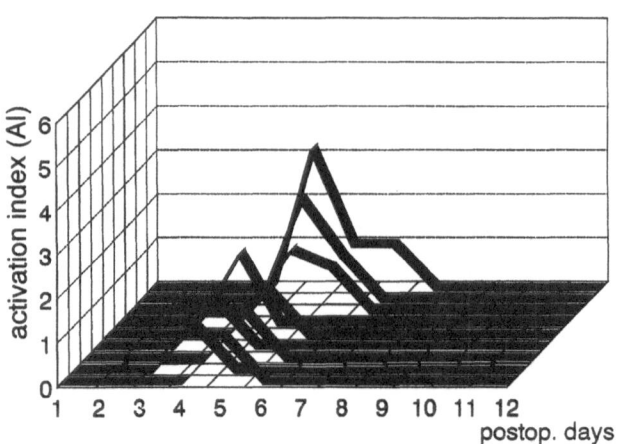

Fig. 4. CIM kinetics after ABO-compatible allograft replacement.

Cryopreserved homograft valves from heart-beating donors showed a regular and morphologically intact tissue structure as observed by light microscopy (Fig. 5). Observations in the scanning electron microscope included an almost intact and confluent endothelium on valve surfaces when the grafts had been cryopreserved within 24 h after harvesting (Fig. 6). An increase of distinct EC loss and damage was observed when the grafts had been stored for more than 24 h in 4 °C nutrient medium before cryopreservation (Fig. 7). Nevertheless, ECs could be detected histologically in all valve specimens after cryopreservation (Fig. 8).

All cryopreserved homograft leaflets showed EC PGI_2 release as well as successful stimulation of secretion with arachidonic acid. As with the histologic findings, the PGI_2 secretion declined when the grafts had been stored at 4 °C for more than 24 h before final storage in liquid nitrogen (Fig. 9). Results obtained with the EZ4U proliferation assay revealed EC viability for proliferation activity in all valve

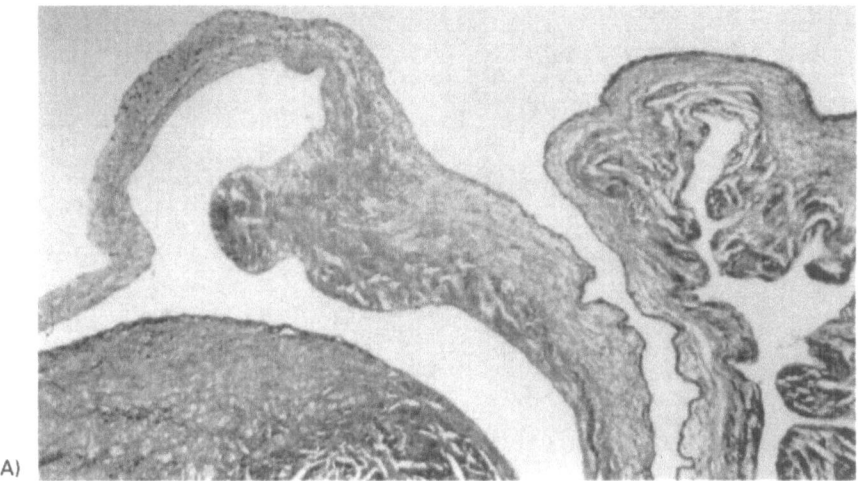

(A)

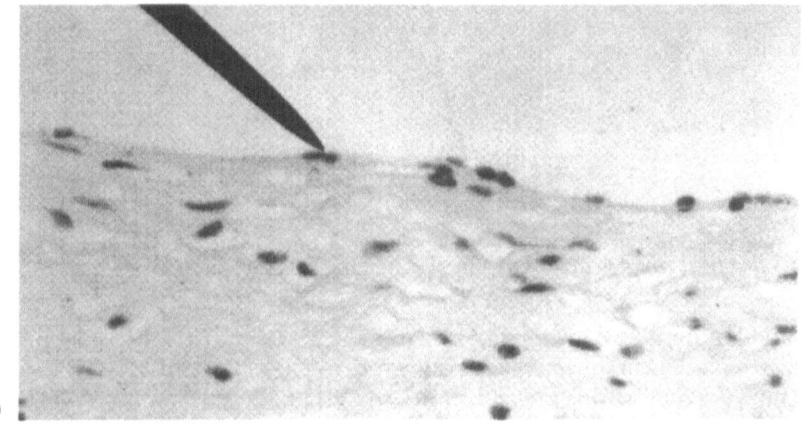

(B)

Fig. 5. Cryopreserved aortic valve from a heart-beating donor shows a properly organized and morphologically intact valvular stroma in **A** and an unbroken coat of endothelial cells (arrow) in **B** under light microscopy.

specimens (0.21 ± 0.13 at 450 nm). However, this proliferation activity can be interpreted as low when compared with the EC viability of fresh harvested grafts before cryopreservation (0.58 ± 0.24).

Discussion

As with much biomedical research, it could be observed that a properly cryopreserved allograft heart valve functions much like a native valve. Its hemodynamic properties are superior to those of mechanical valves and bioprostheses (9). Anticoagulation therapy is not required. It is foreign tissue, yet seems to work as if it were antigen neutral.

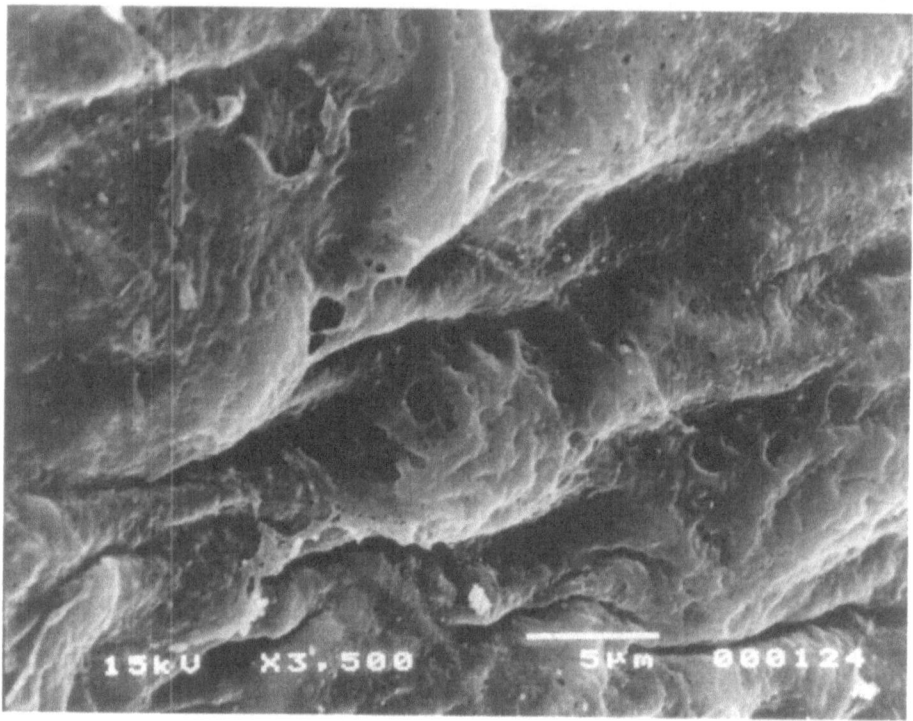

Fig. 6. Scanning electron micrographs of aortic homograft valve surfaces. Intact valve endothelium after graft cryopreservation within 24 h of harvesting (original magnification × 3500).

Examination results concerning immunological reactions following allogeneic heart valve replacement during the early postoperative course are not available at the present time. In contrast to nonvital fresh-wet-stored allografts, cryopreserved heart valves are obviously vital, which means that endothelial cells and fibroblasts remain viable (23). Preimplant viability of the cryopreserved allograft valves was established by O'Brien in 1987 (12). In this context, the question concerning immune responses after implantation is still of importance, particularly in ABO-incompatible valve recipients. It is well known that the endothelial cell membrane of the valve are HLA class I and II positive, even after cryopreservation (21, 22). However, the importance of these immunological cell markers for long-term function of cryopreserved allografts has not been defined up to now. O'Brien was able to isolate donor fibroblasts out of an explanted aortic allograft valve by chromosomal analysis nine years after implantation (13). In experimental studies, Yankah could demonstrate that vital allografts are capable of inducing the production of antidonor-specific antibodies, using direct immuno-fluorescence and immunoperoxidase technique (23). There is some controversy as to what extent one can transfer these facts to human allogeneic valves.

The development of CIM in 1984 by Hammer et al. presents a remarkable advance in immunological rejection diagnosis, particularly following heart transplantation (7). Our experimental work revealed that transmural biventricular biopsy specimens related to the corresponding CIM results on a day-to-day basis. Moreover, the amount of the AI measured by the CIM routine test correlated exactly with the grade of acute rejection (16, 18). Currently, CIM represents one of the few reliable immunological tools to detect acute rejection after allograft transplantation and it is employed

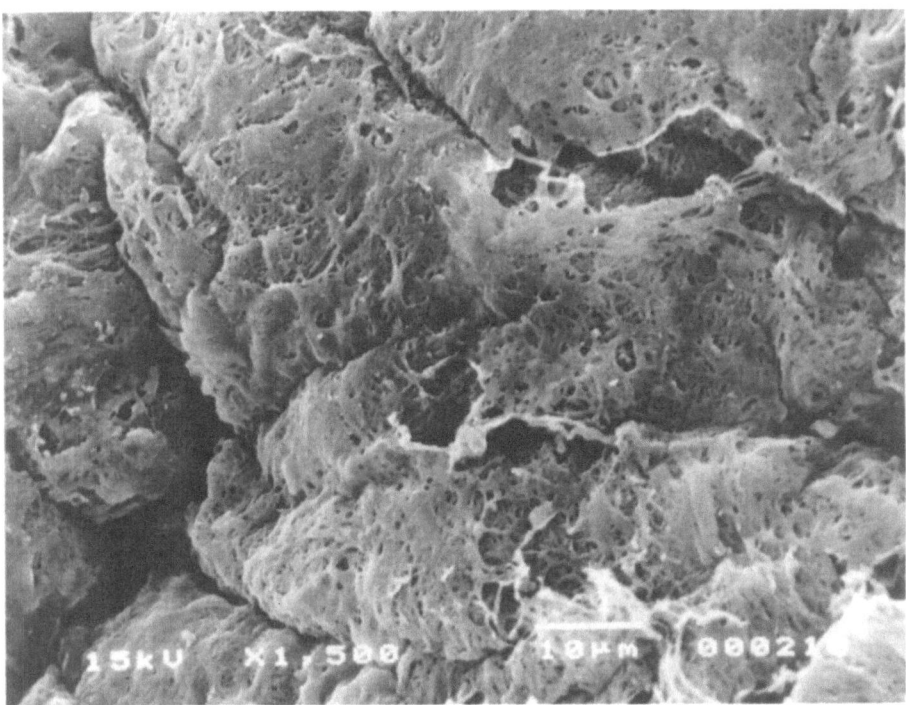

Fig. 7. Scanning electron micrographs of aortic homograft valve surfaces. Graft cryopreservation after 62 h shows severely damaged valve endothelium; collagen fibers are already visible (original magnification × 1500).

successfully in various transplant centers (4, 11). To differentiate acute rejection from viral, bacterial or fungal infections, a detailed CIM cell-subset diagnosis is available, determining the lymphocytic subpopulations of CD4 and CD8 positive cells (8). Nevertheless, the CIM routine test easily allows an efficient statement about a suspected immunological reaction, characterized by an adequate diagnostic accuracy.

The present CIM results, including the determination of the so-called activation index, underline the hypothesis that the allogeneic valve transplantation, using cryopreserved grafts, leads to an immunological reaction almost in the early postoperative course, due to T-cell activation (19). In contrast patients following xenogeneic bioprosthesis replacement did not show a relevant increase of the AI, revealing some activated lymphocytes and, very rarely, lymphoblasts. This observation can be equated with CIM results in patients following cardiopulmonary bypass. The activation of the immune system, proven by a growing number of lymphoblasts in the mononuclear concentrate, starts at day 5 after implantation. This reaction continues for 1–3 days in ABO-compatible allografts and 2–5 days in ABO-incompatible heart valves. Likewise, the intensity of the activation is evidently dependent on ABO-compatibility and can be compared to moderate acute rejection in cases of blood group incompatibility and to mild rejection in ABO-compatible allograft recipients. In all patients, however, a return of the AI to basic level was observed without any specific immunosuppressive therapy. In addition, transesophageal and transthoracal echocardiographic findings after valve replacement reflected graft morphology

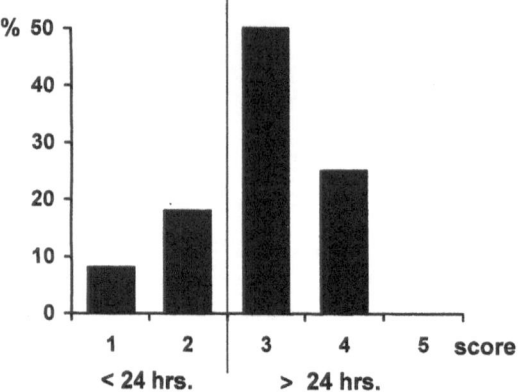

Fig. 8. Observation of endothelium. Assessment of cryopreserved homografts from living donors by scanning electron microscopy. The vertical line separates valves cryopreserved within 24 h and valves processed after 24 h. Portion of investigated specimens is shown in % according to the score system (Table 3).

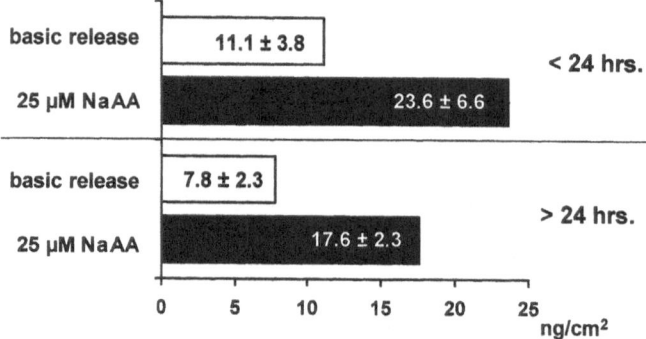

Fig. 9. Amount of prostaglandin I_2 (PGI$_2$) release from homograft valve leaflets when grafts were cryopreserved within 24 h and after more then 24 h (Open bars = basic release; dark bars = after stimulation with 25 µmol/L arachidonic acid [NaAA.]).

without any signs of beginning valve thickening or reduced valve function. So far there are only few experiences regarding the long-term follow-up of cryopreserved allograft valves and, in particular, the effect of the ABO system in valve degeneration and clacification.

Beyond doubt, further detailed investigations should be carried out to clarify the quality of the immunological reactions after allograft valve replacement. An additional approach could be to evaluate the phenotypic profile of peripheral blood lymphocytes and serum levels of the activation state of T-cells, such as the soluble form of the IL-2 receptor and intercellular adhesion molecule-1 (ICAM-1), which is a ligand for the lymphocytic function-associated antigen. The expression of ICAM-1 is regulated by several cytokines, IL-1, TNF-gamma which are produced early during lymphoid and monocyte activation (10, 20).

The question certainly arises whether such a complex and hardly understood system as graft rejection could be detected adequately when examining these very detailed immunological pathways. At least CIM describes a global immunological reaction in allograft valve recipients which is not present in patients after conventional xenogeneic valve replacement.

In this context the importance and role of an intact endothelium to viable allograft performance remains speculative. Viable ECs prevent thrombosis and calcification in the cardiovascular system but are probably the most immunogeneic component of transplanted vascular structures. Our findings indicate that homografts are viable after cryopreservation (5). This viability declines relative to the duration of wet storage nutrient medium at 4°, which was detected by prostaglandin E2 measurement and cell proliferation assay. The storage of homografts for only 48 h prior to cryopreservation already leads to EC damage. All together, cryopreservation proved to be a cell- and tissue-protective preservation method. Even after long storage period, this technique allows preservation of valve ECs, provided that grafts from heart-beating donors had been cryopreserved within 24 h of harvesting and without previous antibiotic sterilization. It is further notable that after a storage period of more than 24 h, EC damage could be demonstrated morphologically by means of scanning electron microscopy as well as by the reduced PGE_2 secretion (6). Thus, a relationship between immunogenicity and degenerative homograft valve changes has been examined, however, with controversial findings. On the other hand, harsh preservation techniques applied in the earlier days of homograft bank systems, such as lyophilization, aldehyde treatment, or irradiation did not result in high clinical durability (2). Cold wet-stored homografts showed an actuarial freedom from valve replacement of 78% and 42% after 10 and 14 years respectively (1). On the contrary, O'Brian and co-workers reported a 92% rate of freedom from valve failure after 10 years in viable cryopreserved homografts after aortic valve replacement (13). These results would, of course, favor the use of viable homografts. Although a loss of donor endothelium may take place already in the early postoperative period, the viable graft tissue could be an optimal prerequisite for stromal cell ingrowth and reendothelialization by host cells after allograft transplantation. Furthermore, viable fibroblasts could be a factor in the renewal of extracellular matrix components.

In conclusion, homograft valves, harvested from recipient hearts of patients undergoing heart transplantation (heart beating donors) are viable after cryopreservation in dependence on the time of final storage. Therefore, it is not surprising that endothelial cell viability generally causes immunological reactions. This immune response of the host due to T-cell activation takes place in the early postoperative course, thereby ABO-incompatible allografts show a more intensive reaction which is reversible as well. The clinical performance of these viable cryopreserved allografts remains unaffected. For this reason it seems that ABO-incompatibility does not affect the outcome of allograft valve durability after cryopreservation. However, the role of ABO tissue matching has not been defined in the long-term follow-up.

References

1. Barratt-Boyes RG, Roche MB, Subramanyan R, Pemperton JR, Whitlock RM (1987) Long-term follow-up patients with the antibiotic-sterilized aortic homograft valve inserted freehand in the aortic position. Circulation 75: 768–777
2. Daly RC, Orszulak TA, Schaff HV, McGovern E, Wallacee RB (1991) Long-term results of aortic valve replacement with non-viable homografts. Circulation 84 (suppl 3): 81–88
3. Feindel CM, David TE, Bos J, Daly PA, Cardella CJ (1991) Recycled heart valves from transplant patients. J Heart Lung Transplant 10: 614–617

4. Fieguth H-G, Haverich A, Schäfers H-J (1988) Cytoimmunologic monitoring in early and late cardiac rejection. J Heart Transplant 7: 95–101
5. Fischlein T, Schütz A, Uhlig A, Frey R, Krupa W, Babic R, Thiery J, Reichart B (1994) Integrity and viability of homograft valves. Eur J Cardio-Thorac Surg 8: 425–430
6. Fischlein T, Schütz A, Haushofer M, Frey R, Uhlig A, Detter Ch, Reichart B (1995) Immunologic reactions and viability of cryopreserved homografts. Ann Thorac Surg 60: 122–126
7. Hammer C, Reichenspurner H, Ertel W, Reichart B, Überfuhr P, Kemkes BM, Gokel M (1984) Cytological and immunological monitoring of cyclosporine-treated human heart recipients. J Heart Transplant 3: 228–231
8. Hammer C (1989) Cytology in transplantation. Schulz Verlag, Percha, Starnberg, Germany, pp 127–154
9. Hopkins RA (1989) Rationale for use of cryopreserved allograft tissues for cardiac reconstruction. In: Hopkins RA (ed) Cardiac Reconstruction with Allograft Valves. Springer Verlag Berlin Heidelberg, pp 15–19
10. Kupiec-Weglinski JW, Diamentstein T, Tilney NL (1988) Interleukin-2 receptor targeted therapy-rationale and applications in organ transplantation. Transplantation 46: 785–792
11. May RM, Cooper DKR, Du Toit Ed, Reichart B (1990) Cytoimmunological monitoring after heart-lung transplantation. J Heart Transplant 9: 133–135
12. O'Brien MF, Stafford EG, Gardur M (1987) The viable cryopreserved allograft aortic valve. J Cardiac Surg 2 (suppl 1): 815–822
13. O'Brien MF, Stafford EG, Gardner AH, Pohner PG, McGrifin DC (1987) A comparison of aortic valve replacement with viable cryopreserved and fresh allograft valves, with a note on chromosomal studies. J Thorac Cardiovasc Surg 94: 812–823
14. O'Brien MF, McGriffin DC, et al. (1991) Allograft aortic valve replacement: long-term comparative clinical analysis of the viable cryopreserved and antibiotic 4 °C stored valves. J Cardiac Surg 6 (suppl): 534–543
15. Ross DN (1991) Technique of aortic valve replacement with a homograft: orthotopic replacement. Ann Thorac Surg 52: 154–156
16. Schütz A, Breuer M, Engelhardt B, Brandl U, Hammer C, Kemkes BM (1991) Comparison of acute rejection in sensitized ("domino") and unsensitized donor hearts. Tex Heart Inst 14: 286–292
17. Schütz A, Pratschke J, Breuer M, Hammer C, Engelhardt M, Brandl U, Babic R, Reichart B, Kemkes BM (1992) Allogeneic heart transplantation following xenogeneic bridging. Transplant Int 5: 307–310
18. Schütz A, Kemkes BM, Breuer M, Brandl U, Engelhardt M, Kugler C, Manz C, Hatz RR, Gockel JM, Hammer C (1992) Kinetics and dynamics of acute rejection after heterotopic heart transplantation. J Heart Lung Transplant 11: 189–300
19. Schütz A, Fischlein T, Breuer M, Haushofer M, Uhlig A, Detter Ch, Kemkes BM, Hammer C, Reichart B (1994) Cytoimmunological monitoring after homograft valve replacement. Eur J Cardio-Thorac Surg 8: 609–612
20. Von Willebrand E, Sandberg M, Salmela K, Isoniemi H, Häyry (1994) Expression of ICAM-1 and HLA class II in acute cellular and vascular rejection of human kidney allografts. Transpl Int 7: 1–3
21. Yacoub HM, Suitters A, Khaghani A, Rose M (1986) Localization of major histocompatibility complex (HLA, ABC, DR) antigens in aortic homografts. In: Bodnar E, Yacoub HM (eds) Biological Bioprosthetic Valves. Yorke Medius Books, New York, pp 64–72
22. Yankah AC, Feller AC, Thiede A, Westphal E, Bernhard A (1986) Identification of surface antigens of endothelial cell of fresh preserved heart allografts. Thorac Cardiovasc Surg 34 (suppl): 1–10
23. Yankah AC, Wottge H-U, Müller-Hermelink HK (1987) Transplantation of aortic and plumonary allografts, enhanced viability of endothelial cells by cryopreservation, importance of histocompatibility. J Cardiac Surg 2 (suppl): 209–220

A. Schütz MD
Department of Cardiac Surgery
Krankenhaus Bogenhausen
Englschalkinger Sr. 77
81925 München
Germany

Immunogenicity of human cardiac valve allografts

E. Simon, N. Zavazava, G. Steinhoff, W. Müller-Ruchholtz, A. Haverich

Depts. of Cardiovascular Surgery and Immunology, Christian-Albrechts-Universität zu Kiel, Germany

Introduction

Since the use of human cadaver tissue was introduced into clinical practice by Gross in 1948 (5), the implantation or transplantation of allogeneic tissue has become an accepted treatment of organ and tissue failure. Lam et al. introduced the concept of allograft heart valve replacement in 1952 (9). Today, the use of allogeneic material for heart valve replacement is an accepted clinical treatment option along with mechanical valve prostheses, which have a better long-term function but require anticoagulation. Also, xenogeneic valve replacements are now widely used, the newest development being stentless xeno-valve prostheses. The two main preclusions to the use of the allograft valve are principally the same as they were in the beginning: Firstly, the complex technique of implantation in the aortic or mitral position and secondly, the limited long-term function of the prosthesis (3). After implantation, allograft valves undergo a process of degeneration, which ultimately leads to their destruction. The factors contributing to this phenomenon are still not clearly understood. While the administration of immunosuppressive drugs is the standard therapy for recipients of whole organs (heart, lung, liver, kidney) and other viable tissues such as pancreatic islet cells and corneas, this concept has not been accepted in the field of allograft valve transplantation. Indeed, it was commonly assumed that no relevant immunological reactions could be triggered by the graft. However, there is growing evidence that, in spite of the widespread belief that "we are implanting dead meat" (D. Ross), there is indeed a very relevant impact of immunological factors in the degeneration of allograft heart valve prostheses.

In animal models, the antigenicity of a heart valve allograft has been shown by other groups (8, 10, 19, 21). In these experiments, it could be demonstrated that allograft valve tissue can sensitize the recipient. Also, it could be shown that cryopreservation does not abolish this immunogenicity.

In clinical practice, the advent of heart valve cryopreservation has led to two improvements. The first one was the steady increase of the availability of allograft valves due to improved storage and shipment options. Secondly, the method of cryopreservation increased the cellular viability of the implant. This tissue viability, which results in the retention of at least a partially viable endothelial lining, has improved the long-term results after valve replacement in human recipients (2, 12). However, since the great immunogenic potential of allogeneic transplants can be attributed to their endothelial cells (1), it appears logical that an increase in viability may cause higher immunogenicity of the graft also. This, in turn, may increase the immunological reaction of the recipient to the graft, which could then reduce the potential benefit gained by implanting a fully viable allograft valve.

Interestingly, the degeneration process observed in allograft valve prostheses has not been observed in valves after heart transplantation, which are, of course, implanted as fully viable organs including a completely preserved endothelial cell lining. The absence of degeneration in these valves could either be a result of the immunosuppression given to the patient or other factors, which are currently unknown.

We sought to address the question of the immunogenicity and allo-stimulatory potential of human cardiac valves with special reference to the valve endothelium and to characterize the expression of molecules which are relevant in the regulation of immunological responses. For this purpose, we used immunohistochemical staining methods to examine cultured human cardiac valve endothelium (HCVE) and cryostat sections of valves obtained during replacement operations and from rejected cardiac grafts at the time of cardiac retransplantation.

Materials and methods

Cell cultures

Human cardiac valve endothelium (HCVE) was harvested via collagenase digestion from aortic valves obtained during replacement operations using a technique described elsewhere (18) and cultured in chamber slide culture chambers (Nunc, DK), and 96 well-microtiter plates at 37 °C and 5% CO_2 until a confluent endothelial monolayer had formed. Cells were fed by exchange of medium when necessary. After the HCVE cultures had been established, several antibodies were used to examine cultured cells and cryostat sections for the expression of endothelial cell markers, MHC class-I and class-II-antigens, selectins, integrins and other adhesion molecules.

Stimulation with IFN-γ

Cells were stimulated with recombinant IFN-γ using routine culture medium supplemented with 250 U/ml of IFN-γ for 5 days as previously described (22).

Explanted valves

Aortic valves were obtained at the time of replacement for insufficiency and stenosis ($N = 6$). Valves from transplanted (TX) hearts were obtained at time of re-TX and/or valve replacement for insufficiency and/or stenosis ($N = 4$, implantation time range 1 to 7 years). Obtained valves were shock-frozen in liquid nitrogen, cut into 5 µm sections and used for immunohistochemical staining.

Antibodies

Primary antibodies

All antibodies used were monoclonal (MoAB). The clone for the W6/32, an anti-HLA-class-I heavy chain antibody was obtained from American Type Cell Cultures (ATCC,

Table 1. Antibodies used

Antigen	Gene superfamily	Primary antigen function
MHC Class-I heavy chain	Ig supergene	Self-nonself recognition
MHC Class-II	Ig supergene	Restriction of immuneresponse
F.-VIII/v. Willebrand Factor		Activation of endogenous coagulation
H/Y		Blood group antigens
CD 31/PECAM-1	Ig supergene	Initiation of EC-EC adhesion
CD 34	Complementary CAMS	
CD 44/ECM R III		Cell homing receptor
CD 49a/VLA-1 α-chain	Integrins	α_1 integrin chain, attachment to and migration through ECM
CD 49b/VLA-2 α-chain	Integrins	α_2 integrin chain, see CD 49a
CD 49c/VLA-3 α-chain	Integrins	α_3 integrin chain, see CD 49a
CD 49d/VLA-4 α-chain	Integrins	α_4 integrin chain, see CD 49a
CD 49e/VLA-5 α-chain	Integrins	α_5 integrin chain, see CD 49a
CD 49f/VLA-6 α-chain	Integrins	α_6 integrin chain, see CD 49a
CD 51/VNR α-chain	Integrins	Cell-matrix adhesion
CD 54/ICAM-1	Ig supergene	Ligand for LFA-1 and Mac-1, leukocyte adhesion
CD 62e/ELAM-1	Selectins	Leukocyte-activated EC adhesion
CD 62p/PADGEM	Selectins	Leukocyte inflammation
CD 102/ICAM-2	Ig supergene	Lymphocyte-EC adhesion
CD 106/VCAM-1	Ig supergene	Leukocyte-activated EC adhesion

USA). The anti-H/Y antibody and the anti-F.-VIII antibody were obtained from Immunotech (France). Additional anti-F.-VIII MoAB were from DAKO (DK). Anti-CD 31, 34, 44, 49b, 49c, 49d, 49e, 49f, 51, 54, 62p, 106 MoAB were purchased from Immunotech. Anti-CD 49b MoAB were from Becton Dickinson (Belgium). The Anti-CD 62e MoAB was obtained from Dianova (FRG). The Anti-CD 102 MoAB was from Bender & Co. GmbH (Austria). Antibodies used and the primary function of their corresponding antigens are listed in Table 1.

Secondary and enzyme coupled MoAB

Anti-phosphatase-anti-alkaline-phosphatase (APAAP) and peroxidase (POD) secondary MoAB were from DAKO. Enzyme-coupled APAAP MoAB were from Dianova.

Immunohistochemical staining of HCVE

Cell cultures were used for immunohistochemical staining as soon as a satisfactory monolayer had developed. Cells were then fixed in acetone at $-20\,°C$ for 10 min and washed in TRIS-buffered saline three times. Cryostat sections or cells adhering to the bottom were then incubated with one of the primary antibodies mentioned above. After the primary incubation, immunohistochemical staining via the APAAP or POD method followed, using a previously described standard protocol (17).

Mixed cell culture

After a confluent monolayer had developed, 10^4 cells were irradiated (20 Gy) and plated on to microtiter plates (Nunc). Cells were fed with RPMI medium containing

15% AB-serum, 2 mM glutamine, 45 µg/ml penicillin and 45 µg/ml streptomycin. 10^4 peripheral blood cells (PBL) from healthy HLA incompatible donors (5 HLA mismatches) were added, and the volume of each well adjusted up to 150 µl. The cells were then kept at 37 °C and 5% CO_2 for 4 days and finally pulsed with ^{3}H-Thymidine (Amersham, UK) for 18 h before harvesting. Thymidine uptake was measured on day 5. PBL and HCVE were used in control experiments as stimulator and responder cells. Cell proliferation was measured in a beta-counter. Cultured HCVE used for this experiment were free of fibroblasts to exclude their influence on the results due to their known immuno-stimulatory potential.

Results

Characterization of HCVE

The in vitro morphology of HCVE was similar to the morphology of vascular endothelium, previously described by others (7, 11, 15). Cells became adherent to the bottom of the culture chambers, slides or microtiter plates within the first 24 h after harvesting from the valve surface. After 5 to 10 days they had either sufficiently multiplied to form a confluent monolayer or, if the initial cell number was too small, cells became dispersed, large and polygonal with a central nucleolus and multiple

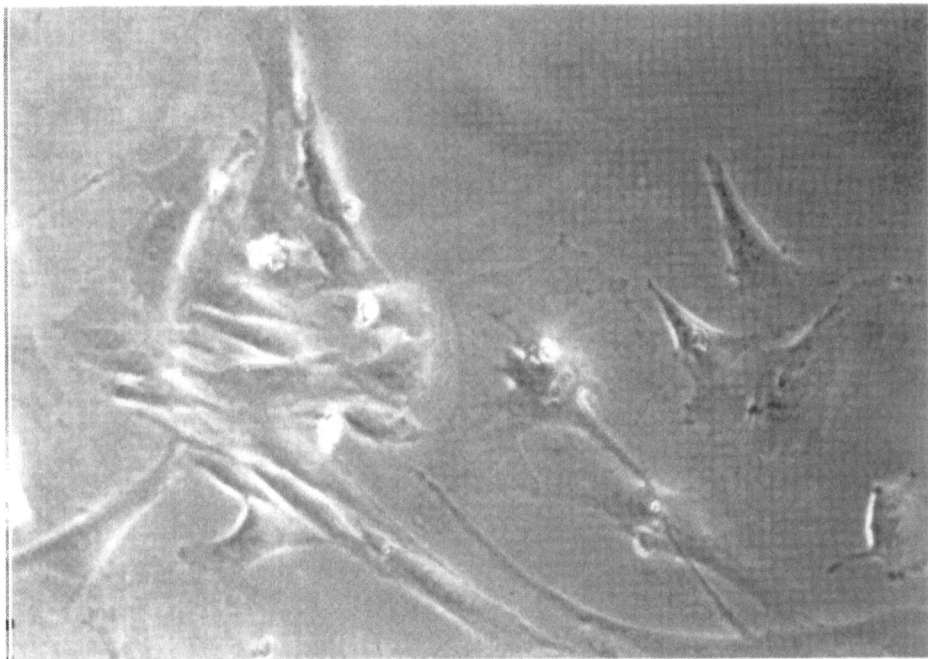

Fig. 1. Dispersed HCVE in vitro. Singular cells, appearing large and polygonal, similar to a fried egg. The central nuclei possess several nucleoli. Within the spread cytoplasm tension striae are visible.

nucleoli. At this time "tension striae" or myofilaments could be detected in singular cells by light-microscopy. Also, perinuclear vacuoles became visible. Sometimes, monolayer patches formed, covering only small areas of the bottom of the flasks or culture chambers. Singular, dispersed cells such as the ones described above sometimes became extremely large, giving the overall appearance of a fried egg (Fig. 1). Within the monolayers of cultures with sufficient initial cell number the cells grew in a confluent fashion, covering the whole bottom of the culture vessel and leaving out only small areas known as "stigmata" (Fig. 2). This phenomenon has also been described for endothelium derived from the vasculature. Individual cell borders within monolayers could be detected by routine light-microscopy only with difficulty. They could, however, be visualized using phase-contrast-microscopy. In cells growing in monolayers, no tension striae or perinuclear vacuoles could be detected.

Expression of cell surface molecules

It could be shown that non-stimulated HCVE strongly express MHC class-I and weakly express class-II-antigens (Figs. 3, 4). They also express H/Y antigens (Fig. 5) but lack expression of F.-VIII. This result is in contrast to results published for endothelial cells of different origin (6, 16). Also, HCVE were found to express the integrins CD 49a–f, the CD 34 and the CD 54 (ICAM-I) antigens. Expression of the selectin CD 62e (ELAM-I), the F.-VIII (v. Willebrand factor) and increased expression of CD 54 molecules could be observed after IFN-γ stimulation. In addition, HCVE was negative for CD 62p (PADGEM), CD 102 (ICAM-II) and CD 106 (VCAM). Cells were not examined for expression of these molecules after stimulation (see Table 2).

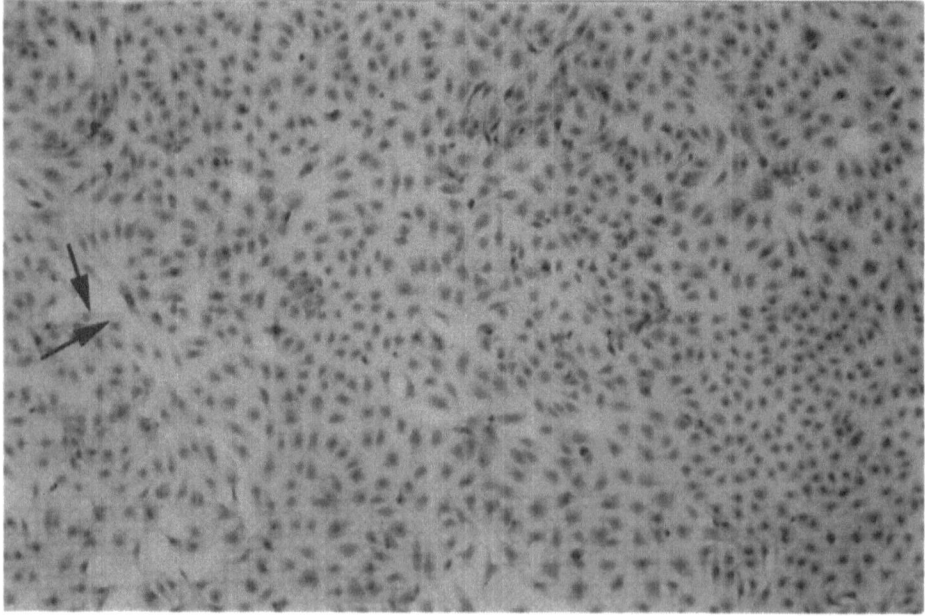

Fig. 2. Confluent monolayer of HCVE in vitro that originated from a culture with sufficient initial cell number. Polygonal cells; no cell borders are visible. In this monolayer, stigmata can be seen.

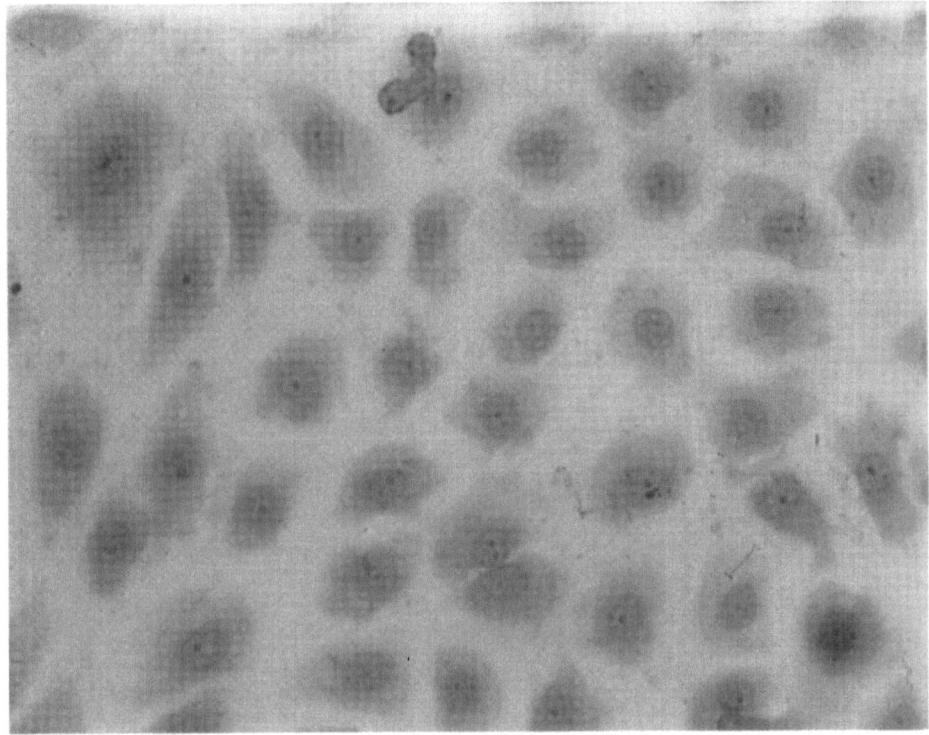

Fig. 3. Immunohistochemical staining of valvular endothelium with the anti-MHC class-I antibody. The picture shows a high level of expression of MHC-class-I antigen.

On cryostat sections of valves obtained during replacement operation or TX hearts at the time of re-TX, a discontinuous positive monolayer could be detected when using the same panel of antibodies which were positive on HCVE in vitro (Fig. 6). Cells on the surface of those valves which stained positive for the panel mentioned above, partially stained positive for F.-VIII also.

In vitro analysis of immunostimulatory capacity of HCVE

Since the expression of MHC or adhesion molecules does not necessarily correlate with immunogenicity, we compared the allo-stimulatory potential of HCVE to that of peripheral blood lymphocytes. To do this, we used a conventional mixed endothelial-lymphocyte cell culture in which PBL from two HLA incompatible blood donors and HCVE were used as stimulator cells. The stimulatory effect observed with HCVE was 2–3 times higher than that observed when using PBL for co-cultivation (Fig. 7). The incorporation of ^{3}H-thymidine during the co-stimulation of PBL in these experiments falls within the average of 20 different stimulator-responder lymphocyte combinations examined earlier in the laboratory of Dr. Zavazava (Inst. Immunology, CAU, Kiel, results not shown).

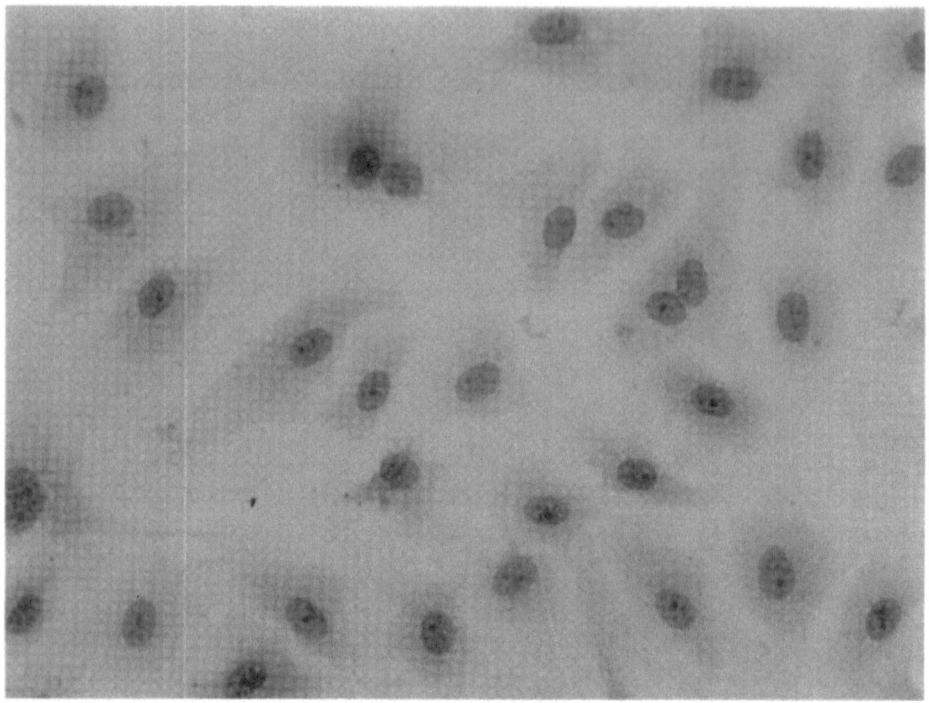

Fig. 4. Immunohistochemical staining of HCVE in vitro with the anti-MHC class-II antibody. Note the difference in level of expression of class-I and -II molecules.

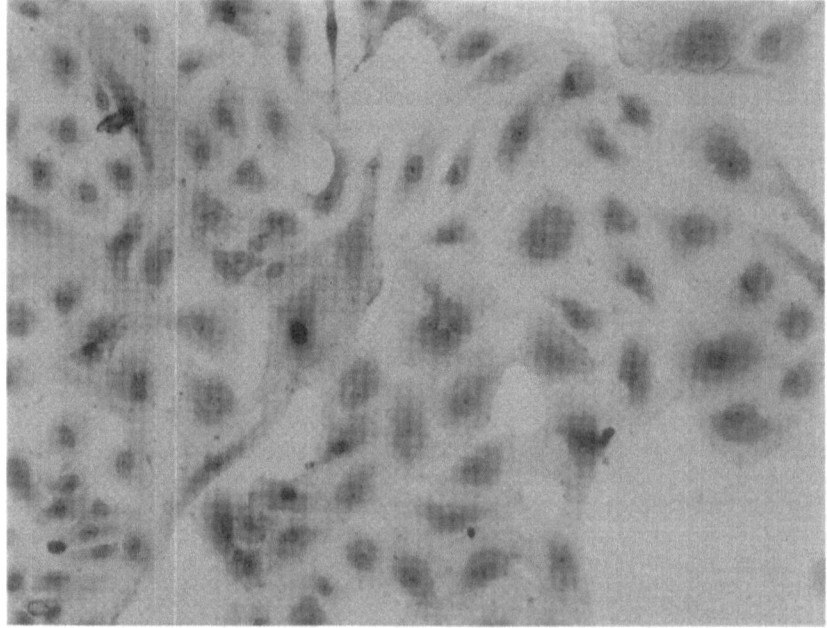

Fig. 5. In vitro culture of valvular endothelium stained with the anti-H/Y endothelial cell marker. There is high level of expression, comparable to that of MHC class-I antigen expression.

Table 2. Expression of cell surface molecules

Antigen	Expression	After IFN-γ-stimulation
MHC Class-I heavy chain	+ +	n.d.
MHC Class-II	+	+ +
F.-VIIIr	−	+
H/Y	+ +	n.d.
CD 49a/VLA-1 α-chain	+	n.d.
CD 49b/VLA-2 α-chain	+	n.d.
CD 49c/VLA-3 α-chain	+	n.d.
CD 49d/VLA-4 α-chain	+	n.d.
CD 49e/VLA-5 α-chain	+	n.d.
CD 49f/VLA-6 α-chain	+	n.d.
CD 51/VNR α-chain	+	n.d.
CD 62e/ELAM-1	−	+
CD 62p/PADGEM	−	n.d.
CD 34	+	n.d.
CD 54/ICAM-1	+ +	n.d.
CD 102/ICAM-2	−	n.d.
CD 106/VCAM-1	−	n.d.
CD 31/PECAM-1	−	n.d.

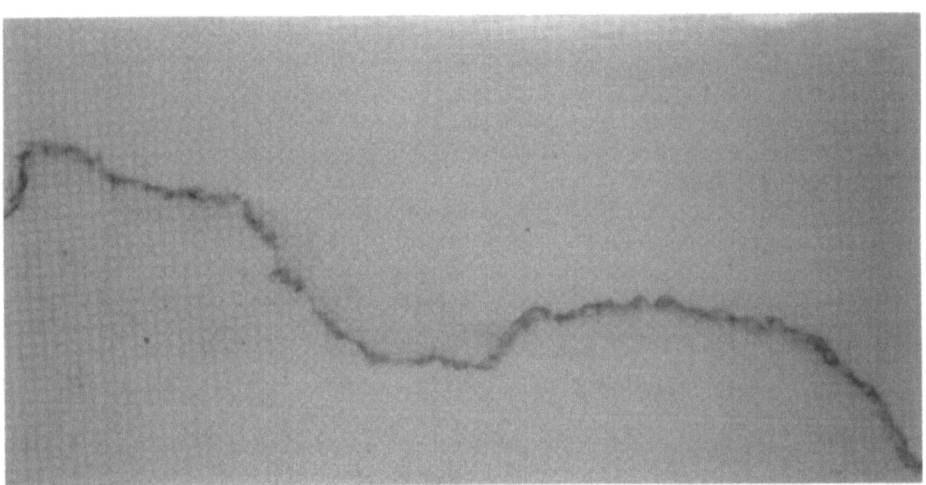

Fig. 6. Immunohistochemical staining of a valve cryostat section obtained at the time of re-TX with the anti-H/Y endothelial cell marker. Note that the region of stain is confined to the surface lining.

Discussion

The morphology of vascular endothelial cells has been previously described by others (7, 11, 15). Although the cells were cultured and of completely different origin, not only within the species but also across species barriers (e.g. porcine cardiac valves, human umbilical vein), no significant differences in their morphological appearance could be

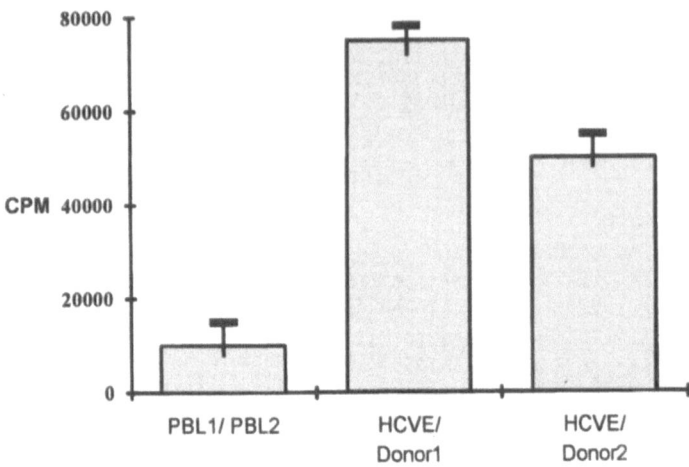

Fig. 7. Mixed endothelial lymphocyte culture. PBL and HCVE were used as stimulator cells. Responder cells were taken from two healthy MHC incompatible donors. Response against HCVE is two to three times higher than response against PBL, which is within the normal range. The data show the high immunostimulatory potential of HCVE. (Results previously published (18).)

detected. The morphology of HCVE is comparable to that of all other vascular endothelial cells in vitro. Beyond the results presented in this study, some important observations were made with respect to HCVE in vitro. During the course of experiments in a previous study (18), it was sometimes necessary to remove fibroblasts from the endothelial cell cultures. After this had been accomplished, an interesting effect could be observed. Cultured cells remained viable only for a few more days after which they ceased to proliferate and subsequently died. This observation suggests that fibroblasts may produce growth factors which may be required for the maintenance of HCVE. An additional observation was made in cultures containing only a small number of HCVE. Singular HCVE seemed to be mobile, moving across the bottom of their culture vessel. The capability of HCVE to move might play an important role in reendothelialization processes which might take place after implantation of allograft tissues.

Human cardiac valvular endothelial cells express both MHC-class-I and -II antigens in vitro. This is felt to be one of the most important findings of the current series of experiments. While the expression of MHC-class-I antigens on cryostat sections of fresh valves has been reported before (20), no in vitro expression of class-II molecules could be shown by the authors. The reason for this particular difference could well be that HCVE do behave differently in vitro than in vivo. However, during the course of these experiments, class-II expression could be shown on cryostat sections of fresh valves, too. Still, there was a remarkable difference between class-I and -II expression with respect to the intensity of the staining. Stimulation with IFN-γ has been shown to upregulate MHC expression in vitro (14). HCVE also show increased MHC-molecule expression after stimulation. This is a very interesting observation, because cytokines locally released during inflammatory processes or rejection might induce this up-regulation of MHC-class-II-molecules in vivo, thereby increasing the immunogenicity and antigenicity of the graft-endothelium and potentially initiating a host reaction to the graft. The expression of MHC antigens by valvular endothelium suggests that a viable allogenic valve might sensitize the patient, thus provoking immunological reactions which could then cause inflammation and the loss of the endothelium. These mechanisms may well shorten the functional lifespan of the implant. Alloantibodies which might contribute to such a process have been demonstrated in allograft recipients (13). It is, however, difficult to determine whether such an antibody production was primarily induced by the implant or by earlier contact with allogenic tissues (e.g. blood transfusion). Nonetheless, in an earlier study by our group using a murine model, we were able to demonstrate vascular grafts to induce both humoral and cellular immune responses (19).

In order to directly demonstrate the immunogenicity of HCVE in vitro, we used a conventional mixed endothelial-lymphocyte reaction. These experiments directly compared the immunostimulatory potential of HCVE to that of PBL, showing that the allostimulation by HCVE was more intense than that by PBL. The results of this experiment strongly support the hypothesis that HCVE is immunogenic.

In addition to MHC expression and allostimulatory potential, we also studied the expression of the F.-VIII and H/Y molecules, conventionally used as endothelial markers. In contrast to most other endothelial cells, we found HCVE to be negative for F.-VIII. It was, however, positive for H/Y antigens, which was subsequently used by us for cell type differentiation. After IFN-γ stimulation, HCVE did express F.-VIII molecules. Since F.-VIII is an important factor in the cascade leading to coagulation, these findings suggest that among the changes imposed by the immunological reaction to HCVE there may be an increase in valve thrombogenicity. Support of this theory may be drawn from clinical findings such as thrombotic material on the surfaces of valves during endocarditis or allograft valve prostheses removed during second replacement operations.

Lastly, we could show that HCVE do express a broad panel of adhesion molecules necessary to regulate not only leukocyte or lymphocyte adhesive binding to their surface, but also subsequent migration of these immunocompetent cells through the endothelial lining. Allograft valve degeneration not only leads to a loss of valvular endothelium but also irreversibly disrupts the internal structure of the valves including subsequent calcification. This observation suggests that the endothelial cells detectable on the surface of the graft after implantation may play a role in the initiation of an internally disrupting processes, also.

Valves taken from transplanted hearts always showed a largely intact layer of HCVE. Also, the internal structure of valves from transplanted hearts appeared to be intact. Still, infiltration of host lymphocytes has been shown by us suggesting that valves are targeted by the immune system during rejection after cardiac transplantation. This observation has been supported by a study recently published (4). In contrast, allograft valves examined after explanation during a second replacement operation appeared to be largely destroyed, denuded of endothelium, and void of stromal cells. The only difference between the tissue of the cryopreserved allograft valve and its counterpart in the whole organ heart transplant is the superior viability of the TX-heart valve. Patient treatment in both groups is similar after implantation except for the immunosuppression of the whole-organ recipient. Since heart valves in these hearts seem to be largely immune to the degenerating process affecting allograft valves, the differences concerning the long-term performances of the two valves has been attributed to both factors.

However the animal experiments mentioned above (8, 10, 19, 21) and the data shown here strongly suggest that implantation of a fully viable valve is not the way to solve the problem leading to the final loss of function of allograft valve prostheses. If further improvements are to be made in long-term function after allograft valve replacement, the immunologic side of the degeneration process has to be addressed too. One possible method to accomplish this is continuous immunosuppression of the patient after valve transplantation. This, of course, is not really acceptable due to the substantial negative side-effects of such a therapy. However, HLA-matching of the donor and recipient, which could be feasible, could have a similar beneficial effect in reduction of immunological reaction of the host to the graft without the negative aspects of immunosuppression.

We therefore propose that HLA-matching should be done prior to implantation of allogenic heart valve prostheses in order to further increase the long-term function of these grafts.

References

1. Allen MD, Thomas O, Mc Donald BS et al. (1992) Endothelial adhesion molecules in heart transplantation. J Heart Lung Transpl 3 (Vol. 11): 8–13
2. Angell WW, Angell JP, Oury JH et al. (1987) Long term function of viable frozen aortic homografts: a viable homograft valve bank. J Thor Cardvasc Surg 93: 815–822
3. Barratt-Boyse BG, Roche AHG, Subramanya R et al. (1987) Long term follow-up of patients with the antibiotic-sterilized aortic homograft valve inserted freehand in the aortic position. Circulation 75: 768–777
4. Breuer M, Schütz A, Brandl U et al. (1994) Acute Rejection in Heart Valves. ECC Int 6, 2nd ed.: 83–90
5. Gross RE, Hurwit ES, Bill AH et al. (1947) Preliminary observations on the use of human arterial grafts in the treatment of certain cardiovascular defects. N Engl J Med 239: 587
6. Hoyer LW, de los Santos RP, Hoyer JR (1973) Antihemophilic factor antigen: Localization in endothelial cells by immunofluorescent microscopy. J Clin Invest 52: 2737–2744
7. Jaffe EA, Nachman RL, Becker CG et al. (1973) Culture of human endothelial cells derived from umbilical veins. J Clin Invest 52: 2745–2756
8. Kathib HE, Thompson SA, Luppinetti FM (1990) Effect of storage at 4 °C in a nutrient medium on antigenic properties of rat valve allografts. Ann Thorac Surg 49: 762–796
9. Lam CR, Aram HH, Munnell ER (1952) An experimental study of aortic valve homografts. Surg Gynaecol Obstets 94: 129–135
10. Lupinetti FM, Christy JP, King DM et al. (1991) Immunogenicity, antigenicity, and endothelial viability aortic valves preserved at 4 °C in a nutrient medium. J Card Surg 6, 454–461
11. Maruyama U (1963) The human endothelial cell in tissue culture. Zeitschr. für Zellforsch 60: 69–79
12. Matzuki O, Robles A, Gibbs S et al. (1988) Long term performance of 555 aortic homografts in the aortic position. Ann Thorac Surg 46: 187
13. Moraes JR, Stanstny T (1977) A new antigen system expressed in human endothelial cells. J Clin Invest 60: 449
14. Pober JS, Collins T, Gimbrone MA et al. (1986) Inducible expression of class II major histocompatibility complex antigens and the immunogenicity of vascular endothelium. Transplantation 14: 141
15. Pollak OJ, Kasai T (1964) Appearance and behaviour of aortic cells in vitro. Am J Med Sci 248: 105–112
16. Santos de los RP, Hoyer LW (1972) Antihemophelic factor in tissue: Localization by immunofluorescence. Fed Proc 31: 262 (Abstract)
17. Simon A (1995) Immunologische Bedeutung von humanem Herzklappenendothelium für die langfristige Funktion von biologischen Ersatzklappen, Thesis
18. Simon A, Zavazava N, Sievers HH, Müller-Ruchholz W (1993) In vitro cultivation and immunogenicity of human cardiac valve endothelium. J Card Surg 8: 656–665
19. Thiede A, Timm C, Bernhard A, Müller-Ruchholz W (1978) Studies on the antigenicity of vital allogeneic valve leaflets in immunogenetically controlled strain combinations. Transplantation 26: 391
20. Yacoub MH (1987) Cardiac Valve Allografts 1962–1987, Steinkopf Verlag Darmstadt/Springer Verlag New York, pp 95–102

21. Yankah AC, Wottge HU, Müller-Ruchholtz W (1987) Cardiac Valve Allografts 1962–1987, Steinkopf Verlag Darmstadt/Springer Verlag New York, pp 77–87
22. Zavazava N, Halene M, Westphal E, Müller-Ruchholtz W (1991) Expression of MHC class I and class II molecules by cadaver retinal pigment epithelial cells: optimization of post-mortem HLA typing. Clin Exp Immunol 84: 163–166

E. Simon, MD
Dept. of Cardiovascular Surgery, CAU, Kiel
Arnold-Heller Str 7
24106 Kiel
Germany

Immune response and calcification of allografts

F. M. Lupinetti

Associate Professor of Surgery, University of Washington, Chief,
Division of Cardiac Surgery, Children's Hospital and Medical Center,
Seattle, Washington, USA

Aside from the cornea, a structure that is not vascularized, the aortic and pulmonary valves are the only tissues that can be successfully transplanted without immunosuppression of the recipient. This has led to speculation as to whether the transplanted heart valve is immunologically privileged in a manner analogous to the cornea. This chapter will discuss the evidence for an immunologic capacity of the allograft valve, the response of the recipient to allograft implantation, and the pathologic consequences. Also discussed are the possible therapeutic manipulations that may alter these properties.

The immunology of the allograft heart valve is unlikely to be fundamentally different from that of other tissues. That is to say that the concept of "immunologic privilege," as applied to cornea transplantation, is probably not of significance in a tissue residing within the blood stream of the recipient and subject to interaction with the recipient's cellular and humoral immune mediators. Accordingly, in an analysis of the immune response to allograft valves it is necessary to consider the degree to which the graft retains the immune characteristics of the donor. This requires an inquiry as to the presence of donor cells, their persistence, their ability to present an antigenic stimulus, and the nature of the recipient response. Considerations of the aortic and pulmonary valves in the transplanted heart are unlikely to provide important information regarding the isolated valve allograft. Aortic and pulmonary valves in the whole-heart transplant rarely demonstrate dysfunction, calcification, or histologic evidence of degeneration (18). Whether this is attributable to methods of heart preservation, immunosuppression, or vascularization of the tissue is unknown, but probably makes it impossible to draw parallels between these disparate clinical settings.

Persistence of donor cells and antigen expression

The cell types composing the allograft valve include endothelial cells, fibroblasts, vascular smooth muscle, and cardiac muscle. Although all of these distinct cell populations have some potential as immune stimuli, the endothelium is perhaps the most powerful determinant of the host response. Endothelium expresses the major histocompatibility antigens as well as the adhesion molecules required for interaction with recipient leukocytes. Therefore the presence of endothelium on the allograft, both at the time of implantation and subsequently, may be of prime importance in determining the immunologic events that follow. The presence of endothelium can be determined based on the use of specific antibodies, such as those directed at von Willebrand's factor and factor VIII, or lectins with a strong affinity for residues of the endothelial cell membrane.

This leads to the logical question of whether endothelium is preserved after various methods of allograft harvest, sterilization, and storage. Christy and coauthors examined the degree of endothelial cell viability in allografts subjected to storage at 4 °C in a nutrient medium. Using flow cytometry and a double-labeling fluorescent dye technique, they showed that endothelial cell viability substantially diminishes over a 3-week period of storage (3).

Fibroblasts, on the other hand, clearly appear to be preserved after storage and implantation, at least to some degree. The duration of fibroblast viability in storage may be as little as 24 h (1) or considerably longer. The demonstration by O'Brien of persistent donor cells more than 8 years after allograft aortic valve implantation indicates that long-term fibroblast viability is possible (14). Contrary studies include those of Mitchell and associates that suggest cryopreserved valves contain few if any viable cells within a short time after implantation (12).

Other cell populations within the allograft valve are also capable of expressing antigens. Salomon and colleagues studied the vascular smooth muscle cells within the aorta of human allograft valves that had previously been cryopreserved and were thawed in preparation for implant (15). Smooth muscle cells were obtained and grown in culture from four grafts out of eight attempts. These cells were cultured both in an unstimulated state and after incubation with interferon gamma. The smooth muscle constitutively expressed class I HLA. Stimulation with interferon gamma resulted in expression of both class I and class II HLA. This study indicates both the persistence of smooth cell viability, and perhaps more importantly, the ability of these cells to present histocompatibility antigens that may result in a host immune response.

Recipient sensitization

If allograft valves have immunologic properties, it would seem logical that recipient sensitization could be demonstrated. Heslop and associates studied production of hemagglutinins and lymphocytotoxic antibodies after implantation of partial or complete aortic valve grafts in rats (8). They concluded that aortic valve grafts were immunogenic, but that the cardiac muscle was the most important contributor to this immunogenicity. They further concluded that the aortic valve leaflets were not immunogenic. In contrast, Cochran and Kunzelman demonstrated in rats that subcutaneous implantation of aortic valve leaflets from weakly allogeneic donors produced accelerated rejection of skin grafts obtained from rats of the same strain as the valve donor (4). Furthermore, the acceleration in skin graft rejection was nearly identical whether the aortic valve tissue was implanted in the fresh state or after cryopreservation. Some of the discrepancies in these studies may be explained by the use of models in which the aortic valve graft is not implanted in a normal intravascular fashion.

The model of aortic valve transplantation heterotopically into the abdominal aorta may permit more accurate and clinically analogous observations. This model, as described by Yankah and colleagues (22), is likely to produce an immunologic response that will not necessarily be achieved by subcutaneous implantation. With the use of the intravascular aortic valve graft model, studies of recipient sensitization have been more consistent in their demonstration of immune stimulation. Specific class II antibodies directed against the donor have been demonstrated using this model (22).

The work of El Khatib and Lupinetti used the intravascular model of rat aortic valve transplantation to examine the immunogenicity of grafts of varying degrees of histocompatibility (5). This investigation showed that mildly, moderately, and strongly allogeneic grafts had proportionally potent effects on the acceleration of second-set skin graft rejection. Furthermore, cryopreservation of these grafts did not reduce the sensitization of the recipient animals. A subsequent study from this laboratory, however, demonstrated that storage of allograft valves at 4 °C in a nutrient medium for progressively longer periods of time was associated with a delayed rejection of the skin graft (6). This prolongation of cold storage was associated with a progressive loss of endothelium as evaluated by scanning electron microscopy. Even when all endothelium was lost, however, the resulting valve grafts caused some acceleration of skin graft rejection compared to sham-operated controls. These findings support the hypothesis that endothelium is a strong immunologic stimulus, but that even in the absence of endothelium the allograft valve retains immunologic potency.

Perhaps the most focused and sensitive assessment of host immune response to experimental allograft valves was reported by Zhao and associates (23). These investigators used mixed lymphocyte cultures, cytotoxic T-cell precursor assay, and flow cytometric detection of donor-specific antibodies to examine the response to implantation of fresh aortic valve grafts in rats. The mixed lymphocyte culture stimulation index showed a marked increase at seven, 14, and 28 days after aortic valve allograft implant. This increase was to a level between that following aortic valve isograft implant and skin allograft placement. Limiting dilution analysis of splenocytes also showed an increase in cytotoxic T-lymphocyte precursor frequency after allograft aortic valve implant that was similar to that following skin allograft placement. Finally, flow cytometry demonstrated an increase in donor-specific anti-T-cell antibodies in valve allograft recipients. These observations therefore indicate the activation of both cellular and humoral immune responses of a specific nature in response to fresh aortic valve allografts. This response occurs early after grafting and is sustained for at least 3 weeks thereafter.

The capacity of allograft valves to sensitize human recipients has only recently been established. One study that suggests sensitization does occur clinically was reported by Schutz and colleagues (16). This study employed cytoimmunological monitoring of patients on a daily basis for 3 weeks after implantation of cryopreserved allograft valves. The cytoimmunologic monitoring technique used consisted of counting lymphoblasts and total lymphoid cells from a peripheral blood sample. The "activation index," the ratio of lymphoblasts to total lymphoid cells, was calculated, and an index exceeding 1 was considered to be demonstrative of an immunologic response. Patients with ABO-incompatible grafts demonstrated a significantly higher and more sustained increase in the activation index than did recipients of ABO-compatible allografts. In turn, the ABO-compatible graft recipients showed significantly higher activation indices than recipients of xenograft bioprosthetic valves. In less than 2 weeks after allograft implantation, however, the activation index fell to less than one in all patients without treatment. Furthermore, postoperative echocardiographic examinations of the valve grafts showed no evidence of dysfunction.

Smith and associates prospectively studied allograft recipients as well as recipients of porcine valves for the formation of panel-reactive antibodies (PRA). Only 20% of porcine valve recipients demonstrated PRA postoperatively, compared with none in the preoperative period. Among recipients of "homovital" valves – grafts implanted without antibiotic preservation – the percentage demonstrating PRA increased from 20% preoperatively to 100% within the first postoperative year. Recipients of antibiotic sterilized valve grafts showed PRA in 20% of cases preoperatively compared to 56% postoperatively. Because "homovital" allograft valves undergo minimal manipulation and may have enhanced cellular viability, the capacity for eliciting recipient sensitization may be enhanced as well. Furthermore, Smith demonstrated that among 11 cases of identifiable HLA-specific antibody expression for which the donor HLA type was known, in 10 cases the antibodies were directed against donor antigens (17).

Effects of sterilization and storage methods

It is possible that methods of allograft harvest, sterilization, and storage can be therapeutically manipulated in a manner that modulates immune response. The endothelium is the site of the greatest expression of histocompatibility antigens. It is logical, therefore, to expect that allograft valve storage methods that reduce the number and viability of endothelial cells will correspondingly decrease the antigen expression of the graft. This seems to be the case. Lupinetti and associates demonstrated that allograft valves studied in the fresh state or after 24 h of storage at 4 °C expressed class I histocompatibility antigens (10). Grafts stored at 4 °C for longer periods did not express class I antigens, however (Figs. 1 and 2). Duration of storage at 4 °C also correlated with a decrease in endothelial cell viability and extended longevity of second-set skin graft survival. Class II antigens were not expressed by any of these unimplanted tissues. This work confirmed the study of Yacoub and colleagues, who examined aortic valves obtained from patients undergoing cardiac transplant (20). Untreated tissues showed the presence of class I antigen, but sterilization and increasing periods of storage resulted in a progressive loss of antigen. The only identifiable class II antigen presence in the aortic valves was associated with leukocytes that disappeared within 48 h of harvest.

  Whether specific storage media can affect immune response was investigated by Bodnar and associates, who implanted allograft aortic segments subcutaneously in recipient rabbits that had been immunized previously with fetal calf serum (2). Each rabbit received two aortic segments, one of which was stored in a solution containing fetal calf serum. By 3 weeks after implantation, the segments stored with fetal calf serum displayed substantially greater disruption of elastic fibers and medial necrosis. A much more intense lymphocytic response was also present in the fetal calf serum-stored specimens. These observations were interpreted as demonstrating an increased potential for immunologically mediated allograft destruction when grafts are treated with fetal calf serum. This study, however, uses a model of presensitization that is of doubtful applicability to the clinical use of calf serum in the cryopreservation process.

  More compelling evidence for the potential of storage methodology to affect immune response comes from the work of Hoekstra and coauthors (9). These investigators studied matched aortic valve leaflets obtained from the same human donor. One leaflet was studied after antibiotic sterilization only, whereas the other was treated with an identical sterilization process and then cryopreserved. Each leaflet was incubated with two human lymphocyte populations, one mismatched for HLA-A, -B, and -DR antigens and the other matched for HLA-DR alone. Immune response was characterized by the stimulation index reflecting incorporation of tritiated thymidine

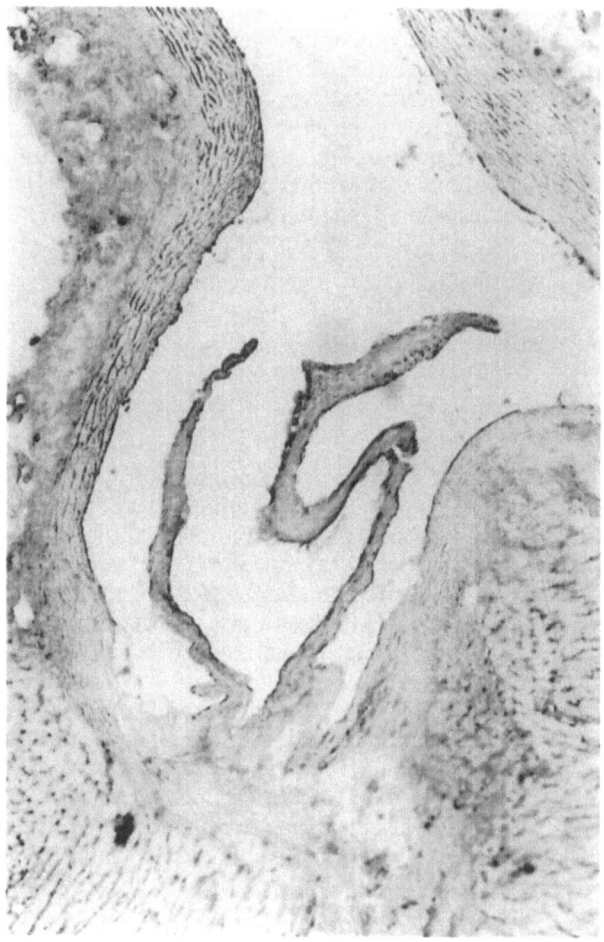

Fig. 1. Immunocytochemical staining for class I antigen in a fresh rat aortic valve graft. The dark precipitate indicates presence of class I antigen.

by the activated lymphocytes. The HLA-DR mismatched lymphocytes showed significant lymphocyte proliferation in response to both the fresh and the cryopreserved valve leaflets, demonstrating the capacity of the valve to elicit an immune response. The stimulation index in the fresh group, however, was significantly greater than that in the cryopreserved group, suggesting the attenuation of the immune stimulus by the storage method. Furthermore, among lymphocytes exposed to HLA-DR matched valve leaflets, the stimulation index was significantly reduced compared to lymphocytes incubated with HLA-DR mismatched leaflets. This study may serve as support for HLA-DR matching valve donors and recipients if possible.

Leukocyte adhesion molecules are a recently discovered class of compounds that are of great importance in inflammatory responses of many types including the host immune response. Leukocyte adhesion molecules mediate neutrophil and lymphocyte chemotaxis in such diverse settings as cardiac transplantation, autoimmune disorders, infection, and other phenomena. The expression of leukocyte adhesion molecules by allograft valves may predict the host inflammatory response and predispose to tissue

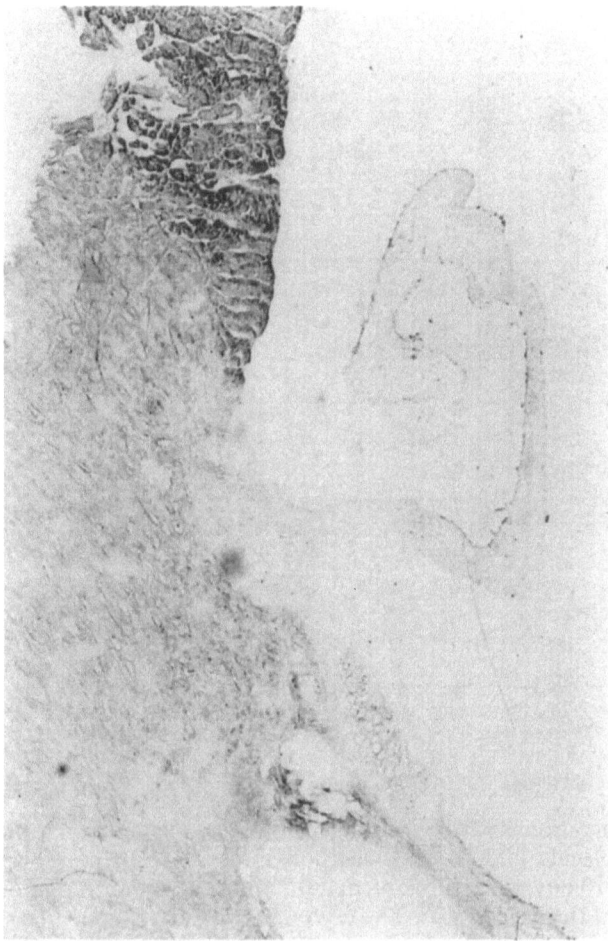

Fig. 2. Immunocytochemical staining for class I antigen in a cryopreserved rat aortic valve graft. The absence of a dark precipitate indicates absence of class I antigen.

injury. Mulligan and associates, using the heterotopic aortic valve graft model in the rat, determined the expression of E-selectin, intercellular adhesion molecule-1 (ICAM-1), and vascular cell adhesion molecule-1 (VCAM-1) by the allograft valve (13). This study examined both syngeneic and allogeneic grafts, including tissues implanted in the fresh state, those subjected to cryopreservation, and those preserved at 4 °C in a nutrient medium for 1–21 days. Grafts were explanted 4 h to 21-days after implantation and subjected to immunocytochemical analysis with monoclonal antibodies to the respective adhesion molecules. Syngeneic valves showed little or no adhesion molecule expression at any time after implantation. This was observed regardless of storage methods employed. This indicates that many of the potential stimuli to adhesion molecule expression, such as surgical trauma, ischemia and reperfusion, or the storage media are insufficient to elicit production of these inflammatory mediators. In contract, allogeneic valves implanted freshly after harvest exhibited intense expression of all adhesion molecules within 4 h of implant. This expression continued without attenuation throughout the 21-day period of late

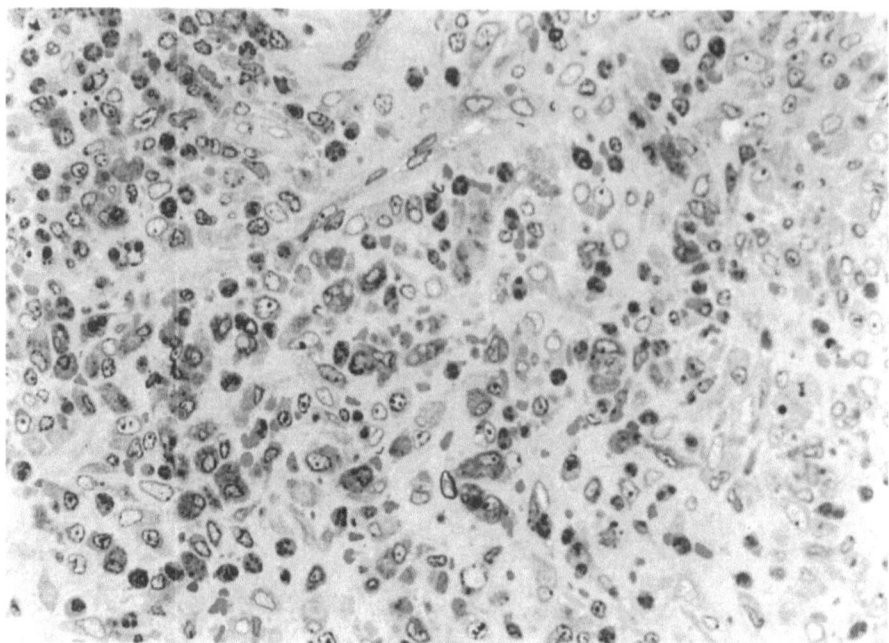

Fig. 3. Micrograph of a fresh rat aortic valve allograft removed 10 days after implant. An intense inflammatory infiltrate is present. This tissue also exhibited abundant staining for the leuko-cyte adhesion molecules E-selectin, intercellular adhesion molecule-1, and vascular cell adhesion molecule-1.

observation. Both cryopreservation and 4 °C storage, however, produced marked attenuation of adhesion molecule expression. Adhesion molecule expression was delayed, not appearing until 10 days after implant, and diminished, not reflecting the intensity of response found in the fresh grafts. The cryopreserved grafts appeared to have a somewhat lessened expression of adhesion molecules than the 4 °C stored valves even as far as 21 days after implant. The grafts demonstrated acute inflamma-tory infiltrates that were roughly proportional to the intensity of adhesion molecule expression (Figs. 3 and 4). This study provides compelling evidence that all storage methods currently used in clinical practice are likely to produce a graft that is less of a stimulus to host immune response.

Evidence of immunologically mediated graft degeneration

If the host immunologic response causes accelerated allograft deterioration, it would be expected that deterioration would be most rapid in ABO incompatible tissues. Although many authorities advise the use of ABO compatible valves when possible, the data to support this recommendation are sparse. Studies have failed to demon-strate any influence of ABO compatibility on allograft survival (19). Yankah and

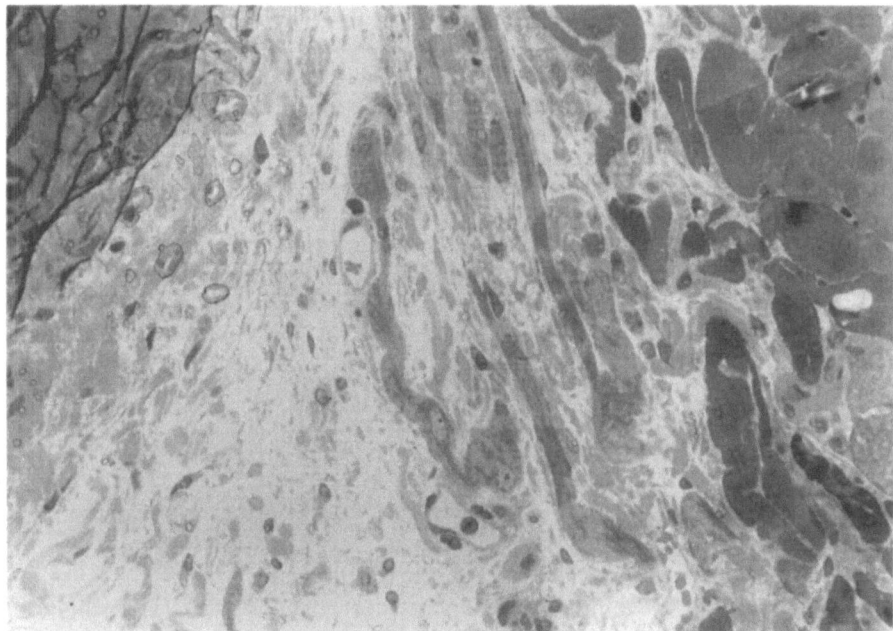

Fig. 4. Micrograph of a cryopreserved rat aortic valve allograft removed 10 days after implant. A minimal inflammatory infiltrate is present. This tissue exhibited no staining for leukocyte adhesion molecules.

colleagues, reviewing allografts implanted in patients less than 2 years old, found allograft dysfunction in seven of 17 recipients of compatible tissues, with replacement required in four cases. However, none of nine patients receiving ABO-incompatible allografts exhibited valve dysfunction or required reoperation (21).

Calcification

The relationship of allograft immunogenicity and calcification is far from resolved. Calcification is a complex process that may reflect multiple factors other than immunology. Some factors that could influence calcification, such as cellular viability, age, and storage methodology, may be covariate influences on immunology as well, further clouding the issue.

One of the first studies to draw a link between immunology and calcification was performed by Gonzalez-Lavin and coinvestigators (7). This study used dogs that underwent reconstruction of the right ventricular outflow tract with an aortic valve allograft. Grafts were obtained from littermates or unrelated donors. Over a period of up to 4 months, grafts were retrieved and examined histologically and chemically for calcium content. The grafts from related donors showed significantly less calcification than those from unrelated donors. Although even tissue from littermate canines may be strongly allogeneic, this study suggests the possibility of immunologic influences on calcium deposition.

A study with a greater degree of immunologic control was reported by Lupinetti and associates (11). This investigation used the heterotopic rat aortic valve graft model, allowing examination of syngeneic grafts as well as grafts obtained from weakly allogeneic, moderately allogeneic, and strongly allogeneic donors. Calcium content within the valve graft leaflets was evaluated with energy dispersion x-ray microanalysis. Calcium deposition was significantly less in syngeneic grafts compared to all allogeneic groups. There was nearly identical calcium deposition in the weakly, moderately, and strongly allogeneic grafts. This lack of difference in calcification among grafts with differing degrees of histocompatibility is somewhat surprising. This observation suggests that calcification, although to some degree inevitable in allogeneic tissue, is not likely to be influenced by weak manipulations of the immune system, incomplete matching of donor and recipient, or ABO blood group matching alone.

Summary

That allograft valves are immunologically potent seems certain. That allografts sensitize recipients seems probable. Whether the host immunologic response results in adverse consequences, however, remains in doubt. Accordingly, efforts at tissue matching should not take precedence over insuring the implantation of a properly sized, structurally intact valve. Immunosuppression of recipients cannot currently be justified, given the known adverse effects of immunosuppressive drugs and the low probability of achieving a desirable response.

References

1. Armiger LC (1995) Viability studies of human valves prepared for use as allografts. Ann Thorac Surg 60: S118–S121
2. Bodnar E, Olsen EGJ, Florio R, Guerreiro D, Ross DN (1988) Heterologous antigenicity induced in human aortic homografts during preservation. Eur J Cardio-thorac Surg 2: 43–47
3. Christy JP, Lupinetti FM, Mardan AH, Thompson SA (1991) Endothelial viability in the rat aortic wall. Ann Thorac Surg 51: 204–207
4. Cochran RP, Kunzelman KS (1989) Cryopreservation does not alter antigenic expression of aortic allografts. J Surg Res 46: 597–599
5. El Khatib H, Lupinetti FM (1990) Antigenicity of fresh and cryopreserved rat valve allografts. Transplantation 49: 765–767
6. El Khatib H, Thompson SA, Lupinetti FM (1990) Effect of storage at 4 °C in a nutrient medium on antigenic properties of rat aortic valve allografts. Ann Thorac Surg 49: 792–796
7. Gonzalez-Lavin L, Bianchi J, Graf D, Amini S, Gordon CI (1988) Degenerative changes in fresh aortic root homografts in a canine model: evidence of an immunologic influence. Transplant Proc 20: 815–819
8. Heslop BF, Wilson SE, Hardy BE (1973) Antigenicity of aortic valve allografts. Ann Surg 177: 301–306
9. Hoekstra F, Knoop C, Jutte N, Wassenaar C, Mochtar B, Bos E, Weimar W (1993) Effect of cryopreservation and HLA-DR matching on the cellular immunogenicity of human cardiac valve allografts. J Heart Lung Transplant 13: 1095–1098
10. Lupinetti FM, Christy JP, King DM, El Khatib H, Thompson SA (1991) Immunogenicity, antigenicity, and endothelial viability of aortic valves preserved at 4 °C in a nutrient medium. J Cardiac Surg 6: 454–461

11. Lupinetti FM, Cobb S, Kioschos HC, Thompson SA, Walters KS, Moore KC (1992) Effect of immunological differences on rat aortic valve allograft calcification. J Cardiac Surg 7: 65–70

12. Mitchell RN, Jonas RA, Schoen FJ (1995) Structure-function correlations in cryopreserved allograft cardiac valves. Ann Thorac Surg 60: S108–S113

13. Mulligan MS, Tsai TT, Kneebone JM, Ward PA, Lupinetti FM (1994) Effects of preservation techniques on in vivo expression of adhesion molecules by aortic valve allografts. J Thorac Cardiovasc Surg 107: 717–723

14. O'Brien MF, Stafford EG, Gardner MAH, Pohlner PG, McGiffin DC (1987) A comparison of aortic valve replacement with viable cryopreserved and fresh allograft valves, with a note on chromosomal studies. J Thorac Cardiovasc Surg 94: 812–823

15. Salomon RN, Friedman GB, Callow AD, Payne DD, Libby P (1993) Cryopreserved aortic homografts contain viable smooth muscle cells capable of expressing transplantation antigens. J Thorac Cardiovasc Surg 106: 1173–1180

16. Schutz A, Fischlein T, Breuer M, Haushofer M, Uhlig A, Detter Ch, Kemkes BM, Hammer C, Reichart B (1994) Cytoimmunological monitoring after homograft valve replacement. Eur J Cardio-thorac Surg 8: 609–612

17. Smith JD, Ogino H, Hunt D, Laylor RM, Rose ML, Yacoub MH (1995) Humoral immune response to human aortic valve homografts. Ann Thorac Surg 60: S127–S130

18. Valente M, Faggian G, Billingham ME, Talenti E, Calabrese F, Casula R, Shumway NE, Thiene G (1995) The aortic valve after heart transplantation. Ann Thorac Surg 60: S135–S140

19. Weipert J, Meisner H, Mendler N, Haehnel JC, Homann M, Paek S-U, Sebening F (1995) Allograft implantation in pediatric cardiac surgery: Experience from 1982 to 1994. Ann Thorac Surg 60: S101–S104

20. Yacoub M, Suitters A, Khaghani A, Rose M (1986) Localization of major histocompatibility complex (HLA, ABC, and DR) antigens in aortic homografts. In Bodnar E, Yacoub M (eds). Biologic and Bioprosthetic Valves. New York, Yorke Medical Books, pp 65–72

21. Yankah AC, Alexi-Meskhishvili V, Weng Y, Schorn K, Lange PE, Hetzer R (1995) Accelerated degeneration of allografts in the first two years of life. Ann Thorac Surg 60: S71–S77

22. Yankah AC, Wottge HU, Muller-Ruchholtz W (1988) Prognostic importance of viability and a study of a second set allograft valve: an experimental study. J Cardiac Surg 3: 263–270

23. Zhao X, Green M, Frazer IH, Hogan P, O'Brien MF (1994) Donor-specific immune response after aortic valve allografting in the rat. Ann Thorac Surg 57: 1158–1163

Author's address:
F. M. Lupinetti, MD
Children's Hospital and Medical Center
4800 Sand Point Way N.E.
Seattle, Washington 98105
U.S.A.

The allograft valve in aortic valve replacement and in transplanted patients

T. Ramos, J. Neves[1], S. Gulbenkian[2], C. Monteiro[2], R. Santos, A. Martins, S. Ramos, J. Q. Melo

Instituto do Coração/Hospital de Santa Cruz, Carnaxide, Portugal
[1] Departamento de Biologia Celular Instituto Gulbenkian de Ciência, Oeiras, Portugal
[2] Departamento de Genética, Faculdade de Ciências Médicas UNL, Lisboa, Portugal

Introduction

Mechanical and biological heart valve substitutes have evolved in parallel, since, in 1951, Hufnagel implanted the first mechanical prosthesis in the descending aorta and attempted, although without success, to implant valve allografts in the same position (reviewed in 35). Five years later, Murray, following the experimental work by Lam and colleages (20), succeeded where Hufnagel had failed, when by placing an allograft in the descending aorta succeeded in reducing an aortic valve insufficiency (29).

In the early 1960s, new developments took place in both fields, with the introduction of the ball valves by Starr (43) and the first replacement of the aortic valve with an allograft in orthotopic position, performed independently by Ross (36) and Barratt-Boyes (4), using the technique developed by Duran and Gunning (10).

At this stage the choice between mechanical valves and allografts depended, above all, upon the skillfulness of the surgeon. Extracorporeal circulation was at its infancy, and only experienced hands could insert an allograft. The limited access to fresh human cadaveric material and the need for specific sizing for recipients were additional factors that conditioned the decision. Therefore, methods for disinfection and extended storage, were explored. Chlorhexidine (36), ethylene oxide (16, 21), β-propiolactone (33), formaldehyde (44) and γ-irradiation (24) were introduced for sterilization. Long-term storage involved freeze-drying or fast-freezing and preservation in a carbon-dioxide freezer at $-70\,°C$ (33). Later, all these methods were shown to render the cellular component of the cusps nonviable and to denature proteins, leading to a substantial alteration of the extracellular matrix (ECM). As a result, soon after implantation, rupture and calcification of the cusps occurred in the allografts, bringing the rate of reoperation to unacceptable levels (5, 28, 41). At this point, mechanical valves with improved hemodynamic conditions (7, 18), and stented xenogeneic porcine valves (17, 34) that had been developed after the first successful implants of xenografts (6, 31) became popular.

Stented allografts had been introduced in the late 1960s (3) when the effects of prolonged cardiopulmonary bypass were prevalent and myocardial protection poorly developed. As compared to the freehand sutured allograft, the valve mounted on a rigid support was easier to implant, thus reducing the length of the surgical procedure. As it turned out, the use of the stent proved detrimental for the durability of aortic valve homografts (2). Later, the same was shown for the stented xenografts where degeneration, calcification and cusp rupture occurred earlier than in freehand allografts, particularly in children and young adults (9, 23, 45).

As the hemodynamics of the heart valves became better understood, the mechanism underlying stented valve rupture was also clarified. The rigidity of the stent created pressure gradients far greater than the physiological ones, with the consequent straining of the tissue.

As it stands today, stented prosthetic valves as well as stentless allograft have precise indications; the procurement and storage methods having evolved to give good long-term results (2, 14).

Sterilization of allogeneic valves with antibiotic was introduced by Barratt-Boyes in 1968 (4) and soon it became clear that both the concentration and duration of the treatment, affected cell viability. As increasing evidence accumulated suggesting that durability of the allograft correlated with cell viability, the methods for sterilization and long-term storage were further refined (reviewed in (32)). Of particular relevance were the development of cryopreservation in liquid nitrogen, in the presence of dimethylsulfoxide (1, 27) and the use of low doses of antibiotics (32). These improvements led to the establishment of standard protocols that ensured a high degree of cell survival (25).

Nevertheless, in spite of this enormous progress, degeneration is still the most frequent cause of allograft failure (2). For the past few years, we have focused our research interests on that problem (26, 30) and worked on the hypothesis that in spite of being viable at the time of implantation, donor cells would be destroyed by the immune response triggered by the presence of a foreign tissue. This possibility arose when allograft valves were first used, but was soon discarded for acute rejection episodes did not occur. Nevertheless, a number of studies performed on explanted human valves, as well as experimental animal models, were consistent with the concept that leaflet degeneration might result from the immune response (8, 11, 12, 15, 19, 46–49). The significance of these studies, and in particular of those using allograft valves in dogs and pigs, was however questioned, because, as opposed to the human, valve leaflets in such animals are highly vascularized (cited from 19). Consequently, these early results were deemed insufficiently conclusive to warrant administration of immunosuppressive therapy to heart valve recipients. This assumption was further supported by the aforementioned evidence suggesting that the long-term success of allograft heart valves directly correlated with the viability of the leaflet fibroblast before implantation (32, 42).

The excellent long-term results of pulmonary autografts (37–39) excluded the possibility that failure of the allografts was due to a flow dynamic's disturbance, caused by the reconstruction of the aortic root, since the same technique was used in both cases. On the other hand, the same data was consistent with an immune mediated mechanism of allograft degeneration. Could it be that, in spite of being of viable at the time of implant, the lifespan of the fibroblasts was limited by a subsequent immune response; or were the preparation and cryopreservation methods, which were perfected to warrant cell viability, still affecting the extra cellular matrix (ECM) in such way that it became inappropriate to harbor the donor's cells and, eventually, support homing of those from the recipient?

To assess these questions, two different approaches were used. In the first, we have compared explanted valves from immunocompetent and immunosuppressed patients, such as occurs in valve replacement (VR) and heart transplantation (HTx), respectively. In addition to the immune status, the two groups differ in that the valves in the transplanted hearts were exposed to a much shorter period of cold ischemia and were not subjected to the sterilization and cryopreservation procedures, as were the VR. Although seemingly irrelevant in the present context, considering the results obtained with pulmonary autografts (37–39), the differences in hemodynamics between the two groups, with the HTx having an intact aortic root and the VR having been reconstructed, should also be mentioned. With the second approach, an experimental model in which cryopreserved allografts and autografts, as well as fresh autografts were implanted in the same animal, we have attempted to establish the relative roles played by the immune response and the procurement/cryopreservation procedures, on the mechanism of degeneration.

Histological and genetic assessment of explanted allograft valves

Determination of the cell origin in an allograft can be used to evaluate the status of the matrix as well as the immune response induced by the allogeneic tissue. Thus, in the absence of an immune response, a well-preserved matrix would be expected to retain cells of donor origin and, eventually be repopulated by cells from the recipient. Conversely, in the presence of an immune response, lymphocyte infiltrates and destruction of donor cells as well as damage of the matrix should be anticipated. Once altered, the matrix would no longer support cell adhesion and, consequently, the tissue would become progressively acellular.

The origin of the cells in a transplanted organ can be established by PCR amplification of DNA hypervariable repeat regions and subsequent evaluation of the number of different sized amplimers obtained. Because each size indicates the presence of a particular allele and since each individual has a maximum of two alleles for each locus, a single sized amplimer indicates a homozygous origin of the cells, whereas the presence of two sized amplimers can indicate a single heterozygous or a dual homozygote. The occurrence of three or four sized amplimers precisely indicates a dual (recipient and donor) origin. The distinction between a single heterozygous and a dual homozygote can be made by analyzing donor's and recipient's control DNA. If control DNA is not available, definite confirmation can also be made by increasing the number of markers.

Using this approach as well as histology and immunohistochemistry, we have analyzed the cellular composition of valve leaflets that were explanted from seven VR patients (V1–V7), five HTx (T1-T5) and one valve autograft (AG). Clinical data, valve origin, procurement and storage are summarized in Table 1.

Histological analysis of explanted valves from the VR group showed that leaflets lost their normal structure, with hyalinization being observed in all cases and focal calcification in four (V3, V5, V6 and V7). It is noteworthy that one of these, V3, had only been implanted for 2 months.

With the exception of a small number of fibroblasts that were found in V1, V2 and V3, histologically, all leaflets were devoid of the connective tissue cellular components, and endothelium (Fig. 1a). Polymorphonuclear (PMN) infiltrates were found in three cases (V1–V3), most likely due to nonspecific acute endocarditis and lymphocytes that were identified as T-cells (Figs. 1b and c) were found in cases V2, V4 and V6. As it will be shown, V4 was the sole case containing cells from both donor and recipient.

In contrast to the leaflets in the VR group, those from HTx patients were histologically normal (Fig. 1d). With regard to the cellular component, only a slight decrease in the number of fibroblasts, at the free edge of the leaflets was found (Fig. 1e). The

Table 1. Clinical summary for donors and recipients

Case	Implant Age		Sex		Blood Group		Cold ischemic time (h)	Cryopreservatio (d)	Follow-up (mo)
	D	R	D	R	D	R			
V1	23	72	m	m	A−	A+	48	51	2
V2	21	62	m	f	A+	A+	24	19	6
V3	40	64	m	m	A+	A+	24	30	2
V4	30	44	m	f	A+	A+	48	307	12
V5	46	17	m	m	A+	O+	624	0	73
V6	na	51	na	f	na	A+	na	0	239
V7	na	31	na	m	na	A+	na	0	230
T1	29	53	m	m	O−	O+	2.0	–	1
T2	28	53	m	m	A+	A+	2.2	–	2
T3	19	42	f	m	A−	A+	2.8	–	5
T4	25	60	m	m	A+	A−	1.5	–	46
T5	23	61	m	m	O−	O+	2.0	–	60
A1		64		f		A+	0.1	–	9

All patients in the HTx group received immunosuppression therapy with cyclosporine, azothioprine and prednisone. *V*, VR group; *T*, HTx group; *A*, Autograft; *Age*, Implant age in years; *D*, Donor; *R*, Recipient; *m*, male; *f*, female; *IT*, Ischemic time; *na*, not available (Reproduced with permission by the publisher from refs. 32 and 33.)

endothelium was focally maintained and none of the leaflets revealed inflammatory infiltrations. The AG valve showed conserved structure and cellularity including endothelium, without leukocyte infiltration (Fig. 1f).

The VR group was genetically assessed with markers D5S82, D5S299 and MCC. Detailed results, including the amplification area for each sized amplimer, for cases V4 through V7, using marker D5S299, are shown in Table 2. Genetic profiles indicated donor cells in three valves after 1, 6 and 19 years of implantation (V4, V5, V7). The presence of donor cells in V5 was inferred from the results obtained with marker D5S299, where the size of the amplimer obtained from the leaflets (158) differed from those of the recipient's control DNA (178 and 184 base pair). The cells in V4, V5 and V7 were most likely fibroblasts. However, they were so scarce that they could not be identified histologically. The differences in identification of fibroblast by the two techniques can be explained by the fact that PCR amplification is more sensitive and that larger fragments are used for DNA extraction. Amplification yielding three sized amplimers, and thus conclusive results of mixed cell origin was found only in case V4. However, the histological finding of T-cells in this case raises the question as to whether the cells of recipient origin included fibroblasts as well.

For the remaining cases, the results were not conclusive, since only one or two sized amplimers were found and in one case (V3), control DNA was not available.

For the HTx group, three different sized amplimers were obtained in three samples (T1, T3, and T5), indicating the presence of two cell populations. In case T1 a 10 to 50 fold difference in the area of one amplimer as compared to the other suggested that one of the populations was homozygous and the other heterozygous (26). A summary of histological and genetic results is shown in Table 3.

From the results presented, it can be concluded that the leaflet's cellularity of heart transplanted patients was far better than that of valve replacement patients. Since the former were subjected to immunosuppressive treatment but not the latter, it is

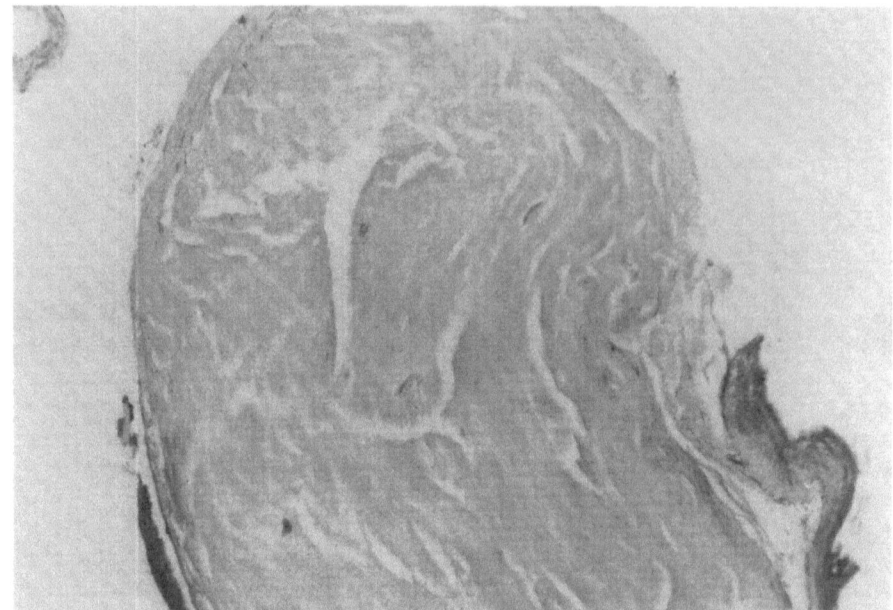

(a)

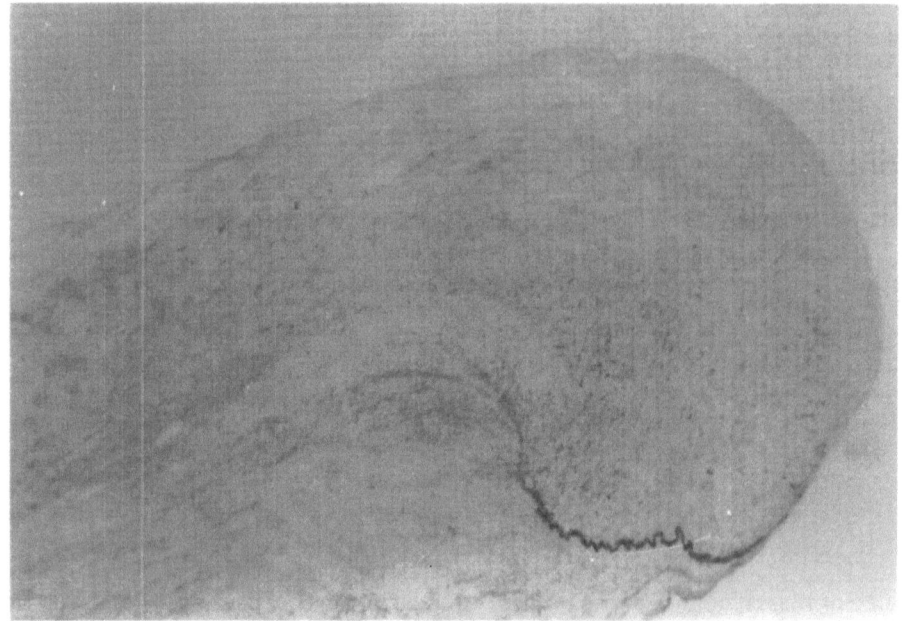

(b)

Fig. 1. (a) and (b)

tempting to conclude that, in the VR patients, cell destruction was mediated by the immune response. However, the possibility that the procedures employed in the preparation of the valves had a long-term effect on the extracellular matrix which led to loss of the appropriate conditions for cell adhesion and homing could not be excluded.

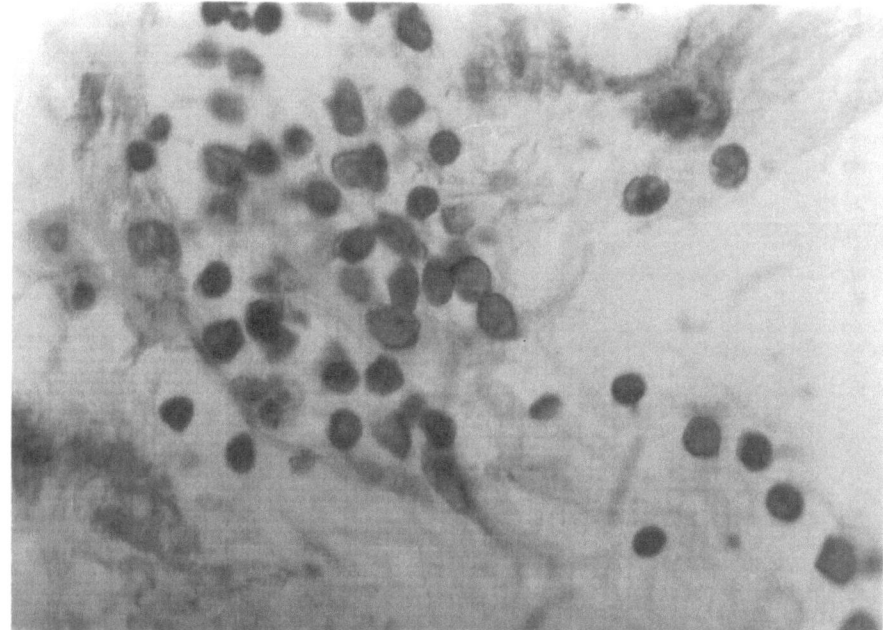

(c)

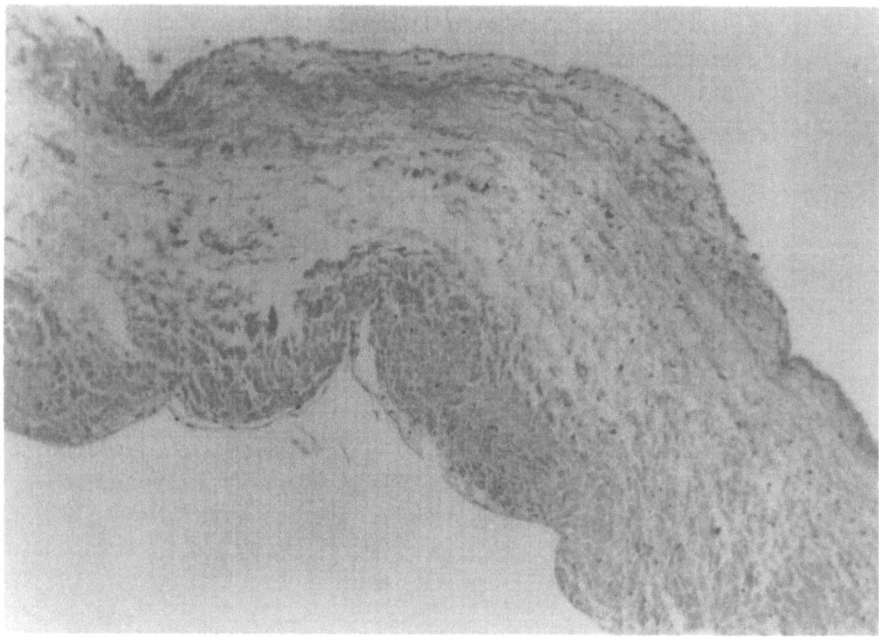

(d)

Fig. 1. a) V4 stained with elastic van Gieson and hematoxylin-eosin (Mag. ×100) showing hyalinization of the connective tissue and absence of fibroblasts and endothelial cells; b) V4 stained with
elastic van Gieson and hematoxylin-eosin (Mag. ×100) showing lymphocytes; c) Peroxidase staining
of T-cells for case V4 using anti-CD45RO Mab (Mag. ×1000); d) T5 stained with elastic van Gieson
and hematoxylin-eosin (Mag. ×100) showing normal histological results; e) T5 stained with elastic

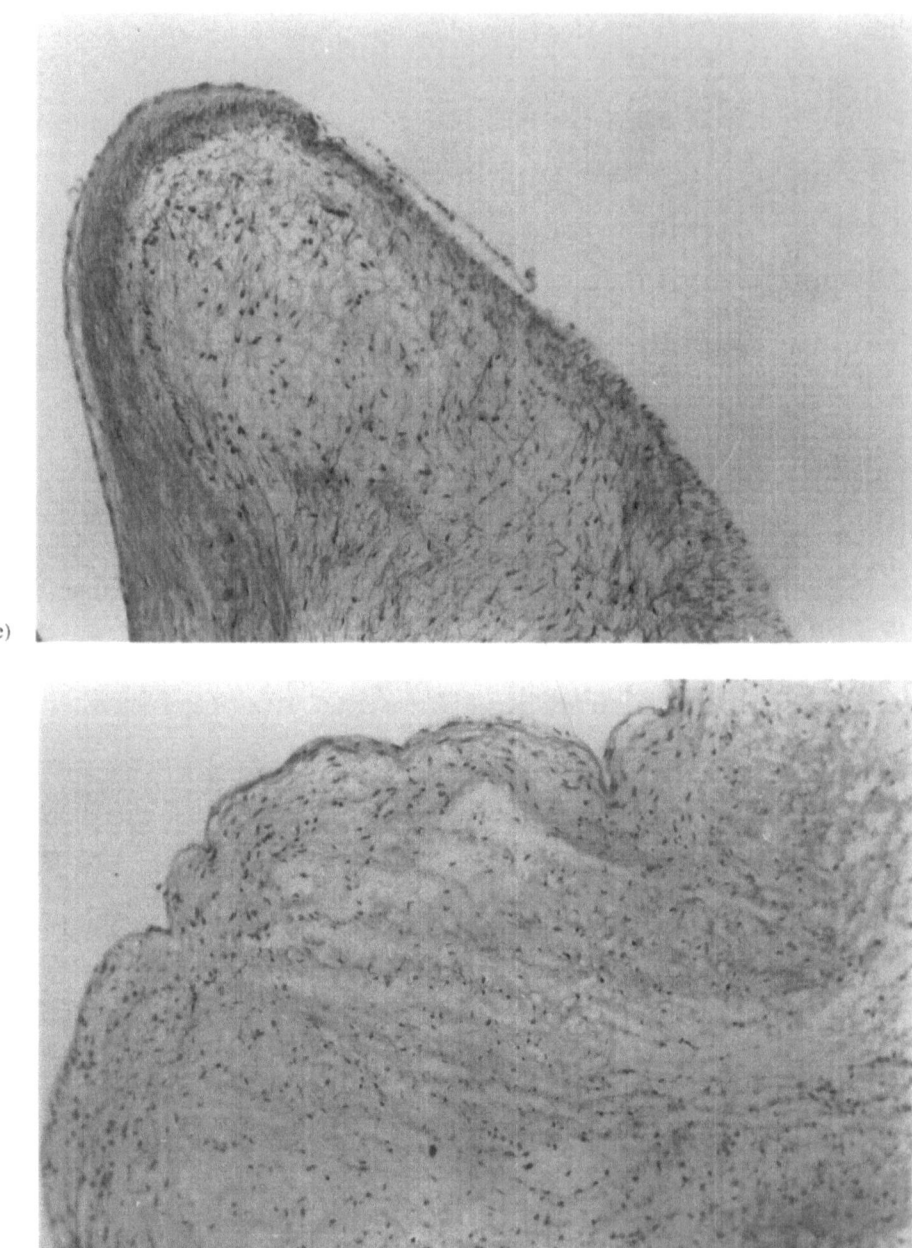

(e)

(f)

van Gieson and hematoxylin-eosin (Mag. ×100) showing a slight decrease in the number of fibroblasts at the free edge and maintained elastic fibers; f) A1 stained with elastic van Gieson and hematoxylin-eosin (Mag. ×100) showing conserved structure and cellularity, including endothelium, without leukocyte infiltration. (Reproduced with permission by the publisher from ref. 33.)

Table 2. VR group genetic results with marker D5S299 indicating PCR amplification area for each size amplimer

Fragment	Amplimer size				
	158	160	178	182	184
V4 A		1979		770	1873
V4 B		13641		3591	6949
V5 A	na				
V5 B	1785				
V5 CONTROL			59879		63170
V6 A			1199		848
V6 CONTROL			36648		29734
V7 A	4551				
V7 C	2086				
V7 CONTROL	11837		6061		

na, no amplification. (Reproduced with permission by the publisher from refs. 32 and 33.)

Immune-mediated mechanism of cryopreserved vascular allograft degeneration

To assess the role of procurement and cryopreservation on the degeneration phenomena, an experimental model was designed in which the behavior of cryopreserved autografts (C-auto) and allografts (C-allo), implanted in the same animal, was compared. Fresh autografts (F-auto) were used to analyze whether denervation and devascularization were relevant elements on the degenerative process (Neves et al. in preparation). Thus, C-allo were implanted in the descending thoracic aorta of 15 sheep. The excised aortic segment was then subject to the same cryopreservation process as used for treatment of the allografts. One to 8 weeks later, the C-auto was implanted, 1 to 2 cm below the C-allo. At this time, the intermediate segment of the native aorta was dissected, thus serving as an F-auto. Animals were sacrificed at different intervals (2 weeks, 1, 3, 6, 12 and 24 months) and the implanted segments harvested together with a portion of the native aorta. Histological and immunohistochemical analysis as well as cell viability assessment was then performed on each of the explanted segments. Similar studies were also conducted on fragments of the C-auto and C-allo, collected before implantation.

With the exception of a partial loss of endothelial cells, prior to implantation, cryopreserved specimens had conserved histology and cell viability. Explanted C-allo, however, showed profound histological changes that affected all strata, as well as decline in cell viability. After an initial period of non-specific inflammatory reaction, which, in most cases, subsided after 1 month, progressive neuronal and smooth muscle degeneration was observed, leading in later stages to the disappearance of perivascular nerves, fibrosis hyalinization and calcification. Most likely due to this process, one C-allo ruptured after 17 months. Lymphocyte infiltrates were found up to 12 months after implantation. Endothelial cells were absent in all cases (Fig. 2a). In contrast, reendothelization occurred in the C-auto (Fig. 2b). After an initial inflammatory

Table 3. Summary of histological and genetic results for the explanted allograft valves.

Case	Fibroblast location free edge	Fibroblast location base	Endoth.	Leuk.	Donor cells	Recp. cells	Number of amplimers D5S82 F	D5S82 C	D5S299 F	D5S299 C	MCC F	MCC C	5S346 F	5S346 C
V1	+	+	no	P	?	?	2	2	0	0	2	2	nd	nd
V2	+	+	no	PT	?	?	1	1	0	0	1	1	nd	nd
V3	0	+	no	P	?	?	1	nc	1	nc	1	nc	nd	nd
V4	0	0	no	T	yes	yes	2	nc	3	nc	3	nc	nd	nd
V5	0	0	no	no	yes	no	1	2	1	2	1	1	nd	nd
V6	0	0	no	T	?	?	2	2	2	2	2	2	nd	nd
V7	0	0	no	no	yes	no	2	1	1	2	1	1	nd	nd
T1	+++	++	yes	no	yes	yes	3	2	2	2	2	2	nd	2
T2	+++	++	yes	no	yes	no	nd	nd	nd	nd	2	2	1	2
T3	+++	++	yes	no	yes	yes	nd	nd	nd	nd	2	nd	3	0
T4	+++	++	yes	no	yes	no	1	2	nd	nd	nd	nd	nd	nd
T5	+++	++	yes	no	yes	yes	nd	nd	3	1	nd	nd	2	2
A1	+++	+++	yes	no	yes	yes								

Endoth., endothelium; Leuk., leukocytes; Recp., recipient; F, fragment; C, control; P, PMN; T, T-cells; nc, no control; nd, not done. Fibroblast scale: 0, acellular; +, few; ++, moderate; +++, normal. (Reproduced with permission by the publisher from refs. 32 and 33.)

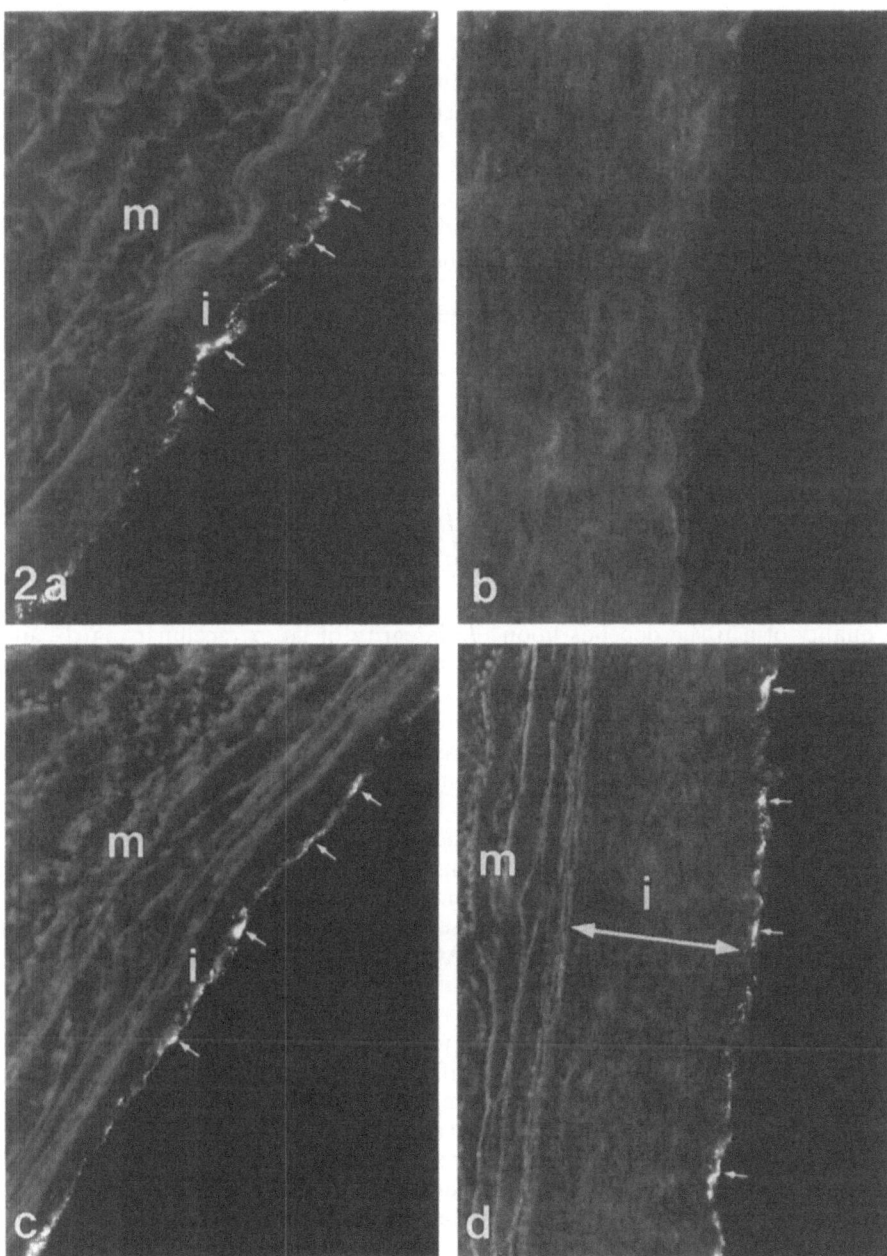

Fig. 2. Cryostat section of a sheep descending thoracic aorta, immunofluorescently stained for the general endothelial marker "von Willebrand factor" (VWF). In native aorta (a), fresh autograft (c) and cryopreserved autograft (d) endothelial cells display strong VWF immunoreactivity (arrows). In the cryopreserved allograft (b), however, no VWF-immunoreactive endothelial cells are observed. Notice the thick intima (i, double headed arrow) of the cryopreserved autograft (d). m, media. Magnification ×280.

reaction, as in all other segments, C-auto showed immunohistochemical signs of nerve degeneration with loss of Schwann cells and axons. After 1 month, however, progressive re-enervation occurred with re-establishment of the normal perivascular innervation pattern being achieved 6 months after surgery. Histologically, a single alteration was patent in these explants, consisting of an intimal thickening. Cell viability was similar to that of native aorta. Histological and immunohistochemical findings with regard to the FA were similar to those of the C-auto, with the exception of the thickening of the intima and the loss of endothelium, which did not occur (Fig. 2c), and were always comparable to those of native aorta (Fig. 2d and Neves et al. in preparation).

In conclusion, it appears that the immunological reaction, rather than the cryopreservation process, was responsible for the degenerative process that occurs in cryopreserved allografts.

Concluding remarks

The quality of a tissue depends upon the integrity of its extracellular matrix and, consequently, of the viability of the cells that are responsible for the continuous degradation and synthesis of its components, the fibroblasts. A well-balanced renewal of the matrix is of particular importance in tissues, such as the heart valves, which are subjected to continuous and vigorous forces. Based on this concept, we have initiated studies aiming at defining the factors that might affect cell survival, in allograft heart valve replacement.

From the three mechanisms that we considered as possible mediators of cell and/or ECM damage, namely, the immune response triggered by the allogeneic tissue, the procurement/cryopreservation processes and the valve hemodynamics disturbance caused by the surgical procedure, the latter could be excluded since, as expected from the excellent long-term viability found for AG valves (36–38), the explanted autograft showed preserved connective tissue and maintained cellularity. In contrast, both the results obtained from the explanted human valves and the experimental work in sheep enforces the argument of the importance of the immune response on the degeneration process. Thus, histologically, three major differences were found between the VR and the HTx groups, the most striking being the amount of fibroblasts, which was nearly normal in the HTx group, but severely reduced in the VR group. Furthermore, the few valves in which fibroblasts were found had been implanted, for only 2 to 6 months (V1, V2 and V3). The two other relevant differences included the preservation of the endothelium in the HTx group but not in the VR, and the hyalinization of the matrix that was observed only in the VR group, sometimes with focal calcification.

Genetic profiles showed dual cell origin in three (60%) cases in the HTx group, while in the VR group cells from both donor and recipient were found only in one (14%) case. Furthermore, the presence of a lymphocyte infiltrate identified by immunohistochemistry as T-cells, in this single case, raised the question as to whether the cells of recipient origin were both lymphocytes and fibroblasts or the former only.

From the results obtained it could, thus, be concluded that the leaflet's cellularity of the HTx and AG patients was superior to that of the VR patients and that, by a mechanism(s) yet to be clarified, homing of fibroblasts occurred in the HTx group but not in the VR.

Generally, the presence of T-cells in a non-lymphoid organ indicates that an immune response is taking place. Although the differences between the two groups were consistent with the occurrence of an immune response in the VR group that was prevented or abrogated by immunosuppressive therapy administered to the HTx group, the presence of T-cells in three of the VR cases strongly suggests that an additional factor could be involved in these cases. Indeed, it is of interest to note that in cases V2 and V4, the donor was male and the recipient female. This finding suggests that the immune response, in these patients, was further potentiated by the reactivity against the male histocompatibility antigen H-Y (40). Unfortunately, we have not been able to obtain information regarding the donor in case V6. Because of the potential relevance of this type of reactivity, we are presently analyzing, experimentally, the contribution of such incompatibility on the viability of vascular allografts.

By creating conditions in which autologous tissue was treated in the same way as the allogeneic, as was the case in the experimental work with the aortic grafts performed in sheep, the possibility could be excluded that preparation procedures, including ischemic time, antibiotic treatment and cryopreservation, had a long-term effect on the extracellular matrix, leading to deterioration of cell adhesion and homing conditions. Of particular interest were the findings that re-enervation, re-endothelization and regeneration of vasa vasorum occurred both on the cryopreserved autograft and the fresh autograft but not in the cryopreserved allograft (Neves et al., J Thorac Cardiovasc Surg, in press). The lack of vascular and perivascular nerve regeneration in the latter case was not related to the initial degeneration, for this occurred also in the autografts. Most likely, the immune response induced by the allogeneic tissue either led to destruction of progenitor cells or prevented the release of angiogenic and nerve growth factors required for the regeneration process.

The single alteration (thickening of the intima) found in the cryopreserved autologous graft did not occur in the fresh autologous fragment. It is, therefore, tempting to hypothesize that this is the sole transformation induced by cryopreservation. The relevance of this finding, not only for valve allografts but also for the understanding of the mechanism(s) of arteriosclerosis, prompts further research focused on the alterations induced on the ECM by the cryopreservation process and on alternative methods for preserving valves.

The results from our studies led us to believe that the allografts' viability might be improved if the leaflets were depleted of the donor's cellular components, provided the ECM integrity is maintained. Reendothelization with cells of recipient's origin, as suggested by Loose et al. (22) might, in addition to preventing thomboembolic phenomena, provide a source of fibroblasts, since endothelial cells have been shown to retain the capacity to switch on the mesenchymal gene regulatory program and transform into fibroblasts, when exposed to the appropriate matrix (13).

References

1. Angell JD, Cristopher BS, Hawtrey O (1976) Fresh viable human heart valve bank: Sterilisation sterility testing and cryogenic preservation. Transplant Proc 8 (Suppl 1): 139
2. Angell WW, Oury JH, Lamberti JJ, Koziol J (1989) Durability of the viable aortic allograft. J Thorac Cardiovasc Surg 98: 48–56
3. Angell WW, Ibsen AB, Stenson EB, Shumway ME (1968) Fresh aortic homografts for multiple valve replacement. J Thorac Surg 56: 323–28
4. Barratt-Boyes BG (1971) Longterm follow-up of aortic valve grafts. Br Heart J 33(Suppl): 60–65

5. Barratt-Boyes BG (1964) Homograft aortic valve replacement in aortic incompetence and stenosis. Thorax 19: 131–50
6. Binet JP, Carpentier A, Langlois J (1965) Heterologous aortic valve transplantation. Lancet 2: 1275
7. Björk VO, Olin C (1970) A hydrodynamic evaluation of the new tilting disc valve for mitral replacement. Scand J Thorac Cardiovasc Surg 4: 37–41
8. Buch WS, Kosek JC, Angell WW (1971) The role of rejection and mechanical trauma in valve graft viability. J Thorac Cardiovasc Surg 62: 696–706
9. Dunn JM (1991) Porcine valve durability in children. Ann Thorac Surg 32: 357–68
10. Duran CG, Gunning AJ (1962) A method of placing a total homologous aortic valve in the subcoronary position. Lancet 2: 488–89
11. El Khatib H, Lupinetti F (1990) Antigenicity of fresh and cryopreserved rat valve allografts. Transplantation 49: 765–67
12. Gonzalez-Lavin L, Bianchi J, Graf D, Amini S, Gordon CI (1988) Degenerative changes in fresh aortic root homografts in a canine model: evidence of an immunologic influence. Transplant Proc 20(Suppl): 815
13. Greenburg G, Hay ED (1982) Endothelia suspended in collagen gels can lose polarity and express characteristics of migrating mesenchymal cells. J Cell Biol 95: 333–39
14. Grunkemeier GL, Bodnar E (1995) Comparative assessment of bioprosthesis durability in aortic position. J Heart Valve Dis 4: 49–55
15. Heslop BF, Wilson SE, Hardy BE (1973) Antigenicity of aortic valve allografts. Ann Surg 177: 301–67
16. Hudson REB (1966) Pathology of the human aortic valve homograft. Br Heart J 28: 291–301
17. Kaiser GA, Hancock WD, Lukban SB, Litwak RS (1969) Clinical use of a new design stented xenograft heart valve prosthesis. Surg Forum 20: 137–38
18. Kay JH, Kawashima Y, Kagawa Y (1966) Experimental mitral valve replacement with a new disc valve. Ann Thorac Surg 2: 485–89
19. Kwong K-H, Paton BC, Hill RB (1967) Experimental use of immunosuppression in aortic valve homografts and heterografts. J Thorac Cardiovasc Surg 54: 199–212
20. Lam CR, Aram HH, Munnell ER (1952) An experimental study of aortic valve homografts. Surg Gyn Obst 94: 129–35
21. Longmore DB, Lokey E, Ross DN, Pickiring BN (1966) The preparation of aortic valve homografts. Lancet ii: 463–64
22. Loose R, Schultze-Rhonhof H, Sievers H, Bernhard A (1993) Preparing heart valve allografts for endothelial cell seeding. Transp Proc 25: 3244–46
23. Magilligan DJ, Lewis JW, Tilley B, Peterson E (1985) The porcine bioprosthesis valve. J Thorac Cardiovasc Surg 89: 499–507
24. Malm J, Bowman F (1967) An evaluation of aortic homografts by electron beam energy. J Thorac Cardiovasc Surg 54: 471–75
25. McNally RT, Brockbank KG (1992) Issues surrounding the preservation of viable allograft heart valves. J Med Eng & Tech 16: 34–38
26. Melo JQ, Monteiro C, Neves J, Santos R, Martins A, Ramos S, Calta C, Matoso-Ferreira A, Viana J, Rueff J, Macedo MM (1995) The allograft valve in aortic valve replacement and heart transplant patients – Genetic assessment of the origin of the cells using DNA profiles. J Thorac Cardiovasc Surg 109(2): 218–23
27. Mermet B, Buch WS, Angell WW (1970) Viable heart grafts: Preservation in the frozen state. Surg Forum 21: 156–57
28. Missen GAK, Roberts GI (1979) Calcification and cusp rupture in human aortic valve homografts sterilised by ethylene oxide and freeze-dried. Lancet ii: 962–64
29. Murray G (1956) Homologous aortic valve segment transplant as surgical treatment for aortic and mitral insufficiency. Angiology 7: 446–71
30. Neves J, Monteiro C, Santos R, Martins A, Ramos S, Ramos T, Calta C, Rueff J, Melo JQ (1995) Histological and genetic assessment of explanted allografts valves. Ann Thorac Surg 60: 5141–45
31. O'Brien MF (1967) Heterograft aortic valves for human use. Valve Bank. Techniques of measurements and implantation. J Thorac Cardiovasc Surg 53: 392–97
32. O'Brien MF, Stafford G, Gardner M, Pohlner P, McGiffin D, Johnston N, Brosnan A, Duffy P (1987) The viable cryopreserved allograft aortic valve. J Cardiac Surg 2(suppl): 153–67
33. Rains ATH, Crawford N, Sharp SH, Shrewsbury JFD, Barson GJ (1956) Management of an artery graft bank with special reference to sterilisation by beta-propiolactone. Lancet ii: 830–32

34. Reis RL, Hancock WD, Yarbrough JW, Glancy DL, Morrow AG (1971) The flexible stent. A new concept in the fabrication of tissue heart valve prosthesis. J Thorac Cardivasc Surg 62: 683–89
35. Robicsek F (1994) The application of biological tissues in cardiac surgery. The history of the first two decades. J Heart Valve Dis 3: 613–26
36. Ross DN (1967) Replacement of the aortic and mitral valves with a pulmonary autograft. Lancet 58: 859
37. Ross DN (1988) Pulmonary valve autotransplantation. J Cardiac Surg 3(Suppl): 313–18
38. Ross DN, Jackson M, Davis J (1992) The pulmonary autograft – a permanent aortic valve. Eur J Cardiothorac Surg 6: 113–17
39. Ross DN (1962) Homograft replacement of the aortic valve. Lancet 2: 487
40. Simpson E, Gordon RD (1977) Responsiveness to H-Y antigen, Ir gene complementation and target cell specificity. Immunol Rev 35: 59–75
41. Smith JC (1967) The pathology of human aortic valve homografts. Thorax 22: 114–38
42. Stark J (1987) Do we really correct congenital heart defects? J Thorac Cardiovasc Surg 97: 1–9
43. Starr A, Edwards ML (1961) Mitral replacement: the shield ball valve prosthesis. J Thorac Cardiovasc Surg 42: 673–77
44. Wallace RB, Giuliani ER, Titus LJ (1971) Use of aortic valve homografts for aortic valve replacement. Circulation 43: 365–73
45. Williams DB, Danielson GK, McGoon DC, Danielson GK, McGoon DC, Puga F, Mair DD, Edwards DW (1982) Porcine heterograft valve replacement in children. J Thorac Cardiovasc Surg 84: 446–50
46. Yankah AC, Wottge HU, Müller-Hermelink HK, Feller AC, Lange P, Wessel U, Drey H, Bernhard A, Müller-Ruchholtz W (1987) Transplantation of aortic and pulmonary allografts, enhanced viability of endothelial cells by cryopreservation, importance of cryopreservation. J Cardiac Surg 2(Suppl): 209–20
47. Yankah AC, Wottge HU, Müller-Ruchholtz W (1988) Antigenicity and fate of cellular components of heart valve allografts: In: Yankah AC, Hetzer R, Yacoub Mh, eds. Cardiac Valve Allografts 1962–1987. Current concepts on the use of aortic and pulmonary allografts for heart valve substitutes. Darmstadt: Steinkopff Verlag, 77–78
48. Yankah AC, Wottge HU, Muller-Ruchholtz W (1988) Prognostic importance of viability and a study of a second set allograft valve: an experimental study. J Cardiac Surg 3: 263–70
49. Zhao X, Green M, Frazer IH, Hogan P, O'Brien MF (1994) Donor-specific immune response after aortic valve allograft in rat. Ann Thorac Surg 57: 1158–63

Author's address:
Prof. J. Q. Melo, MD, PhD
Hospital de Santa Cruz
Department of Cardiothoracic Surgery
Avenida Professor Reinaldo dos Santos
Carnaxide 2795 LINDA-A-VELHA
PORTUGAL

Allograft conduit wall calcification in a model of chronic arterial graft rejection

A. C. Yankah, H-U. Wottge*

German Heart Institute Berlin, Institute of Immunology,
University of Kiel*, Germany

Introduction

Early allograft vascular wall degeneration has emerged as a major important complication in young patients.

It develops in 30% of young patients with allograft conduits in the pulmonary circulation and it is seen as early as 4 months after implantation by x-ray as focal or diffused calcification without traces of calcification in the valve cusps (5, 15). Proliferation and migration of smooth muscle cells and deposition of extra cellular matrix accounts for much of the vascular intimal hyperplasia and calcific stenosis. Cytokine or cytokine-receptor expression and production of growth factors and T-cell activation following an immune response might be causes for fibro-proliferative processes and calcification in allograft vascular wall (9, 17). This mechanism by which rejection may lead to calcification of the vascular conduit is poorly understood. A method of arresting the fibroproliferative process in allograft conduits is therefore urgently needed for improving its durability. For this purpose, we evaluated explants of aortic allograft valved conduits implanted heterotopically into the infrarenal aorta of inbred rats to explain the pathogenesis and the mechanism of allograft vasculopathy.

Materials and method

Animal model: Male and female inbred CAP (RT1^c) rat strains weighing 250–350 g served as valved couduit and skin donors. LEW rat strains weighing 300–400 g were exclusively used as recipients. They were housed in wire bottom cages with controlled light/dark cycles and allowed free access to water and rat chow. Experimental group: Experimental rat models were established from a combination of: CAP > LEW (strongly allogenic, RT1- and non-RT1-incompatible) rat strains. The allovital (fresh) and viable (antibiotic treated) valved conduits were retrieved from CAP rats. In our previous studies on immunological aspects of allograft valve transplantation more than two control groups were used (27, 29). The two control groups selected for this study were: LEW > LEW, syngeneic and AS > LEW, weakly allogeneic (RT1-compatible and non-RT1-ncompatible combinations. Only the strongly allogeneic strains were used in this study.

Donor heart explantation, harvesting and preparation of valved conduits: Under ether anesthesia the donor heart was exposed via median sternotomy and explanted with a 4–5 mm segment of ascending aorta. The donor heart was placed in a container with cold (4 °C) Ringer solution to avoid warm ischemia. 4–5 mm long aortic root valved conduits with a segment of ascending aorta were dissected at operation day for immediate use as fresh, allovital conduits. The allovital valves were composed of living cellular components viz. endothelial cells and fibroblasts.

Viable Allografts: the dissected valved conduits were treated with antibiotic solution in nutrient medium (RPMI 1640, Roswell Park Memorial Institute) with fetal calf serum (20%) for 7 days after which the endothelial cells were identified to be non-viable and being detached from the valve surfaces as well as the inner surface of the conduits when the conduits were gently rinsed in the nutrient medium for a few minutes. The antibiotic treated valved conduits are then composed of viable fibroblasts (28, 30).

Heterotopic implantation of valved allograft conduit into the infrarenal aorta: Under ether anesthesia, median laparatomy was performed and the infrarenal abdominal aorta was exposed. The prepared valved allograft conduits of aortic root segments were trimmed of excess myocardium, the two coronary arterial segments were ligated. The conduits were implanted into the infrarenal aorta by interposition with 8-0 Prolene sutures between two special bulldog clamps beginning with the posteriolateral and then the anterior proximal end-to-end anastomosis. The ventricular side of the aortic valve was placed against the antegrade blood stream and the valve cusps were made incompetent by sutures at the base of the cusps when the proximal anastomosis was being performed. After the distal anastomosis the aortic clamps were released for antegrade blood flow. The patency of the anastomoses was controlled by digital palpation. The laparatomy wound was closed and dressed with soft wire gauze and the allograft recipients were taken into their cages (28, 29).

Explantation of the valved allograft conduits: The allografts were explanted from the hosts humanely under anesthesia on days 20, 30, 50, 100 after heterotopic implant for Immunofluorescence (IF) study and scanning electron microscopy (SEM).

Immunofluorescence staining technique: Identification of antibodies against graft endothelial cells using direct immunofluorescence technique: Four micro thick cryostat sections mounted on carbon stubs at −20 °C from freeze-dried specimens were incubated with 50 microliter fluorescein isothiocynate (FITC) conjugated anti-rat immunoglobulin G (IgG) and placed in a dark refrigerator for 30 min, washed two times in phosphate-buffered saline solution (pH 7.4), air-dried and with a drop of buffered glycerin and with a cover slip viewed under Zeiss microscope. Antigenicity of allografts was determined by indirect immunofluorescence technique using first mouse monoclonal antibodies (0X6, Medac, Hamburg, Germany) directed at class II rat antigens and then fluorescein isothiocynate (FITC) conjugated anti-rat immune globulin G (IgG) as described above. Immunogenicity of the graft, i.e., the capability to elicit immune response was demonstrated by identifying production of anti-graft antibodies immune globulin G (IgG) by direct immunofluorescence (IF) with FITC-conjugated anti-rat monoclonal antibodies (Camon, Wiesbaden, Germany). Immunoperoxidase staining techniques were used (22). Anti-Ulex europaeus I lectin (anti-UEA I, Ey-Laboratories, San Mateo, CA, USA) was used for identifying endothelial cells (8). Since smooth muscle cells showed reactivities with anti-UEA I lectin, we used more specific v. Willebrand antibodies anti-Factor VIII (Camon, Wiesbaden, Germany) to confirm the presence of endothelial cells (2, 29). In this way, we could also differentiate the endothelial cells from the smooth muscle cells in the vascular wall of the conduits. For the evaluation of a state of presensitization of the host induced by the first-set valved allograft conduit, a second-set skin grafting (skin graft harvested from the same valved conduit donor strain) was performed 3 weeks after heterotopic transplantation of a valved allograft conduits. Presensitization of the recipient was confirmed by accelerated rejection times of the skin graft. The results have been previously reported (27, 29, 30). Identification of cell origin from LEW and CAP rat strains: Preparation of alloantisera. LEW, CAP rats received from each other two separate abdominal skin grafts at 10 days interval for four successive times CAP > LEW, LEW > CAP. After the fourth skin grafting each rat received intraperitoneal (ip) innoculation of 5×10^7 spleen cells every week for four successive times. A week after the fourth ip innoculation the rats were exsanguinated and the anti-CAP and anti-LEW sera were retrieved and cryopreserved for the experimental studies. The anti-sera were tested with BN (RTI^n) strains to exclude cross reactions. The anti-sera were used to differentiate cells from the host and donor grafts.

Light microscopy: Tissue was postfixed in 10% buffered formalin for 24 h and processed for paraffin wax embedding (Lancer, Ireland). Four micro thick sections were cut on a Leitz base sledge microtome and stained with Haematoxylin and Eosin and elastic tissue van Gieson. For calcium phosphates von Kossa staining was used and counterstained with Eosin. Scanning electron microscopy (SEM): Specimens were postfixed in a 4% Glutaraldehyde solution in 0.05 molar sodium cacodylate buffer (pH 7.4) for 18 h. The specimens were dehydrated through graded alcohol (10–90%, cleared in frigen and flat embedded on aluminum carrier stub sprayed with gold particles and viewed under scanning electron microscope (SEM S4-10, Sterosan Cambridge).

Results

Allovital (fresh) aortic conduits

Donor-specific endothelial cells were regularly organized on day 20 but became disorganized on day 30 showing partly loosened bindings and sloughing. Neointima was visible on day 50 with calcific deposits. In the media and adventitia there was a moderate infiltration of mononuclear cells which were mostly macrophages and a few T-lymphocytes on day 20 (Fig. 1). On day 30 the cellular infiltrates were diminishing, leaving a minority of macrophages and smooth muscle cells. The anti-UEA I demonstrated the presence of endothelial cells and presumably medial smooth muscle cells which are presumably of donor origin on day 30 (Fig. 2). Medial cellular infiltrates disappeared on day 50, while the elastic fibers and the collagens became moderately disorganized showing calcific degeneration (Fig. 3). A few adventitial infiltrates were still present while neocapillaries were formed (Fig. 3b). Graft calcific degeneration with clefts and large gaps between the collagen bundles became prominent on day 100. Expression of class II antigens with 0X6 (directed at RT1-Class II-Antigens) in the intima and the neointima, and deposition of IgG around the smooth muscle cells and in the areas of smooth muscle cell necrosis in the media was demonstrated at 50 and 100 days after operation (Fig. 2a, 2b) was an evidence of recipient anti-graft antibody response against the graft endothelial cells and medial structures.

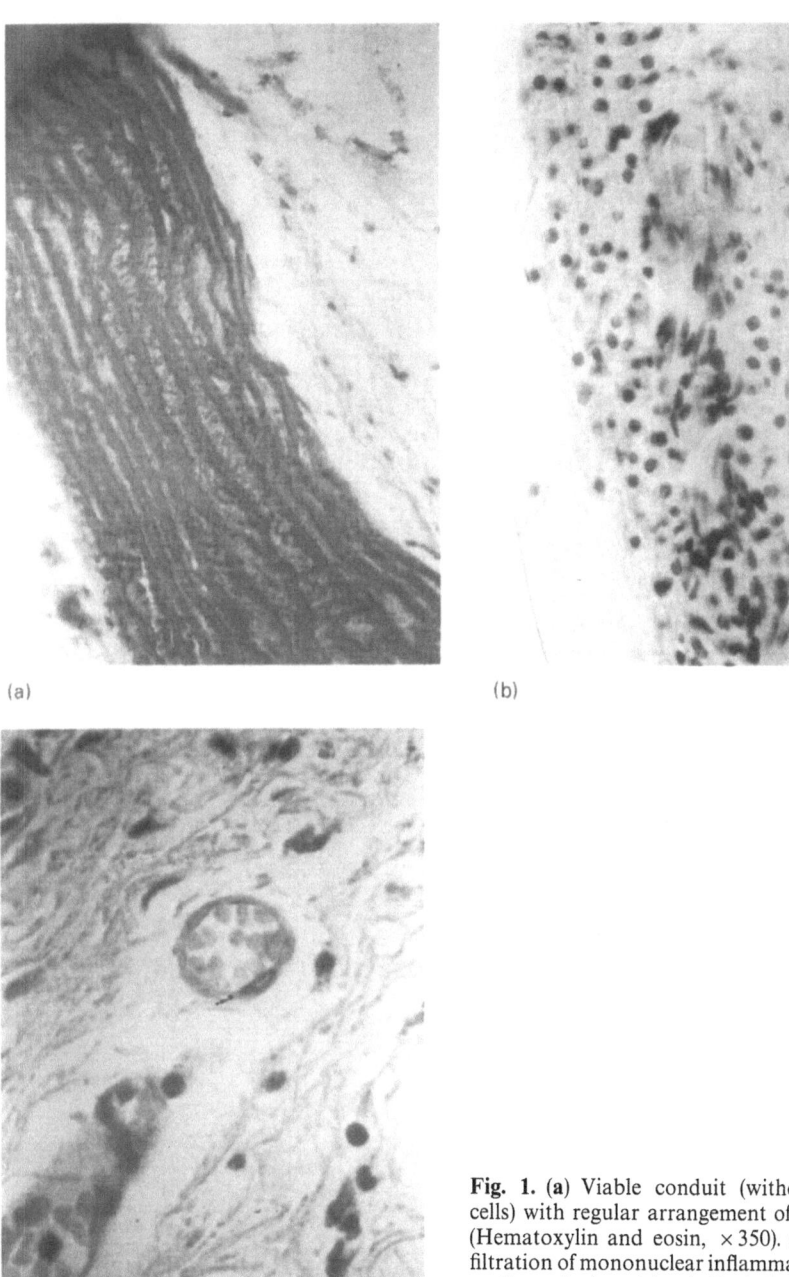

(a)

(b)

(c)

Fig. 1. (a) Viable conduit (without endothelial cells) with regular arrangement of collagen fibers (Hematoxylin and eosin, × 350). (b) Massive infiltration of mononuclear inflammatory cells in the media and adventitia of allovital vascular conduit on days 20 and 30 (Giemsa, × 400). (c) Formation of neocapillaries in the adventitial tissue on day 50 in viable vascular conduit (Giemsa, × 700).

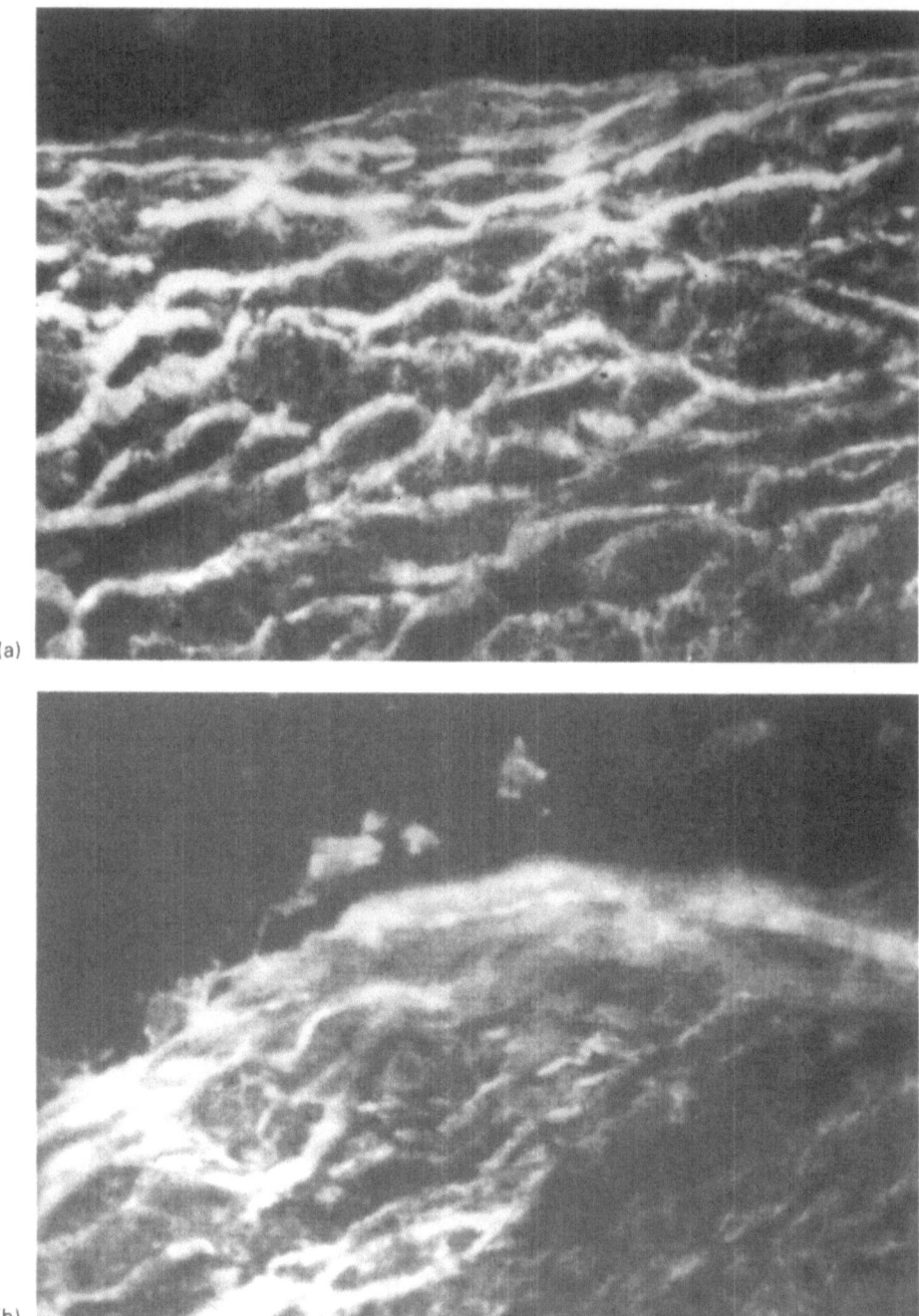

Fig. 2. (**a**) Collagen breaks and clefts with large gaps between the collagen bundles and deposits of IgG in the media and neointima in the vascular wall of an allovital conduit on day 50 (indirect immunofluorescence, × 700). (**b**) Increased collagen and elastic fibers which are disorderly organized on day 100 and deposition of IgG in media and neointima of allovital vascular conduit presumably elastin gene expression as well (indirect immunofluorescence, × 700).

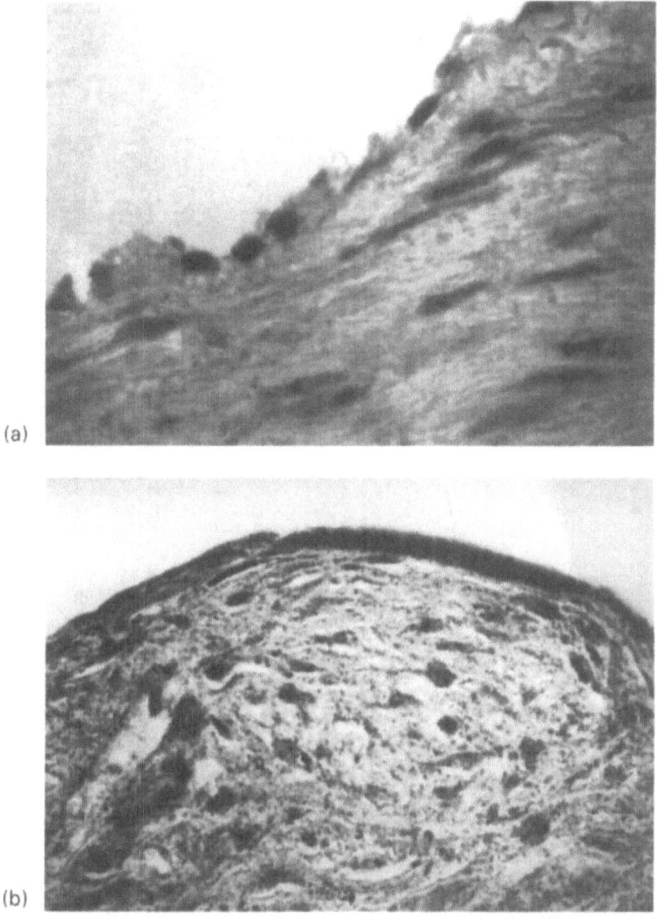

Fig. 3. (a) Disappearance of mononuclear cell infiltrates. Donor endothelial and migrated smooth cells on the intima. Demonstration of residual nests of smooth muscle cells as remnants of the original allovital conduit cells on day 30 using anti-Ulex europaeus I lectin antibodies (indirect immuno-peroxidase staining, × 700). **(b)** Neointimal and medial calcification of allovital conduit on day 50. Scattered foci of macrophages and loss of normal population of smooth muscle cells in the media (v. Kossa and eosin, × 700).

Viable aortic conduits

The media of the vascular wall appeared normal on day 20. A thin layer of neointima and focal infiltration of mononuclear cells consisting of macrophages and T-lympho-cytes were seen in the media and adventitia on day 30 which disappeared on day 50. The smooth muscle cells were still present while the collagen and elastic fibers were preserved. On day 50 host cells and some migrated smooth muscle cells were found in the neointima. Endothelial cells were not identified by immune peroxidase staining using anti-Ulex europaeus 1 lectin and anti-factor VIII (2, 8, 16, 22). On day 100 the elastic and collagen fibers were still preserved. IgG deposits were identified by direct IF in the neointima (Fig. 4b) and in the media around the smooth muscle cells as well as in the areas of necrosis on day 30 through day 100. The second-set skin graft

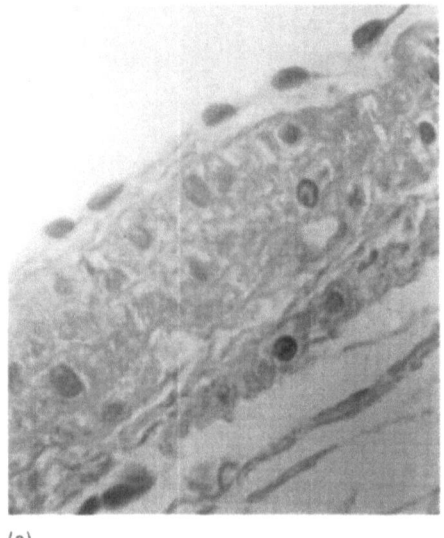
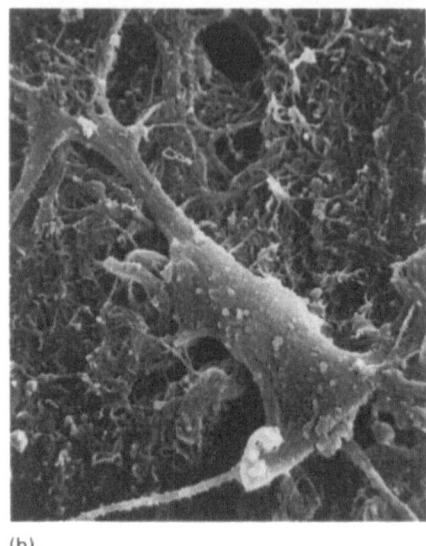

(a)   (b)

Fig. 4. (a) Demonstration of endothelial cells of vascular allograft conduit (indirect immun-peroxidase staining with anti-Ulex europaeus I lectin, × 700). (b) Formation of neointima in a viable allograft conduit with a host cell on day 100 (SEM, × 5000).

challenge however was rejected earlier than the control graft indicating a state of presensitization.

Discussion

The objective of allograft conduit procurement and processing should be the preservation of viability which ensures the structural integrity of the conduit at implantation. In animal experimental model as well as in young patients aortic allografts present a greater challenge to the recipient than do allograft veins (23). We studied the fibroproliferative processes in allograft aortic conduits to establish its importance and future role in clinical allograft valve transplantation. This process is seen in young patients with clinical allograft implants (4, 5, 12, 15, 21) and is reproducible in a rat heterotopic model.

The results of the study indicate that fresh conduits were consistently more viable than the antibiotic treated conduits. The advantages of the allovital conduits appear to be balanced by the disadvantage of early intimal thickening, medial fibrosis and retraction. Besides hypertension or mechanical injury fibroproliferative process in intima and media of allograft conduits is caused by rejection. Immune response initiates release of cytokines and growth factors which induce proliferation and migration of fibroblasts and smooth muscle cells to the intima and adventitia (9, 17). Subsequently, production and deposition of antigraft antibodies (IgG) in the media and neointima occur which were recognized by direct immunofluorescence. Among the neointimal cells are smooth muscle cells which have migrated from the media of the conduit wall during the arterial graft rejection (9). The fibroproliferative process in the allograft conduit leads to intimal hyperplasia and medial, adventitial fibrosis and thickening and finally to luminal narrowing, stenosis and calcification.

Neointimal hyperplasia and increased production of collagens and elastin in response to humoral immune reaction is a structural behavior of allograft conduits to resist dilatational degradation. In strong allogeneic strain grafts dilational aneurysm of vascular conduits were common and occurred in most cases before neointimal hyperplasia and calcification (24). These findings suggest that conduit dilatation and rejection play a significant role in the pathogenesis of structural deterioration of allograft vascular wall. This is supported by the findings in the isografts in which fibrocalcification did not develop (9, 20, 24). Formation of neocapillaries in the adventitia and around the conduit presented ongoing chronic rejection which was a risk factor for subsequent development of medial fibrosis and calcification. Loss of vasa vasorum of the adventitial tissue in arterial allografts could cause ischemic damage such as collagen dissections which is associated with a great diffusion barrier to oxygen delivery. As implantation time lengthened, the collagen became increasingly abnormal, with large gaps and clefts between bundles resulting in medial necrosis. One could speculate that in viable conduits if smooth muscle cells in the allograft conduit maintain normal function after implantation the conduit will depend on the original collagenous and elastic framework in the media for their continued function. Re-endothelization of the vascular conduit would maintain the function of the viable structures in the media further.

The endothelium of allovital valve as well as the vascular conduit is the initial source of sensitizing antigen, since it is readily available to the host circulation (3, 13, 17, 24, 26–30). Endothelial injury is the *sine qua non* of rejection of allograft valved conduit (13, 27, 28, 30). This fact explains the continuing loss of endothelium from allograft conduit after implantation which is replaced by neointima. Formation of host endothelial coverage in the viable conduits without chronic rejection provided immune tolerance or a condition for prolonged durability (30). This observation might explain prolonged patency and function of viable valved conduits in patients with histocompatible grafts. This fact emphasizes the need for histocompatible viable grafts for maintaining the viable structures of the allograft conduit. The findings in our present report on the pattern of vascular wall degeneration confirms the sequential structural deterioration and tissue calcification observed in allograft vascular walls and valves in patients (27, 29). Others have shown that the noninflammatory cells involved in the intimal thickening seemed to be smooth muscle cells (9, 18, 19). They demonstrated these cells to be immunostained by anti-alpha-actin, anti-desmin and anti-vimentin monoclonal antibodies. These findings are not consistent with allograft valves in humans although endothelial repopulation has been observed in humans with bioprosthetic porcine valve leaflets (28, 32). It seems that endothelial repopulation of the neointima by the host did not occur in allovital conduits in which accelerated calcification occurred in contrast to viable conduits. These findings have been proved by direct immunofluorescence studies with anti-UEA-1 (16).

In comparison to the results of viable valves the durability of allovital valves was influenced by the endothelial cells present at the time of implantation and by antibodies (IgG) produced against the endothelial cells (6, 11, 13, 27, 29) and structures in the media. Direct immunofluorescence studies and skin graft challenge demonstrated the state of responsiveness of the host to produce antibody against the endothelial surface antigens therefore confirmed the immunogenic potential of aortic allografts (3, 13, 20, 24, 25, 29, 30). The allograft rejection and the sequelae were also confirmed by the earlier appearance of structural deterioration of the endothelium and the media in scanning electron microscopy. The recipients with viable allograft valved conduits demonstrated, in spite of absence of endothelial cells, a state of presensitization. These findings might be associated with presence of elastin in the media and neointima as demonstrated by experimental work by others (19). The search for a pharmacological approach to minimize fibroproliferative process in the graft in view of achieving prolonged graft durability is still a challenge. In our experimental model as well as others it has been shown that CSA suppresses the humoral response against non-Rt1-compatible alloantigens in rats to achieve immune tolerance (7, 14, 20, 30, 31) while the Rt1 and non-Rt1-incompatible grafts in strongly allogeneic strains underwent chronic or subacute rejection under the same dosage of immunosuppression. Subsequently, focal fibroproliferative changes and calcification occurred sequentially in the conduit and in the valves (20, 30). On the other hand, our previous studies on allograft valves and reports from others showed that inflammatory cells were commonly present in viable valves in contrast to allovital valves in which deposition of immunoglobulins, activated compliment (C3C), and T-lymphocytes with CD4 subtypes were demonstrated (1, 16, 20, 21, 30). The histocompatible viable grafts survived longer as the allovital valves while allovital valves from the syngeneic strains (isografts) could survive indefinitely. Laboratory experimental experience showed that optimal therapeutic dosis of initial 10 mg/kg immunosuppressants would arrest or delay rejection process in allovital valves and vascular conduits (20, 30). Under this therapy cellular proliferation was arrested and fibroproliferation with production of abnormal collagens and deposition of IgG and abnormal elastin in the media and neointima could be prevented. A short-course non-toxic dosis of immunosuppressive therapy might therefore be an alternative approach to achieving prolonged graft durability in allovital grafts. In contrast, viable conduits might need anti-inflammatory drugs such as aspirin to prevent infiltration of inflammatory cells, thus minimizing or arresting pathological proliferation of smooth muscle cells.

In conclusion, intimal hyperplasia, medial and adventitial fibrosis ultimately developed into a fibroproliferative graft arteriosclerosis. The process has been attributed to rejection or mechanical trauma (damage to intima and vasa vasorum) during processing of allografts. In order to minimize or prevent this fibroproliferative process in allograft conduits one should aim at preserving the vaso vasorum and eliminate the viable endothelial cells. Elimination of endothelial cells can be achieved by applying in vitro non-toxic medication to inactivate the cells. While postoperative infiltrating inflammatory cells in allograft conduits can be arrested by anti-inflammation drugs such as aspirin, the rejection process in allograft conduit might need systemic treatment of the host with non-toxic immunosuppressants. These approaches might provide improvement in the durability of allograft conduits. Whether in vitro treatment of the allograft conduits with immunosuppressants might also serve this purpose still remains speculative.

Acknowledgement

The authors are grateful to Prof. Dr. W. Müller-Ruchholtz former Director of Institute of Immunology of the University of Kiel, Germany for his initial encouragement and support.

References

1. Angell WW, Oury JH, Lamberti JJ, Koziol J (1989) Durability of the viable allograft. J Thorac Cardiovasc Surg 98: 48–56

2. Burgdorf WHC, Mukai K, Rosai J (1981) Immunohistochemical identification of factor VIII related-antigen in endothelial cells of cutaneous lesions of alleged vascular nature. Am J Clin Pathol 76: 197–200
3. Caforio ALP, Bottazo GF, McKenna WJ (1990) Class II MHC antigens on cardiac endothelium: an early biopsy marker of rejection in the transplanted human heart. Transp Proc 22: 1830
4. Clarke DR, Campbell DN, Hayward AR, Bishop DA (1993) Degeneration of aortic valve allografts in young recipients. J Thorac Cardiovasc Surg 105: 934–42
5. Cleveland DC, Williams WG, Razouk AJ, Trusler GA, Rebeyka IM, Duffy L, Kan Z, Coles JG, Freedom RM (1992) Failure of cryopreserved homograft valved conduits in the pulmonary circulation. Circulation 86: (Suppl. II): II-150–153
6. Gonzalez-Lavin L, Bianchi J, Graf D et al. (1988) Degenerative changes in fresh aortic root homografts in a canine model: evidence of an immunologic influence. Transplant Proc 20 (Suppl. 1) 815
7. Gregory CR, Huie P, Billingham ME, Morris RE (1993) Rapamycin inhibits arterial intimal thickening caused by both alloimmune and mechanical injury. Transplantation 55: 1409–1418
8. Holthöfer H, Virtranen I, Kariniemi AL, Hormia M, Linder E, Miettinen A (1982) Ulex europaeus I lectin as a marker for vascular endothelium in human tissues. Lab Invest 47: 60–66
9. Isik FF, Clowes AW, Gordon D (1994) Elastin expression in a model of acute arterial graft rejection. Transplantation 58: 1246–51
10. Ito T, Strepkowski SM, Kahan BD (1990) Soluble antigen and cyclosporin-induced specific unresponsiveness in rats. Transplantation 49: 422–28
11. Jonas RA, Ziemer G, Britton L et al. (1988) Cryopreserved and fresh antibiotic-sterilized valved aortic homograft conduits in a long-term sheep model. Hemodynamic, angiographic and histological comparison. J Thorac Cardiovasc Surg 96: 746
12. Kirklin JK, Smith D, Novick W, Naftel DC, Kirklin JW, Pacifico AD, Nanda NC, Helmcke FR, Bourge RC (1993) Long-term function of cryopreserved aortic homografts. A ten-year study. J Thorac Cardiovasc Surg 106: 154–66
13. Lupinetti FM, Cobb S, Kioschos HC, Thompson SA, Walters KS, Moore KC (1992) Effect of immunological differences on rat aortic valve allograft calcification. J Cardiac Surg 7: 65–70
14. Meiser BM, Billingham ME, Morris RE (1991) Graft vessel disease: the role of rejection and the effect of rejection and the effect of cyclosporine, FK506 and rapamycin. Lancet 338: 1297
15. Monro JL, Salmon AP, Keeton BR (1993) The outcome of antibiotic sterilised homografts used in the Fontan procedure. Eur J Cardio-thorac Surg 7: 360–364
16. Müller-Hermelink HK, Yankah AC (1988) Immunohistopathology of cardiac valve allograft explants. In: Cardiac valve allografts 1962–1987 (eds. Yankah AC, Hetzer R, Miller DC, Ross DN, Somerville J, Yacoub MH), Steinkopff Verlag, Darmstadt, Springer Verlag, New York 89–94
17. Ohno T, Gordon D, San H et al. (1994) Gene therapy for vascular smooth cell proliferation after arterial injury. Science 265: 781–84
18. Plissonier D, Nochy D, Poncet P et al. (1995) Sequential immunological targeting of chronic experimental arterial allograft. Transplantation 60: 414–424
19. Sappino AP, Schürch W, Gabbiani G (1990) Differentiation repertoire of fibroblastic cells expression of cytoskeletal proteins as marker of phenotypic modulations. Lab Invest 63: 144
20. Schmitz-Rixen T, Megerman J, Colvin RB, Williams AM, Abbott WA (1988) Immunosuppressive treatment of aortic allografts. J Vasc Surg 7: 82–92
21. Somerville J (1988) Late results of homograft function used for right ventricular outflow obstruction. In: Cardiac valve allografts 1962–1987 (eds. Yankah AC, Hetzer R, Miller DC, Ross DN, Somerville J, Yacoub MH), Steinkopff Verlag, Darmstadt, Springer Verlag, New York, pp 249–256
22. Stein H, Gerdes J, Schwab U et al. (1982) Identification of Hodgkin Sternberg-Reed cells as in unique cell type derived from a newly detected small-cell population. Int J Cancer 30: 445–59
23. Thiede A, Engemann R, Körner HH et al. (1975) Comparison of the immunologic reactions of arterial transplants in the arterial system and of venous transplants in the venous system using inbred strains of rats. Transp Proc 11: 603–6
24. Thiede A, Timm C, Bernhard A, Müller-Ruchholtz W (1978) Studies on the antigenicity of vital allogeneic valve leaflet transplants in immunogenetically-controlled strain combinations. Transplantation 26: 391–395
25. Yacoub MH (1988) Applications and limitations of histocompatibility in clinical cardiac valve allograft surgery, In: Cardiac valve allografts 1962–1987 (eds. Yankah AC, Hetzer R, Miller DC, Ross DN, Somerville J, Yacoub MH), Steinkopff Verlag, Darmstadt, Springer Verlag, New York, pp 95–102

26. Yankah AC, Feller AC, Thiede A, Westphal E, Bernhard A (1986) Identification of surface antigens of endothelial cells of fresh preserved heart allografts. Thorac Cardiovasc Surgeon 34 (Suppl): 1–108
27. Yankah AC, Wottge HU, Dreyer W, Bernhard A, Müller-Ruchholtz W (1986) Kinetics of endothelial cells of aortic valve allografts transplanted heterotopically in inbred rats. In: Biologic and bioprosthetic valves (eds. Bodnar E, Yacoub MH), Yorke Medical Books, New York, pp 73–84
28. Yankah AC, Wottge HU, Müller-Hermelink HK, Feller AC, Lange P, Wessel U, Dreyer H, Bernhard A, Müller-Ruchholtz W (1987) Transplantation of aortic and pulmonary allografts, enhanced viability of endothelial cells by cryopreservation. Importance of histocompatibility. J Cardiac Surg 1 (Suppl.): 209–220
29. Yankah AC, Wottge HU, Müller-Ruchholtz W (1988) Prognostic importance of viability and a study of second-set allograft valve: An experimental study. J Cardiac Surg 3: 263–70
30. Yankah AC, Wottge HU, Müller-Ruchholtz W (1994) Effect of cyclosporin A on rat aortic valve allograft survival. Delayed or arrest of non-MHC encoded endothelial antigen expression. In: New Horizons and the Future of Heart Valve Prostheses (S. Gabbay, RWM Frater eds.) Silent Partners Inc., Austin, , pp 53–72
31. Yankah AC, Wottge HU, Müller-Ruchholtz W (1995) Short-course cyclosporin-A therapy for definite allograft valve survival. Immunosuppression in allograft valve operations. Ann Thorac Surg 60: S146–50
32. Zavazava N, Simon A, Sievers HH, Bernhard A, Müller-Ruchholtz W (1995) Porcine valves are reendothelized by human recipient endothelium in vivo. J Thorac Cardiovasc Surg 109: 702–6

Author's address:
A. Charles Yankah, MD, PhD
Consultant, Assistant Professor
Deutsches Herzzentrum Berlin and Humboldt University
Dept. Cardiothoracic and Vascular Surgery
Augustenburger Platz 1
D-13353 Berlin
Germany

Immunosuppression in allograft valve surgery.
A study on inbred rat model

A. C. Yankah, H-U. Wottge*

German Heart Institute Berlin, Institute of Immunology, University of Kiel*,
Germany

Introduction

Allograft valves are preferred cardiac valve substitutes because of their superior
hemodynamics and lack of postoperative anticoagulation and resistance to infection
(2, 3, 11, 12, 16). Early structural deterioration due to an immune response in some
groups of patients is now a concern to surgeons and cardiologists (6, 9, 15, 17). This
study was therefore designed to determine the effect of a short-course Cyclosporin
A therapy (8, 10) on allograft valve survival across the histocompatibility barriers on
semiallogeneic (hybrid) rat model.

Materials and method

Animal model: Male and female inbred (CAP × LEW)F1 (RT1 c/1) and CAP (RT1^c,
control group) rat strains weighing 250–350 g were used as donors for valves and skin
allografts. LEW rat strains weighing 300–400 g were exclusively used as recipients.
They were housed in wire bottom cages with controlled light/dark cycles and allowed
free access to water and rat chow. Experimental rat models were established from
a combination of (CAP × LEW)F1 (semi-allogeneic, hybrids) and LEW rat strains
((CAP × LEW)F1 > LEW). For the control study a combination of CAP and LEW
(strongly allogeneic, RTI- and non-RT1-incompatible). Strains and LEW > LEW
syngeneic rat strains (isografts) were used. Two major experimental groups were
established from the rat models: I) cyclosporin A (CSA)-untreated group (with fresh
or allovital valved and antibiotic treated viable conduits) II) CSA-treated group (with
fresh or allovital valved conduits) with oral dosis of Cyclosporin at 10 mg/kg/day for
14 days beginning from the day of operation.

Donor heart explanation and preparation of valved conduits

In ether anesthesia the donor heart was exposed via median sternotomy and explanted with a segment of ascending aorta. The donor heart was placed in a container
with cold (4 °C) Ringer solution to avoid warm ischemia. Allograft valved conduits of
1.0–1.2 cm long with a segment of ascending aorta were dissected at operation day for
immediate use as fresh allovital conduits. Allovital allografts consisted of living
cellular components viz. endothelial cells and fibroblasts. Endothelial cell-free viable

valved conduits were used as control allografts. Viable allografts were prepared by treating fresh allografts with antibiotic solution (16) in nutrient medium (RPMI 1640, Roswell Park Memorial Institute) with fetal calf serum (20%) and stored at 4 °C for up to 7 days. The endothelial cells of the valves and the aortic walls did not survive under these conditions and therefore died and became easily detached from the valve surfaces as well as from the inner surface of the aortic walls when the conduits were vigorously rinsed in the nutrient medium for a few minutes (15, 16). The antibiotic treated conduits are then composed of viable fibroblasts without living endothelial cells.

Preparation of polyclonal allo-antisera

Polyclonal allo-antisera were prepared fro identifying donor-specific endothelial cells before and after transplantation. Donors of skin grafts and spleen cell suspensions were LEW, CAP, AS and (CAP × LEW)F1 rat strains and recipients were LEW and CAP rat strains. LEW, CAP rat strains received at four consecutive times at 10 days interval two skingrafts from each strain (LEW > CAP, CAP > LEW, AS > LEW and (CAP × LEW)F1 > LEW. Subsequently, they received after primary immunization on day 0, three consecutive intraperitoneal (i.p.) booster inoculations of 5×10^7 spleen cell suspensions on days 7, 14 and 21. The cell suspensions were prepared from spleens harvested after splenectomy from rat strains syngeneic to the skin graft donor (LEW > CAP, CAP > LEW, AS > LEW and (CAP × LEW)F1 > LEW). In the following week the recipient rat strains were humanely sacrificed under ether anesthesia for drawing whole blood for extracting the serum. The pooled polyclonal sera were tested for the presence of endothelial surface antigens by indirect immunofluorescence technique and the rest sera were frozen and stored at − 80 °C.

Test for specific rat strain antibodies

Indirect immunofluorescence technique with FITC-labeled sheep-antirat IgG (kindly supplied by Camon, Wiesbaden, Germany) were used to test for the specificity of the rat strain polyclonal anti-sera. Anti-CAP-Sera from LEW rat were tested against the endothelial cells of CAP and LEW valves; anti-LEW-Sera from CAP rat were tested against the endothelial cells of LEW and CAP valves, anti-AS-Sera from LEW rat were tested against the endothelial cells of AS and LEW valves and anti-(CAP × LEW)F1-Sera from LEW rat were tested against the endothelial cells of (CAP × LEW) F1 and LEW valves.

Demonstration of endothelial cell surface antigens of valve allograft by indirect immunofluorescence

Glass slides with "Endothelhäutchen" or cryostat preparations were used for this study. 50 µl each of 1) mouse-anti-rat-anitbodies (0X6, Medac, Hamburg, Germany) directed at rat MHC-Class II-Antigens and 2) polyclonal allo-antisera (anti-LEW, anti-CAP × LEW)F1) (in both sera 1:40 dilution with phosphate buffered saline) were put on the slides and the slides were placed in a moist chamber and incubated in a refrigerator for 30 min. After the incubation time the cells on the slides were gently rinsed in a phosphate buffered saline (pH 7.4) and incubated with 50 µl (1:15 dilution with phosphate buffered saline) of FITC-labeled anti-rat-IgG (Camon, Wiesbaden,

Germany) for 30 min in a dark refrigerator. After the incubation time the preparation was gently rinsed in a phosphate buffered saline two times and rendered dry. A drop of buffered glycerin was placed on the slide for fluorescence microscopy. Positive IF was defined as a weak or strong fluorescence staining.

Demonstration of antibodies against endothelial cells of valve allograft by direct immunofluorescence

Cryostat sections of valve allografts were used for the study. Fifty µl (1:15 dilution with phosphate buffered saline) of FITC-labeled anti-rat-IgG (Camon, Wiesbaden, Germany) for 30 min in a dark refrigerator. At the end of the incubation time the preparation was gently rinsed in a phosphate buffered saline two times. A drop of buffered glycerin was placed on the slide after it was dry for fluorescence microscopy. Positive IF was defined as a weak or strong fluorescence staining.

Skin grafting

Full-thickness skin grafts of a rat strain syngeneic to the donor of allograft valved conduit ((CAP × LEW)F1 > LEW) was taken from a disinfected shaved abdominal skin and transplanted into the place of an excised abdominal skin of an allograft valved conduit CyA-treated and CyA-untreated recipients 3 weeks after heterotopic implantation into the infrarenal aorta (Table 1). The graft was turned about 90 degree at implantation so that the growing hairs would face perpendicular to those of the hosts. The skin grafts were protected by using a soft wire gauze for daily dressing after the wound inspection while detecting for skin rejection times. Grafts which were not rejected showed normal wound healing and scar. The hair growth as well as the blood circulation of the skin grafts also appeared normal. In contrast, the rejected skin grafts showed abnormal hair growth, while the graft tissue appeared edematous with red induration, necrosis and demarcation. When rejection of skin graft was observed the demarcation caused by reduced circulation of the rejected skin graft was confirmed by identifying the region with intravenous injection of 0.3–0.4 ml disulfide blue (0.62%) in the tail or penile vein. The rejected skin showed a weakly blue coloration as indication of reduced local blood circulation as compared to the host viable skin tissue.

Table 1. Median survival times of (CAP × LEW)F1 and CAP second-set skin grafts challenge on allovital valve implant in recipients (LEW) with short course CyA treatment. 14 days CSA therapy at oral dosis of 10 mg/kg. Legends: VG = valve grafts, SG = skin graft

Skin graft donor and recipient	n	Interval VG & SG (days)	Survival of SG (days)	Compared with control
LEW (VG) > LEW + (SG)	5	21	**	**
(CAP × LEW)F1 (VG) > LEW (VG) + (SG)	5	21	60.8 ± 1.4	9.2 ± 0.8
CAP (VG) > LEW + (SG)	5	21	42.5 ± 1.3	7.3 ± 0.8

Heterotopic implantation of valved allograft conduit into the infrarenal aorta

Under ether anesthesia, median laparatomy was made and the infrarenal abdominal aorta was exposed. The prepared valved allograft conduits of aortic root segments were trimmed of excess myocardium, the two coronary arterial segments were ligated. The conduits were implanted into the infrarenal aorta by interposition with 8–0 Prolene sutures between two special bulldog clamps beginning with the posterio-lateral and then the anterior proximal end-to-end anastomosis (15). The ventricular aspect of the aortic valve was placed against the antegrade blood stream and the valve cusps were made incompetent by sutures at the base of the cusps when the proximal anastomosis was being performed. After the distal anastomosis the aortic clamps were released for antegrade blood flow. The patency of the anastomoses was controlled by digital palpation. The laparatomy wound was closed and dressed with soft wire gauze and the allograft recipients were taken into their cages. The allografts were explanted humanely from the hosts under anesthesia on days 20, 50 and 100 and 150 after heterotopic implant for immunofluorescence (IF) study.

Immunosuppression with Cyclosporin A (CSA)

CSA (Sandimmun, crystalline powder for oral application, Sandoz, Basel, Switzerland) was dissolved in pure olive oil at 500 ug/15 ml by stirring constantly for 40–60 min at 30 °C. The CSA-treated animals in Experiment II received daily 10 mg/kg dose of CSA orally, beginning from the day of operation for 14 days. Whole blood was obtained on day 1, 3, 7, 11, and 14 during the CyA treatment and at the termination of the CSA treatment on days 18, 22 and 28 from the tails of the recipient rat strains (LEW) for determining the CSA serum levels (Fig. 1).

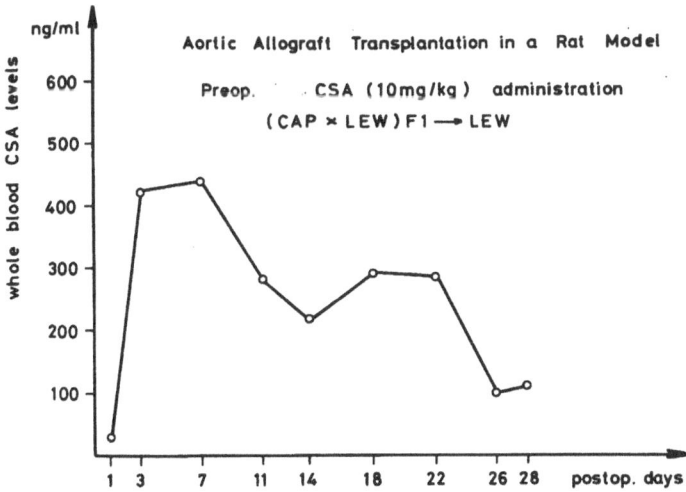

Fig. 1. Pharmacokinetics of oral CyA dosis in rats. Whole blood CyA levels after administration of 10 mg/kg CyA for 14 days starting from the operation day.

Results

Allograft valves with the semiallogeneic F_1 hybrid encoded endothelial cells showed no humoral response under a short-course immunosuppression as compared to the valves in the untreated group. There was a prolonged survival of the second-set skin graft therefore an indication of temporary unresponsivenes of the host under short-term immunosuppression (Table 1). The untreated allovital valves, on the other hand, as compared to viable valves, demonstrated early fibrocalcification on the 100th postoperative day. Syngeneic isografts did not elicit immune response and showed no structural deterioration (Table 2).

Comments

Longer-term allograft valve durability could be achieved with MHC-compatible than with MHC-incompatible valves. This is confirmed clinically in corneal transplantation (14, Table 3). Alternatively, allograft valve survival across a MHC-incompatibility barrier could be prolonged by a short-course immunosuppression. The study showed that CSA inhibits humoral response to MHC endothelial antigens in rats. The dose of 10 mg CSA/kg/day given orally for 14 days appears to be sufficient to induce unresponsiveness, hence improve valve durability (1, 5, 7, 13, 14). As shown in the

Table 2. Graft survival in treated and untreated recipients

Strain combination	Allovital grafts				Viable grafts		Skin graft survival (d)	
	NoCSA		CSA					
	50d	100d	50d	100d	50d	100d	NoCSA	CSA
LEW → LEW	–	–	–	–	–	–	0	0
(CAP × LEW) F1 → LEW	–	+	–	–	–	+	8.1	61
CAP → LEW	+ + +	c	–	+	–	+ +	3.8	28.7

(Symbols: + + + = severe, + + = moderate, + = mild, – = no rejection, d = days, c = fibrocalcification)

Table 3. Survival of histocompatible corneal transplant D'Amaro et al. 1992 (17)

HLA-DR	n	24-month survival
Matched graft	51	90%
Unmatched graft	101	52%
HLA, A, B	n	15-year survival
Matched graft	459	80%
Unmatched graft	266	55%

direct immunofluorescence studies, the state of unresponsiveness and absence of antibody production against the endothelial surface antigens in CSA-treated group appeared to be the proper alternative approach to prevent allograft valve endothelial destruction.

Conclusion: CSA could arrest or delay allograft rejection, thus prevent early degeneration of allografts with semiallogeneic F1 hybrid encoded endothelial cells. It appears that the use of histocompatible allograft valves alone and short-course non-toxic immunosuppression are the two alternative approaches to improve the durability of allograft valves in high-risk patients, particularly in children. This study represents an experimental foundation for a more successful clinical allograft valve surgery.

References

1. Brent L, Rayfield S (1983) Fully allogeneic cells are less effective in inducing neonatal tolerance than semiallogeneic F1 hybrid cells. Transplant Proc 15: 864
2. Clarke DR, Campbell DN, Hayward AR, Bishop DA (1993) Degeneration of aortic valve allografts in young recipients. J Thorac Cardiovasc Surg 105: 934–42
3. Cleveland DC, Williams WG, Razouk AJ, Trusler GA, Rebeyka IM, Duffy L, Kan Z, Coles JG, Freedom RM (1992) Failure of cryopreserved homograft valved conduits in the pulmonary circulation. Circulation 86: (suppl. II) : II–150–153
4. D'amaro J, Völker-Dieben HJ, Kruit PJ, de Lange P, Schipper R (1992) HLA matching and other factors in corneal transplantation: a single-center experience with more than 1800 consecutive transplants in 15 years. In: HLA 1991 (K. Tsuji, M. Aizawa, T. Sasazuki eds.) Vol. 2, Oxford University Press, Oxford, New York, Tokyo, pp 478–479
5. Dunn DC, White DJG, Wade J (1978) Survival of first and second kidney allografts after withdrawal of cyclosporin A therapy. IRCS Med Sci 6: 464
6. Gerosa G, McKay R, Davies J, Ross DN (1991) Comparison of the aortic homograft and the pulmonary autograft for aortic valve or root replacement in children. J Thorac Cardiovasc Surg 102: 5161
7. Green CJ, Allison AC (1978) Extensive prolongation of rabbit kidney allograft survival after short-term cyclosporin A treatment. Lancet 1: 1182
8. Gregory CR, Huie P, Billingham ME, Morris RE (1993) Rapamycin inhibits arterial intimal thickening caused by both alloimmune and mechanical injury. Transplantation 55: 1409–1418
9. Lupinetti FM, Cobb S, Kioschos HC, Thompson SA, Walters KS, Moore KC (1992) Effect of immunological differences on rat aortic valve allograft calcification. J Cardiac Surg 7: 65–70
10. Meiser BM, Billingham ME, Morris RE (1991) Graft vessel disease: the role of rejection and the effect of rejection and the effect of cyclosporine, FK506 and rapamycin. Lancet 338: 1297
11. Monro JL, Salmon AP, Keeton BR (1993) The outcome of antibiotic sterilised homografts used in the Fontan procedure. Eur J Cardio-thorac Surg 7: 360–364
12. Radley-Smith R, Yacoub MH (1986) Aortic homograft replacement in children. A 15 year experience. In: Biologic and bioprosthetic valves. (eds. Bodnar E, Yacoub MH), Yorke Medical Books, New York, pp 299–304
13. Takeshi N, White DJG, Calne RY (1982) Kinetics of unresponsiveness induced by a short course of cyclosporin A. Transplantation 33: 31–35
14. Tutschka PJ, Belanger R, Hess AD, Beschorner WE, Santos GW (1983) Suppressor cells in transplantation tolerance to self and non-self. Transplant Proc 15: 853
15. Yankah AC, Wottge HU, Dreyer W, Bernhard A, Müller-Ruchholtz W (1986) Kinetics of endothelial cells of aortic valve allografts transplanted heterotopically in inbred rats. In: Biologic and bioprosthetic valves. (eds. Bodnar E, Yacoub MH), Yorke Medical Books, New York, pp 73–84
16. Yankah AC, Wottage HU, Müller-Hermelink HE, Feller AC, Lange P, Wessel U, Dreyer H, Bernhard A, Müller-Ruchholtz W (1987) Transplantation of aortic and pulmonary allografts, enhanced viability of endothelial cells by cryopreservation. Importance of histocompatibility. J Cardic Surg 1 (suppl.): 209–220

17. Yacoub MH. Applications and limitations of histocompatibility in clinical cardiac valve allograft surgery. In: Cardiac valve allografts 1962–1987 (eds. Yankah AC, Hetzer R, Miller DC, Ross DN, Somerville J, Yacoub MH), Steinkopff Verlag, Darmstadt, Springer Verlag, New York. 1988; 95–102

A. Charles Yankah, MD, PhD
Consultant, Assistant Professor
Deutsches Herzzentrum Berlin and Humboldt University
Dept. Cardiothoracic and Vascular Surgery
Augustenburger Platz 1
D-13353 Berlin
Germany

Clinical results of freehand subcoronary aortic valve and root replacement with cryopreserved homografts (allografts)

A. C. Yankah, Y. Weng, J. Hofmeister, V. Alexi-Meskhishvili, H. Siniawski, P. E. Lange, R. Hetzer

German Heart Institute Berlin, Germany

Introduction

The homograft valve as a biologic valve substitute has gone through three major developmental phases, namely, 1) chemical sterilization (6, 7, 11), irradiation and freeze drying, 2) antibiotic sterilization (13, 16) and 3) cryopreservation (19, 23) since its introduction into clinical surgery in 1962 (2, 20). Antibiotic sterilization and cryopreservation methods have improved the allograft tissue quality and therefore the long-term durability. This was confirmed at the international Homograft meeting held in Berlin in 1987 and by others (13, 17, 18, 22, 24). The turning point in the era of allograft surgery in the 1990s has been a controversy about a particular implantation technique to achieve a longer-term allograft valve durability (3, 5, 12–14, 17, 18, 22). The clinical results and durability of cryopreserved aortic homografts in the aortic position might not depend on the quality of the tissue alone, but on other factors such as specific implantation technique in a specific patient group and in a specific aortic root if one assumes an immunological factor as a common hazard for the AVR and ARR techniques. The purpose of this report therefore is to review our 9-year experience with the freehand subcoronary aortic valve implantation and root replacement techniques with cryopreserved homograft valves.

Patients and methods

Cryopreserved homografts have been used at the German Heart Institute Berlin since October 1986 for reconstruction of the right and left ventricular out-flow tract obstructions, and since then 495 homograft operations have been performed. 208 patients underwent allograft replacement of the aortic valve (freehand subcoronary technique, $n = 147$) and root ($n = 61$) with concomitant procedures between January 1987 and March 1996. The age of the patients ranged between 1.5 and 78 years with a mean age of 41 years (Fig. 2). There were 55 females and 153 males. The major indications for particular implantation technique are summarized in Table 1. The diagnoses of the aortic valve and root diseases were classified into two major groups (Table 1); active infective aortic root ($n = 94$) with 47 ring abscesses and non-infective aortic root ($n = 114$). 197 patients have been followed between 2 and 111 months ending on March 31, 1996.

Indications for a specific allograft valve implantation technique are shown in Table 1. Since allograft valves in absence of immunosuppressive treatment of the

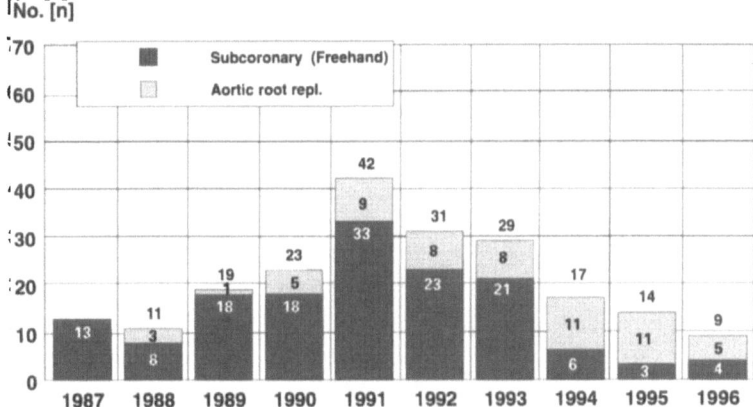

Fig. 1. Annual distribution of subcoronary freehand homograft aortic valve and root operations. Reproduction by permission (ref. 28).

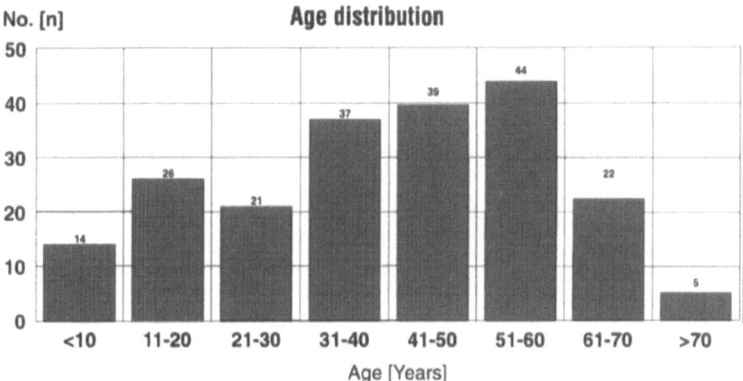

Fig. 2. Age distribution of patients who underwent subcoronary freehand aortic valve and root operations. Reproduction by permission (ref. 28).

recipient will become non-viable and therefore have no potential to grow, aortic root replacement with an appropriate adult size allograft to match the native root is recommended in patients under 30 years of age if pulmonary autograft is not preferred (8–10). Further indications for aortic root replacement are (Table 1): distorted aortic root (acquired or congenital), endocarditis with annular and subannular abscesses (41), aortic root disease in Marfan patients, short allografts (4–5 cm in length) or undersized allografts (more than 3 mm smaller than the recipient's annulus internal diameter), recurrent prosthetic endocarditis, recurrent paraprosthetic valvular leaks, aneurysm of the ascending aorta and severe poststenotic dilatation of the ascending aorta. Adult patients beyond 30 years of age with annulus diameter of 23–26 mm will receive subcoronary freehand valve replacement if their root pathology and geometry are normal. This will hold for aortic valve infection without localized annular abscess formation.

Allograft valve data: Allograft valves were harvested from heart transplant recipients (Fig. 3) or during multiorgandonation from unsuitable donor hearts for heart

Table 1. Aortic root diseases, etiology and indications for subcoronary freehand aortic valve and root replacement (reproduction by permission, ref. 28)

Aortic root diseases, etiology and indications for aortic root and valve replacement	Specific allograft valve implantation technique	
	Root repl. n	Freehand AVR n
Small or distorted aortic root ($n = 5$)		
a) hypoplastic tunnel obstruction	2	–
b) bicuspid aortic valve	2	–
c) prosthetic valve	1	–
Normal aortic root ($n = 91$)		
a) arteriosclerosis	–	58
b) bicuspid aortic valve	–	23
b) rheumatic valve	–	10
Dilated aortic root and aneurysm ($n = 5$)		
a) Marfan disease	1	–
c) aneurysm of sinus Valsalva	–	2
d) ascending aneurysm	2	–
Prosthetic valve dysfunction ($n = 13$)		
a) recurrent paravalvular leakage	2	2
b) mechanical valve thrombosis		2
c) bioprosthetic valve degeneration		3
d) allograft (homograft) valve degeneration	4	
Active infection of the aortic root with and without ring abscesses ($n = 94$)		
a) native valve	35	42
b) aortic allograft	–	
c) prosthetic valve	12	5
	61	147

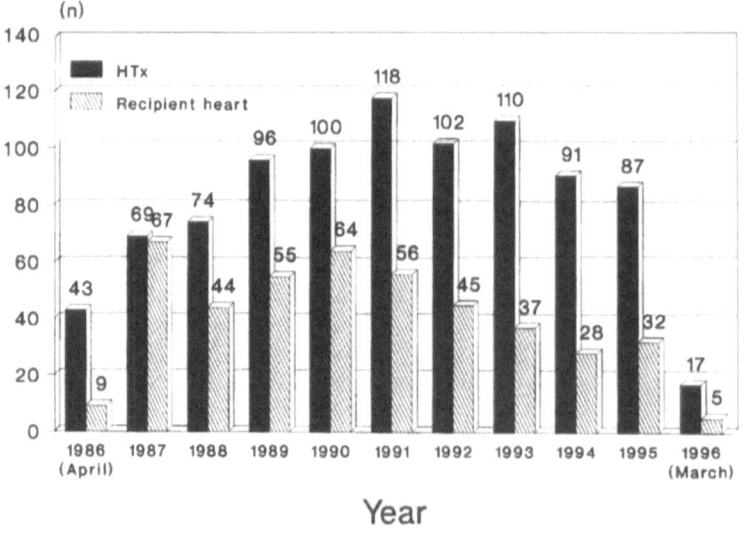

Fig. 3. Annual distribution of heart transplantation and number of recipients hearts harvested for allograft valve procurement (Htx = heart transplant). Reproduction by permission (ref. 28).

transplantation. Donors ages were between 12 and 56 years (mean 40.8 ± 14 years). Aortic and pulmonary valves were dissected, processed and cryopreserved as described elsewhere (1, 16, 17, 24, 25, 26). The allograft valves details of underlying diseases of the cardiac transplant recipients and multiorgan donors and allograft valve sizes are shown in Table 2. Allograft valve sizes were between 16 and 29 mm (mean 22.5 ± 3 mm). The implanted homograft valves were obtained from our Institution-based bank in Berlin, BioImplant service of EuroTransplant in Rotterdamm, the European Homograft Bank in Brussels and Homograft bank in Barcelona.

Echocardiographic assessment

Preoperative transesophageal or transthoracal echocardiography is routinely performed to measure the annulus diameter and assess the root morphology. The findings have been helpful in the selection of proper allograft valve size (internal diameter in mm) and in the preoperative decision making on particular implantation technique. Echo Doppler studies, including color-flow mapping, were performed at intervals of 3, 6 and 12 months postoperatively (Table 3).

Table 2. Annular dimensions of aortic and pulmonary valve homografts harvested during heart transplantation and at multiorgan donation. Diagnoses of heart transplant recipients and multiorgan donors

Annular dimensions of aortic and pulmonary valves in adults			
Diagnosis of heart donors	Aortic annulus (mm)	Sino tubular ridge (mm)	Pulmonary annulus (mm)
Non-cardiac diseases $n = 171$	22.1 17–25 (range)	19.3 15–22 (range)	25.2 16–29 (range)
Ischemic heart diseases, $n = 114$	23.5 23–27 (range)	20.4 21–24 (range)	28.8 23–31 (range)
Dilating Cardiomyopathy, $n = 285$	26.0 23.29 (range)	23.5 21–26 (range)	29.7 25–33 (range)

Table 3. Echocardiographic results 1 to 8 years after freehand subcoronary aortic valve and root replacement

Echocardiographic data 1-12 months postop.						
Implantation technique		LV-Ao ΔP mmHg x̄			Regurgitation	
	n	1-2	3-5	>5	0-1	III
Subcoro. "Freehand"	140	138	2	-	136	4
ARR+coronary reimpl.	48	46	2	-	48	-
Reop.: 4 (1-11 months)						
Echocardiographic data 1-8 years postop.						
	n	1-2	3-5	>5	0-1 II	III
Subcoro. "Freehand"	138	135	3	-	129 2	7
ARR+coronary reimpl.	46	44	1	1	44 1	1
Reop.: 9 (22-50 months)						

Operative technique

Through a median sternotomy cardiopulmonary bypass is established with hypothermic perfusion at 30–32 °C and myocardial preservation is achieved with cold cardioplegic arrest with crystalloid cardioplegic solution. In all cases transatrial left ventricular vent is inserted. Two implantation techniques: the subcoronary freehand aortic valve and root replacements were used in the series. Allograft valve preparation for different types of aortic roots and the implantation techniques are described in detail elsewhere (22, 24, 26) and in Figs. 4–7.

Different implantation techniques of homograft aortic value and root replacement in a noninfectious aortic root

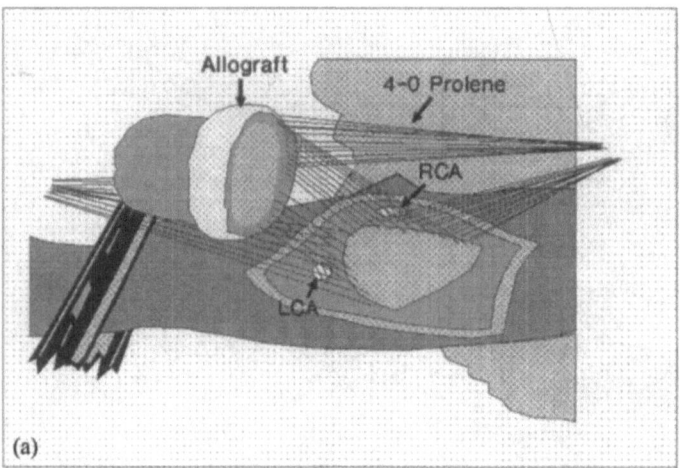

(a)

Fig. 4a–d. Technique of performing a standard proximal suture line: a) The unscalloped allograft is held outside the pericardium placing horizontal multiple single interrupted 4/0 prolene sutures beginning at the midpoint of the annulus below the left coronary ostium; firstly the sutures are placed through the allograft skirt below the cusps from outside (aortic) towards inside (ventricular) passing through the annulus of the host from ventricular aspect in a clockwise manner. At the left posterior commissure the sutures are now placed from the aortic to the ventricular aspect of the host annulus and then through the allograft wall from inside towards outside along the annulus in a clockwise manner to the non-coronary annulus (RCA and LCA = right and left coronary artery), b) and c) After the allograft is seated on the host annulus and tied down the right and the left coronary sinuses are scalloped leaving 5–7 mm rim of sinus wall. Temporary fixation of the commissures at proper position to achieve alignment with the valve leaflets and leaflets coaptation (RCA and LCA = right and left coronary artery, NCS = non-coronary sinus), d) after confirming proper commissural positions and achieving competent valve closure an interrupted continuous running 4/0 prolene suture is used to fix the graft sinus wall to the host sinus wall beginning from below the left coronary ostium towards the left commissure (RCA and LCA = right and left coronary artery, NCS = non-coronary sinus).

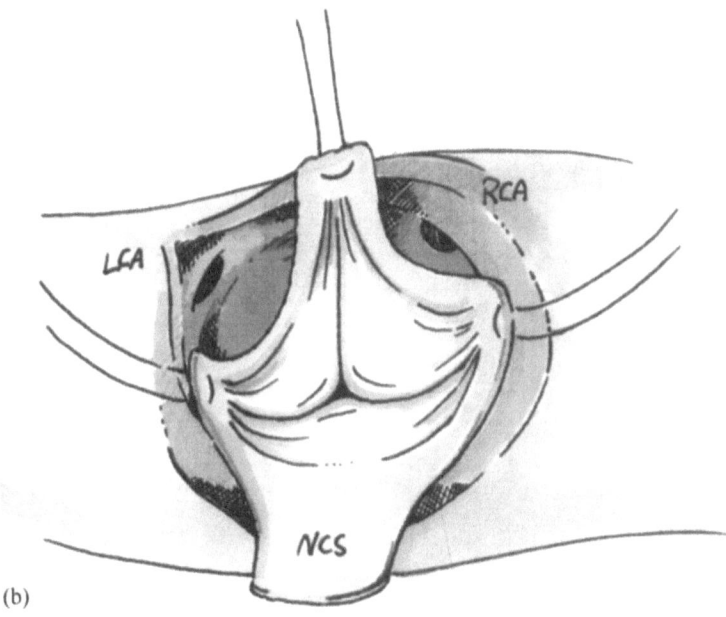

(b)

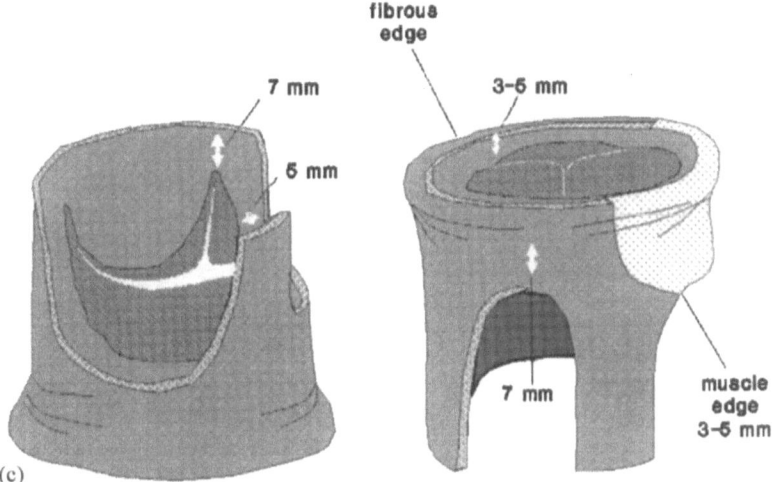

(c)

Fig. 4b and c.

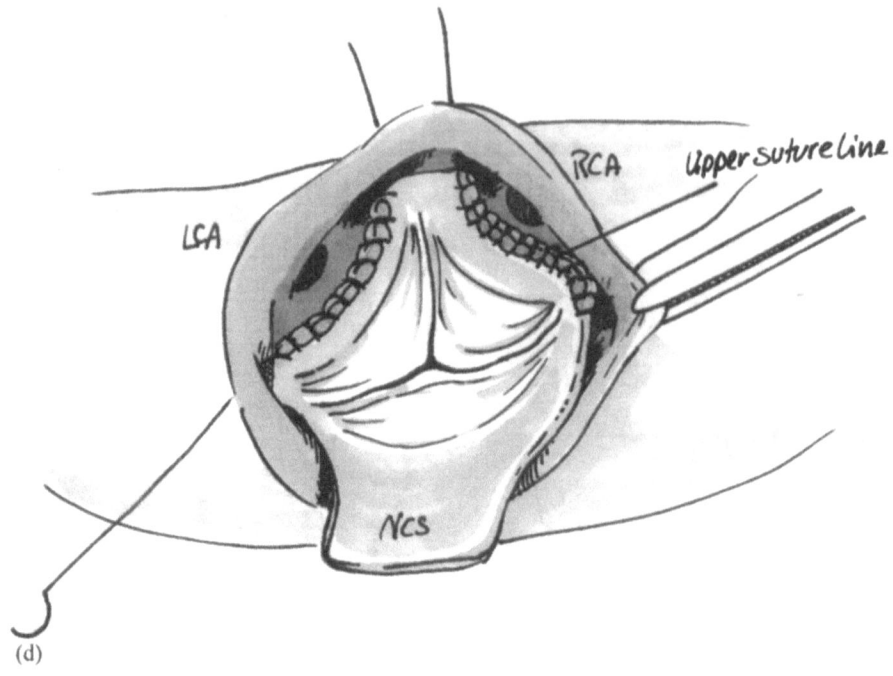

(d)

Fig. 4d.

Results

Early mortality

The mortality in non-infective root group was 2.6% and 8.5% in the infective root group, whereas congestive heart failure in New York Heart Association (NYHA) functional class IV with sepsis was the risk factor for death in these patients. The overall hospital mortality was 5.2%. The hospital mortality in the group with freehand subcoronary technique mainly with degenerative aortic valve diseases was 3.4% as compared to 9.8% in the root replacement group. Complicated endocarditis was the major indication for the root replacement.

Late survival

There were four late deaths (2.0%). Sudden death occurred in two patients 6 weeks and 1 year after surgery, presumably due to arrhythmia respectively. The third patient had kidney cancer and died of renal failure while the fourth patient, a drug addict, died of sepsis following a redo aortic root replacement for recurrent complicated endo-carditis. The actuarial patient survival was 95% ± 2% in patients with freehand subcoronary allograft implantation and $86\% \pm 4\%$ in those patients with root replacement at 8 years respectively (Fig. 8).

Structural and non-structural deterioration and allograft dysfunction

Structural deterioration (SD) in the entire series was 3.5%. It caused early valve regurgitation in six patients with freehand subcoronary valve replacement and in one patient with root replacement due to undersized homograft which led to reoperation 44 and 48 months after the first operation respectively. Actuarial rates for freedom from structural deterioration in patients with the freehand subcoronary implantation technique was $96.5\% \pm 2\%$ and in those patients with root replacement technique

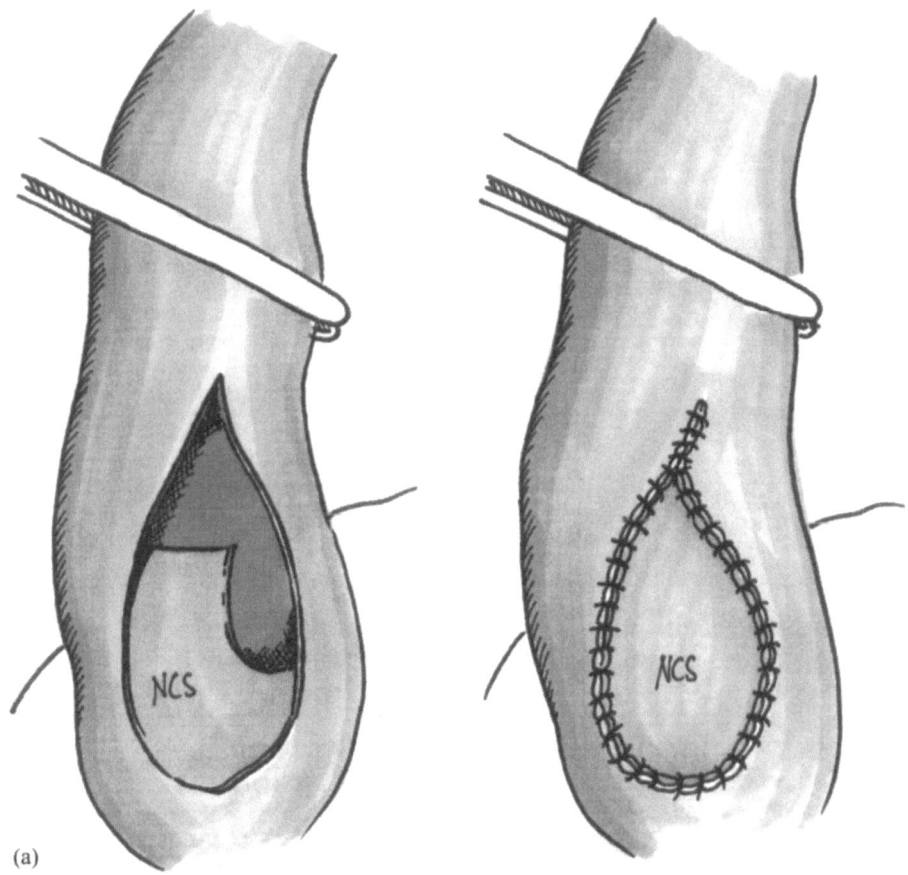

(a)

Fig. 5a and b. Closure of aortotomy. a) The allograft non-coronary sinus is used to enlarge the host non-coronary sinus. b) The allograft non-coronary sinus is incorporated into the aortotomy closure where the dead space is obliterated by three single 4/0 prolene sutures place in a triangular fashion (NCS = non-coronary sinus).

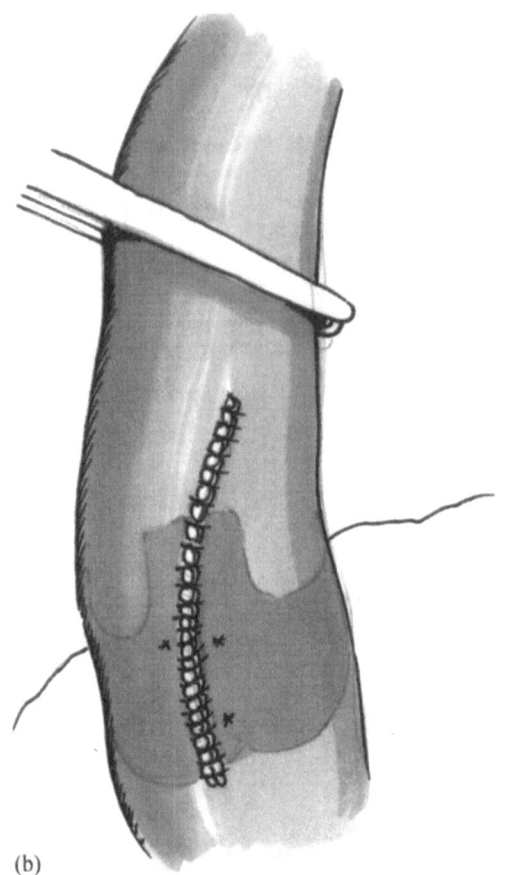

(b)

Fig. 5b.

was 98% ± 2% after 8 years. Non-structural deterioration (paravalvular leak) was observed in one Marfan patient (2.4%) with ARR and in two other patients (4.4%) with AVR who developed pseudoaneurysm formation.

Reoperation

Thirteen patients have been reoperated between 4 and 50 months after the first homograft operation for the following reasons: 1) Paravalvular leakage ($n = 3$). Two of them had previous endocarditis with annular abscesses who received freehand subcoronary valve replacement and developed pseudoaneurysm. They were re-operated 4 and 18 months after the first operation with an uneventful postoperative course. The third was a Marfan patient with a previous degenerated bioprosthesis which was replaced by a homograft as a root and developed paravalvular leakage. The suture dehiscence at the non-coronary aortic annulus could be refixed without necessitating a replacement of the homograft 3 months after the first operation.

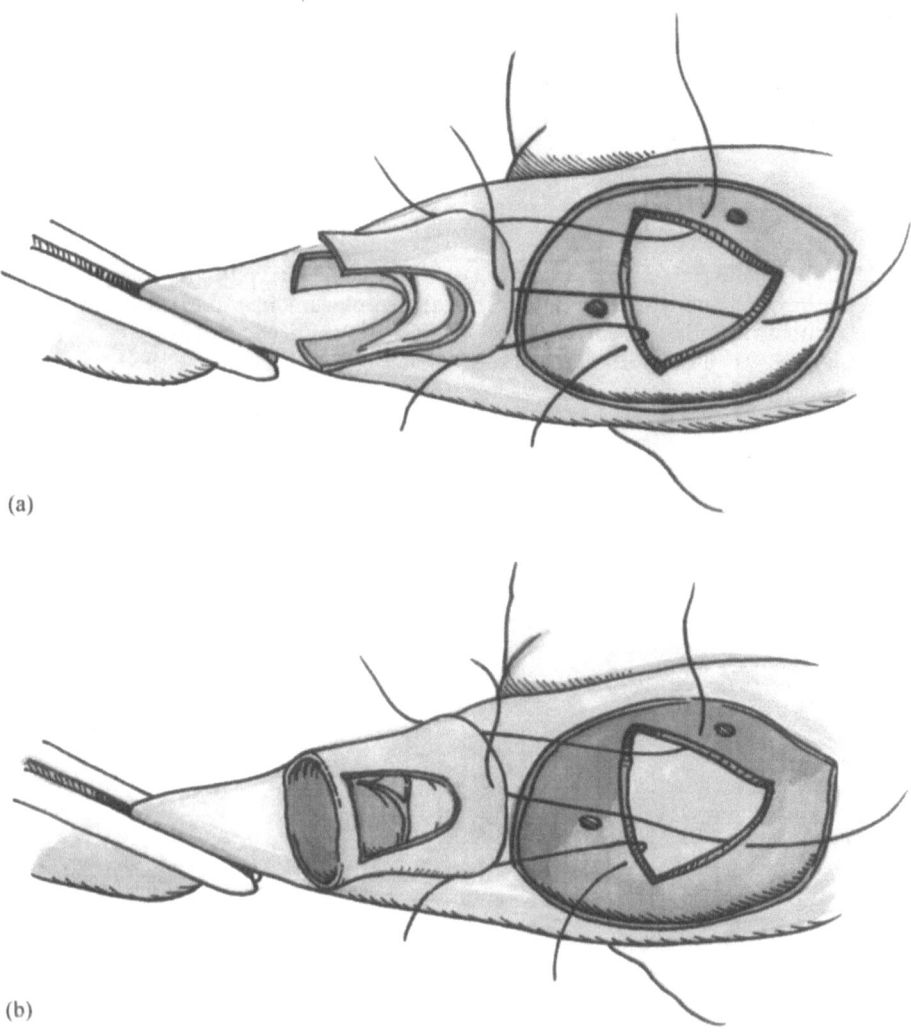

(a)

(b)

Fig. 6a and b. Demonstration of a) scalloped right, left and non-coronary sinuses, the Barratt-Boyes technique before performing the proximal suture line, b) excised button holes in the sinuses before performing the proximal suture line, the Bailey technique.

2) Recurrent complicated allograft endocarditis. The patient who was a drug addict had a reinfection of his allograft root replacement and was reoperated 50 months after surgery and died of sepsis. 3) Allograft degeneration: stenosis of allograft root replacement due to undersizing was observed in one patient 44 months after operation and replaced with another homograft. Allograft valve regurgitation ($n = 6$) in young patients between the ages of 6 and 32 years developed late postoperatively and led to reoperation between 3 to 48 months (mean: 26 months) after surgery. 4) Technically related allograft valve incompetence after freehand subcoronary implantation immediately after surgery ($n = 2$). Freedom from reoperation for the freehand subcoronary valve and root replacement techniques was 94% $\pm$ 2% and 93% $\pm$ 4%,

respectively, which was statistically insignificant (Fig. 10). The rate for freedom from reoperation in children with freehand subcoronary homograft implantation was 73% ± 5% (Fig. 9).

Endocarditis

Postoperative allograft endocarditis occurred in only one patient (0.9%) following a laparatomy 18 months after allograft valve replacement which was successfully treated with antibiotics. Recurrent endocarditis was observed in two patients (4.9%), one of whom was a drug addict and died of sepsis. Both had previous root replacement. Freedom from recurrent endocarditis was 93% at 8 years.

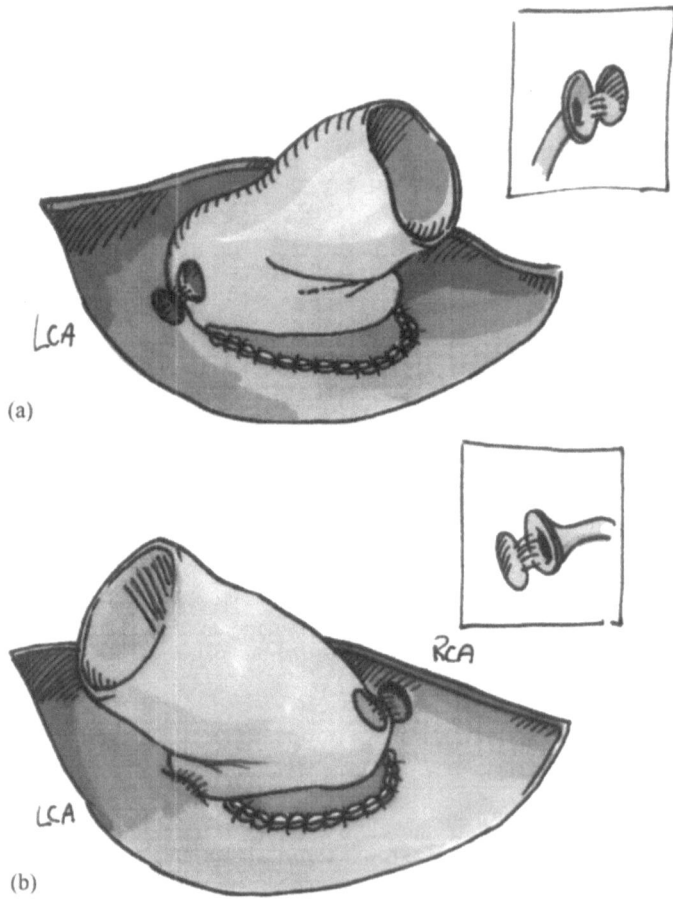

(a)

(b)

Fig. 7a–c. Aortic root replacement in a non-infected root. a) Completion of proximal suture line with single, multiple interrupted 4/0 prolene sutures. Excised left coronary button and reimplantation of the left coronary arteries with 5/0 prolene continuous interrupted suture (direct side-to-side anastomosis). b) direct side-to-side anastomosis of the right coronary ostium, c) completed allograft aortic root replacement with a teflon strip around the proximal anastomosis which might be necessary occasionally to control hemostasis (RCA and LCA = right and left coronary artery).

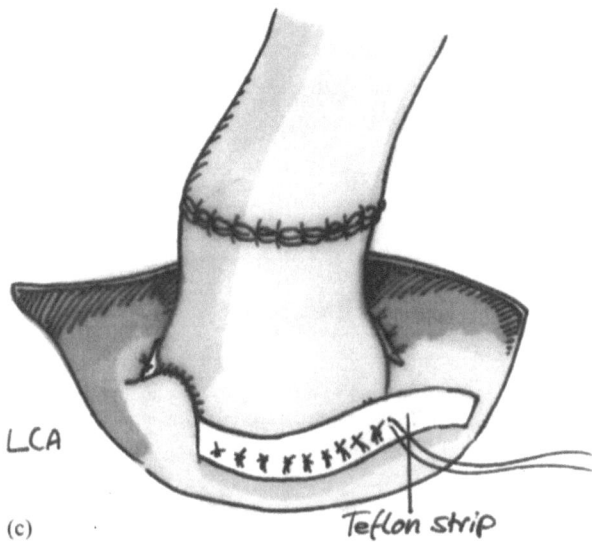

LCA

(c)   Teflon strip

Fig. 7c.

Thromboembolic complication

The patients received beside aspirin for three months no other anticoagulation therapy. During the follow-up period no thromboembolic events were observed in both groups of patient.

Discussion

Appropriate homograft size equivalent to that of the host annulus or even 1–2 mm larger might be a safe method for minimizing early postoperative valve incompetence when using the freehand subcoronary technique with preservation of the non-coronary sinus. The preserved non-coronary sinus wall is freestanding and provides commissural symmetry and alignment with the valve leaflets without being subject to distorsion and is useful for enlargement or replacement of the host's non-coronary sinus.

While subcoronary freehand allograft implants in an aortic root of 23–26 mm annulus diameter provide excellent long-term hemodynamic and functional results (Tables 3–5). Children and adolescents might need adult-size homograft for replacement of their restenotic aortic valve after surgical relief of their left ventricular outflow tract obstruction in infancy, whereas timing and appropriate valve size for homograft replacement at the second procedure might depend on the left ventricular function (26, 27). Children with annulus of 19 mm or below will outgrow their allograft valves, therefore they are potentially suitable candidates for root replacement using adult size allograft or pulmonary autograft switch operation (8–10, 15, 21, 29). Outgrown

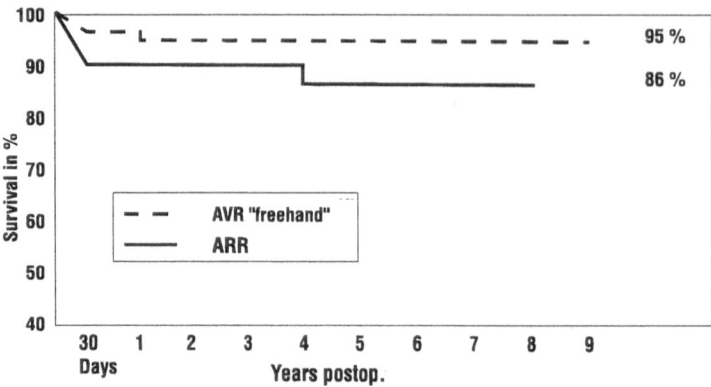

Fig. 8. Actuarial curve showing patients survival after freehand subcoronary aortic valve and root replacement (Kaplan-Meier method). Reproduction by permission (ref. 28).

allograft valves will become relatively stenotic resulting in higher gradients and leaflet stress. The leaflets will loose their expansibility with time, as has been demonstrated by Christie and Barratt-Boyes (5), and therefore pose a potential risk for early structural deterioration, besides the inherent immune response in younger age group (Fig. 9). Allografts implanted by intraaortic cylinder technique in this patient group might undergo the same degenerative process. These patients will therefore benefit from freestanding aortic root replacement with adult size allografts or pulmonary aurografts.

Single multiple interrupted sutures are recommended for the proximal anastomosis in all implantation techniques, at least during the learning phase. With this suturing technique less postoperative valve incompetence and perivalvular leaks have been observed. The above recommended techniques provide proper positioning and seating of the allograft root without distortion, and losing spatial relationship of the aortic root geometry therefore enables the surgeon to position the allograft commissures precisely to maintain the spatial geometry of the valve leaflets and achieve proper coaptation. Although five surgeons wee involved in this program the technical related postoperative valve incompetence was significantly low.

Intraaortic cylinder root replacement technique requires equivalent allograft size in case of poststenotic dilatation or aneurysmal ascending aorta in order to prevent the allograft from being crushed when wrapping it with the host ascending aortic wall. The major disadvantage of the intraaortic cylinder root replacement is the potential risk for coronary artery distorsion either due to blood and clots within the space or during the wrapping of the allograft with the host aortic wall. There is also a potential late problem from allograft aortic wall calcification induced by the organized clots in the dead space between the graft and the host aortic wall. Reoperation might therefore occasionally present some technical problems due to severe wall calcification and rare calcification around the coronary ostial anastomosis. The two root replacement techniques are applicable for large annulus of 27–29 mm.

At present, we believe that freestanding allograft root replacement is the appropriate method for small and distorted aortic, large annulus >27 mm, dilated roots and aneurysm of the ascending aorta as well as infective root with abscesses. In cases of root infection with subannular abscess cavities or ventricular aortic dehiscence a knicker-bocker shaped allograft conduit might be appropriate to fit the left

Table 4. Data on actuarial rates for freedom from morbid events in patients undergoing freehand subcoronary allograft aortic valve replacement

Author	Per cent freedom from events at n years							
	SD	yrs.	Reop.	yrs.	Endocarditis	yrs.	Survival	yrs.
Barratt-Boyes et al.	78	10	79	10	94	10	57	10
1987 (4 °C)	42	15	54	14	–	–	38	15
Matsuki & Ross et al.	60	10	–	–	90	10	85	10
1988 (4 °C)	12	20	–	–	82	20	51	20
O'Brien et al.	80	15	69	15	94	15	62	15
1995 (Cryo)	76	18	66	18	94	18	45	18
O'Brien et al.	45	15	58	15	91	15	56	15
1995 (4 °C)	34	21	49	21	89	21	33	21
Langley &	85	10	87	10	98	10	78	10
Monro et al.	63	15	71	15	96	15	65	15
1995 (4 °C)	41	20	50	20	95	20	55	20
Albertucci & Yacoub	72	10	70	10	88	15	71	10
et al. 1994	61	15	45	15	–		52	15
Yankah et al.	96	8	94	8	100	8	95	8
1995 (Cryo)	73*	8	73*	8	–	–	88*	8

* Results in children

Table 5. Data on actuarial rates for freedom from morbid events in patients undergoing allograft aortic root replacement

Author	Per cent freedom from events at y years							
	SD	yrs.	Reop.	yrs.	Endocarditis		yrs.	Survival	yrs.
Okita & Ross et al. 1988 (4 °C)	91	10	70	10	80		10	66	10
O'Brien et al. 1995 (Cryo)	86	8	82	8	88		8	85	8
Yacoub et al. 1995 (Homovital)	94	10	91	10	94		10	94	10
Yankah et al. 1996 (Cryo)	98	8	93	8	91		8	86	8

ventricular outflow tract in order to prevent angulation and supraannular stenosis (39). The allograft conduit preparation during the processing should be fashioned accordingly to serve this purpose.

If one compares the low-risk patient population of Barratt-Boyes (3) with the series of O'Brien et al. (16, 18) and Langley et al. (14) the rates of reoperation after freehand subcoronary implantation would be identical (Fig. 10). These results demonstrate that the controversial risk factor for postoperative valve incompetence with this implantation technique can be minimized with patient selection and surgical perfection. In the above-mentioned series the allografts were antibiotic sterilized and stored at 4 °C or cryopreserved.

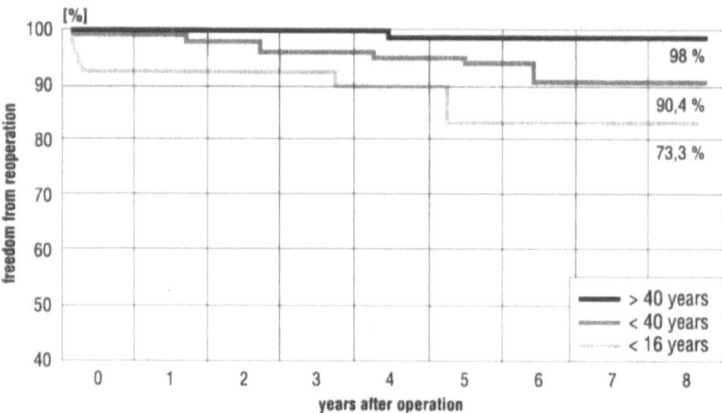

Fig. 9. Actuarial rate for freedom from reoperation according to age groups after subcoronary freehand aortic valve and root replacement with cryopreserved homografts (Kaplan-Meier method). Reproduction by permission (ref. 28).

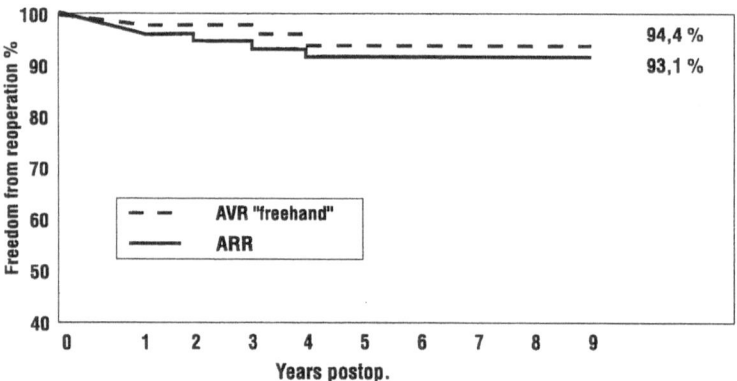

Fig. 10. Actuarial rate for freedom from reoperation after subcoronary freehand aortic valve and root replacement with cryopreserved homografts (Kaplan-Meier method). Reproduction by permission (ref. 28).

The time definition for identifying valve degeneration and determining time for reoperation are usually not identical but variable, due to the fact that many patients tolerate the gradual onset of mild to moderate aortic regurgitation well and not uncommonly postpone elective reoperation until symptoms appear or become worse if the left ventricular end-diastolic dimensions increase. A multicenter studies to assess the values of the two implantation techniques might be the appropriate method to provide objective data for determining proper implantation technique.

The inherent errors of the preoperative echocardiographic measurements of the host annulus have not been great, however, did not exceed the 2–3 mm which were seen more in the calcific small roots where less predictive accuracy was demonstrated.

In conclusion, despite acceptable early low reoperation rate with the AVR technique the mid-term valve survival is identical with that of the ARR technique in our series if one ignores the immunological factor as a common hazard for both techniques and excludes patients under 16 years of age. Since allograft valves have no potential to grow in children and adolescents, they might outgrow the intraaortic subcoronary aortic valve replacement which might lead to accelerated degeneration beginning in the vascular wall. We therefore recommend ARR with adult size homografts in these high-risk patients if pulmonary autograft is not preferred. However, pulmonary autograft aortic root replacement as a viable histocompatible tissue is instead recommended in young patients.

References

1. Angell WW, Angell JD, Oury JD, Oury JH, Lambert JJ, Grehl TM (1987) Long-term follow-up of viable frozen aortic homografts: a viable homograft bank. J Thorac Cardiovasc Surg 93: 815–22
2. Barratt-Boyes BG (1964) Homograft aortic valve replacement in aortic incompetence and stenosis. Thorax 19: 131–150
3. Barratt-Boyes BG, Roche AHG, Subramanyan R, Pemberton JR, Whitlock RML (1987) Long-term follow-up of patients with the antibiotic-sterilized aortic homograft valve inserted freehand in the aortic position. Circulation 75: 768–77
4. Bentall HH, DeBono A (1968) A technique for complete replacement of the ascending aorta. Thorax 23: 338–339
5. Christie GW, Barratt-Boyes BG (1991) Identification of a failure mode of the antibiotic sterilized aortic allograft after 10 years: implications for their long term survival. J Cardiac Surg 6: 462–467
6. Cohen DJ, Myerowitz PD, Young WP et al. (1988) The fate of aortic homografts 12 to 17 years after implantation. Chest 93: 482–4
7. Daly RC, Orszulak TA, Schaff HV, McGovern E, Wallace RB (1991) Long-term results of aortic valve replacement with non-viable homografts. Circulation 84 (5 Suppl): III81–8
8. Elkins RC, Santangelo KL, Randolph JL et al. (1992) Pulmonary autograft replacement in children: the ideal solution? Ann Surg 216: 363–71
9. Elkins RC (1994) Pulmonary autograft – The optimal substitute for the aortic valve? New Eng J Med 330: 59–60
10. Gerosa G, McKay R, Ross DN (1991) Replacement of the aortic valve or root with pulmonary autograft in children. Ann Thorac Surg 51: 424–9
11. Harris PD, Kovilak AJW, Marks JA, Malm JP (1958) Factors modifying homograft structure and function. Surgery 63: 45–51
12. Jones EL (1989) Freehand homograft aortic valve replacement. The learning curve: a technical analysis of the first 31 patients. Ann Thorac Surg 48: 26–32
13. Kirklin JK, Smith D, Nowick W et al. (1993) Long-term function of cryopreserved aortic homografts: a ten-year study. J Thorac Cardiovasc Surg 106: 154–66
14. Langley SM, Barron DJ, Tsang VT, Livesey SA, Lamb RK, Monro JL (1995) Long term results of valve replacement using antibiotic sterilized homografts in the aortic position. In: Proceedings of the 9th Annual Meeting of the European Association for Cardio-Thoracic Surgery; Sept 24–27; 1995; Paris: 218
15. Matsuki O, Okita Y, Almeida RS, Ross DN (1988) Two decades' experience with aortic valve replacement with pulmonary autograft. J Thorac Cardiovasc Surg 95: 705–11
16. O'Brien MF, Stafford EG, Gardner MAH, Pohlner PG, McGiffin DC (1987) A comparison of aortic valve replacement with viable cryopreserved and fresh allograft valves, with a note on chromosomal studies. J Thorac Cardiovasc Surg 94: 812–23
17. O'Brien MF, Finney RS, Stafford EG, Gardner MAH, Pohlner PG, Tesar PJ, Cochrane AD, Gall KL, Smith SE (1995) Root replacement for all allograft aortic valves: preferred technique or too radical? Ann Thorac Surg 60: S87–S91
18. O'Brien MF, Stafford EG, Gardner MAH, Pohlner PG, Tesar PJ, Cochrane AD, Mau TK, Gall KL, Smith SE (1995) Allograft aortic valve replacement: long-term follow-up. Ann Thorac Surg 60: S65–S70
19. Penta A, Qureshi S, Radley-Smith R, Yacoub MH (1984) Patient status 10 or more years after "fresh" homograft replacement of the aortic valve. Circulation 70 (3 Pt.2): II 82–6
20. Ross DN (1962) Homograft replacement of the aortic valve. Lancet 2: 487

21. Ross D, Jackson M, Davies J (1991) Pulmonary autograft aortic valve replacement: long-term results. J Cardiac Surg 6: Suppl: 529–33
22. Yacoub M, Rasmi NRH, Sundt TM, Lund O, Boyland E, Radley-Smith R, Khaghani A, Mitchell A (1995) Fourteen-year experience with homovital homografts for aortic valve replacement. J Thorac Cardiovasc Surg 110: 186–194
23. Yacoub MH, Kittle CF (1970) Sterilization of valve homografts by antibiotic solution. Circulation 41 (Suppl 2): 29
24. Yankah AC, Hetzer R, Miller DC, Ross DN, Somerville J, Yacoub MH (1988) Cardiac Valve Allografts 1962–1987, Steinkopff Verlag, Darmstadt, Springer Verlag, New York, pp 1–391
25. Yankah AC, Wottge HU, Müller-Hermelink HK, Feller AC, Lange P, Wessel U, Dreyer H, Bernhard A, Müller-Ruchholtz W (1987) Transplantation of aortic and pulmonary allografts, enhanced viability of endothelial cells by cryopreservation, importance of histocompatibility. J Cardiac Surg 2 (Suppl): 209–220
26. Yankah AC, Siniawski H, Lange PE, Fleck E, Hetzer R (1995) Connaissances de Base. Allogreffes et autogreffes valvulaires cardiaques. Conservation et chirurgie (D. Metras ed.) Masson, Paris, Milan, Barcelone, pp 49–78
27. Yankah AC, Regensburger D, Lange PE, Bernhard A (1986) Timing for second procedures after surgical relief of left ventricular outflow tract obstruction in infants and children. In: Pediatric Cardiology (EF Doyle, MA Engle, WM Gersony, WJ Rashkind, NS Talner, eds.), Springer-Verlag New York, Berlin, Heidelberg, Tokyo, pp 587–91
28. Yankah AC, Weng Y, Hofmeister J, Alexi-Meskhishvili V, Siniawski H, Lange PE, Hetzer R (1996) Freehand subcoronary aortic valve and aortic root replacement with cryopreserved homografts. Intermediate term results. J Heart Valve Dis 5: 498–504

Author's address:
A. Charles Yankah, MD, PhD
Consultant, Assistant Professor
Deutsches Herzzentrum Berlin and Humboldt University
Dept. Cardiothoracic and Vascular Surgery
Augustenburger Platz 1
D-13353 Berlin
Germany

Results of allograft aortic root replacement in children

D. R. Clarke, D. A. Bishop

The Children's Hospital and University of Colorado Health Sciences Center, Denver, Colorado, USA

Introduction

Left ventricular outflow tract obstruction with its complex pathology remains a challenge for pediatric cardiac surgeons. Isolated aortic valve replacement performed for simple valvar aortic stenosis or insufficiency, often is inadequate due to associated multilevel aortic obstruction or hypoplastic annulus. Cryopreserved aortic valve allografts offer a promising alternative to bioprosthetic or mechanical valve replacements that suffer degeneration or thromboembolic complications and require anticoagulation.

It has been over 20 years since the first aortic root replacement was performed by Donald Ross in 1972. The surgery was intended to relieve left ventricular outflow tract stenosis produced by aortic valvar hypoplasia and multilevel obstruction. A valve allograft was used to replace the aortic root and the coronary arteries were reimplanted into the allograft conduit. In 1982, the first series of surgical patients who underwent aortic root replacement was reported by Somerville and Ross (9). In 1987, McKowen et al. first published results of the extended aortic root replacement technique which they implemented in 1985 (7). The procedure combined Ross's allograft aortic root replacement with the annulus enlarging methods of aortoventriculoplasty, the details of which were described independently in the mid-1970s by Konno et al. and Rastan and Koncz (5, 8).

Patient population

At The Children's Hospital and the University of Colorado Health Sciences Center in Denver, 74 aortic root replacements have been performed using cryopreserved aortic allografts from June 1985, through June 1995. There were 48 male (65%) and 26 female children (35%). At the time of surgery, patient ages ranged from 1 day to 18 years with a mean age of 8.6 years. Fifty-eight children (78%) were older than 1 year of age at operation and 16 (22%) were 12 months of age or younger. Preoperative diagnoses are listed in Table 1, and Table 2 delineates previous cardiac surgeries.

Table 1. Preoperative diagnosis

Diagnosis	Patient age group	
	>1 Year	≤1 Year
Recurrent subvalvar aortic stenosis	20	
Multilevel aortic stenosis with insufficiency	14	7
Aortic insufficiency	13	1
Multilevel aortic stenosis	7	4
Aortic stenosis with hypoplastic annulus	3	1
Truncal valve insufficiency	–	3
Marfans → aortic stenosis and ascending aortic aneurysm	1	–
Total	58	16

Table 2. Previous cardiac surgical procedures

Operation	Patient age group	
	>1 Year	≤1 Year
Aortic valvotomy	24	3
Resect subvalvar membrane/myectomy	23	1
Repair coarctation of the aorta/ interrupted aortic arch	17	5
Aortic valve replacement	5	2
Atrial/ventricular septal defect repair with patent ductus arteriosus ligation	4	–
Ventricular-apical aortic conduit	3	–
Repair double outlet left ventricle	2	–
Repair atrial septal defect	1	1
Complete repair truncus arteriosus	–	2
Portacaval shunt (type II hyperlipidemia)	1	–
Main pulmonary artery → descending thoracic aorta conduit	1	–
No previous surgery	7 (12%)	5 (31%)

Surgical technique

In every case, a cryopreserved aortic valve allograft is used to reconstruct a congenitally anomalous left ventricular outflow tract. One of three variations on the procedure; a standard, extended, or modified aortic root replacement is employed. The chest is entered through a median sternotomy incision. The aorta and inferior and superior venae cavae are cannulated and 24–28 °C hypothermia is implemented. A catheter is positioned in the coronary sinus for retrograde administration of cardioplegia. Cold blood cardioplegia is administered to arrest the heart. Throughout the crossclamp period, a continuous trickle of cold blood cardioplegia is maintained when possible, and bolus doses are infused every 20 to 30 min.

Standard aortic root replacement has been described previously in detail (1, 9). The ascending aorta is transected 1 cm above the valve commissures. The aortic valve left and right coronary ostial buttons and redundant aortic wall are excised. A preselected and thawed aortic allograft valved conduit is prepared by trimming the proximal muscle to 5 mm below the valve and removing the attached anterior leaflet of the mitral valve. The proximal anastomosis between allograft and aortic annulus is performed with simple interrupted sutures tied over a pericardial strip. The coronary ostia are then reimplanted into the allograft conduit and the distal connection completed with running suture.

Extended aortic root replacement (3) is initiated with a vertical incision along the ascending aorta and an oblique incision across the right ventricular outflow tract. The infundibular septum can be incised to relieve the subvalvar component of the obstruction. The donor right coronary stump and recipient left coronary artery are aligned and the proximal allograft connection is begun posteriorly. Running suture continues bilaterally toward the interventricular septum. The donor anterior mitral valve leaflet is incorporated into the septal incision to enlarge the left ventricular outflow tract (Fig. 1).

In the modified aortic root replacement (10), the ascending aorta is transected and closed below the coronary ostia. Coronary and carotid arteries are revascularized via a side-to-side connection between ascending aorta and allograft. The aortic allograft is anastomosed to the descending thoracic aorta and a polytetrafluoroethylene patch augments the previously incised interventricular septum (Fig. 2). The technique is an option in patients with associated aortic hypoplasia or interrupted aortic arch. Table 3 exhibits the number of children who underwent each type of operation. Patient weight at the time of surgery and size of implanted allografts are documented by age group, in Table 4.

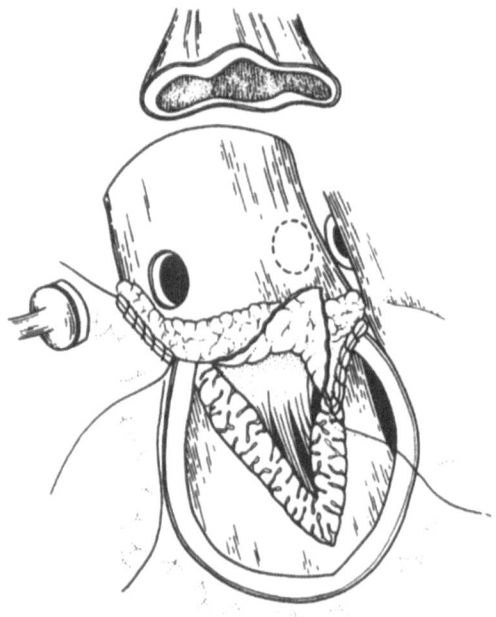

Fig. 1. The anterior mitral leaflet of the donor aortic allograft is sewn into the interventricular septal defect. (From: Clarke DR (1987) Extended aortic root replacement for treatment of left ventricular outflow tract obstruction. J. Cardiac Surg 2 (suppl): 121–128)

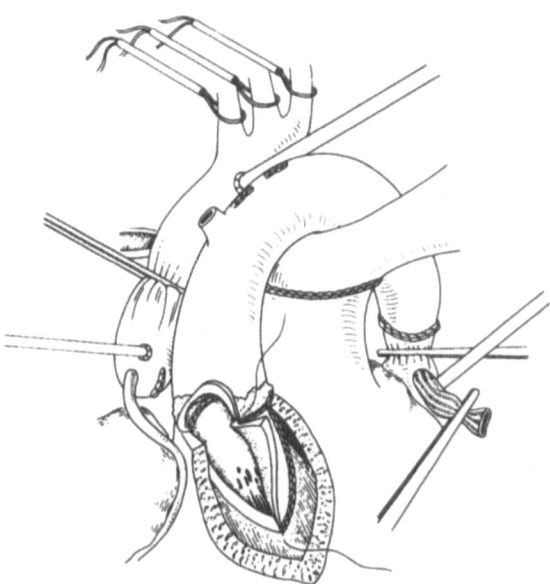

Fig. 2. The modified aortic root replacement utilizes a polytetrafluoroethylene patch extension and includes replacement of the aortic arch. (From: St. Cyr JA, Campbell DN, Fullerton DA, Grosso M, Bishop DA, Clarke DR (1992) Cryopreserved allograft repair of aortic hypoplasia and interrupted aortic arch. Ann Thorac Surg 53: 1110–1113)

Table 3. Operative variations for aortic valve allograft reconstruction of the left ventricular outflow tract

Aortic root replacement technique	Patient age group		
	>1 Year	≤1 Year	Total
Aortic root replacement	22	5	27
Extended aortic root replacement	34	9	43
Aortic root replacement with PTFE patch	2	2	4
Total	58	16	74

PTFE = polytetrafluoroethylene.

Table 4. Patient weight at operation and internal diameter of implanted allograft

Patient age group	Patient weight at operation (kg)	Allograft internal diameter (mm)
>1 Year	Range: 7.8–84.0 Mean: 36.7	Range: 14–25 Mean: 21
≤1 Year	Range: 2.8–8.1 Mean: 4.5	Range: 10–17 Mean: 12

Results

In the group of patients older than 1 year of age, mean transaortic gradient was 55 mmHg and 50 of 58 patients (86%) demonstrated the presence of moderate to severe aortic valvar insufficiency. Mean transaortic gradient in the infant group was 68 mmHg and 10 of 16 patients or 62%, exhibited associated aortic valve insufficiency. T-test for independent samples and chi square for independent samples respectively revealed no statistically significant difference between the mean transaortic gradient ($p > 0.10$) or the percentage of children in each group with aortic insufficiency ($p > 0.10$).

Mean age of the 58 children who were greater than 1 year old at the time of surgery was 10.9 years with a range of 1.8 years to 17.9 years. There were three perioperative deaths (5%). A 3-year-old boy with aortic subvalvar tunnel stenosis and supravalvar mitral stenosis both of which had required previous surgical resection, underwent aortic root replacement and mitral valve replacement. Disseminated Candidiasis developed and the child expired 11 days postoperatively. A 3-year-old girl had undergone aortic valvotomy at 20 months of age and presented with severe aortic valvar stenosis and insufficiency. Intraoperatively, the patient suffered ischemic contracture following extended aortic root replacement and was unable to be weaned from cardiopulmonary bypass. The third hospital death occurred in a 9-year-old boy with multilevel aortic stenosis. He had undergone repair of coarctation of the aorta and left ventricular outflow tract myectomy at 2 years of age. An uneventful extended aortic root replacement was followed by gradual hemodynamic deterioration and the child succumbed to left ventricular failure 7 days postoperatively. While 19 (34%) of the 55 older operative survivors experienced a benign postoperative course, a variety of manageable, early, postoperative complications were observed in 36 children (Table 5).

Postpericardiotomy syndrome was most prevalent occurring in 18% of children. Transient heart block or arrhythmias and pulmonary sequelae were also frequently observed. Early cardiac transplantation was necessary for one 5-year-old boy with

Table 5. Early postoperative complications

Complication	Patient age group	
	>1 Year	≤1 Year
Postpericardiotomy syndrome	10	2
Pulmonary	8	3
Transient heart block, arrhythmia	7	1
Endocarditis, mediastinitis, sepsis	3	6
Pericardial effusion	3	1
Hemorrhage	2	2
Neurologic impairment	2	1
Right phrenic palsy	1	2
Left ventricular failure (LVAD) → cardiac transplant	1	–
Miscellaneous	4	1
No complications	19/55 (34%)	2/12 (17%)

LVAD = left ventricular assist device.

Shone's syndrome. At 4 days of age, he underwent repair of coarctation of the aorta followed at 8 months of age, with aortic valvotomy and subvalvar resection. Concomitant extended aortic root replacement and St. Jude mitral valve replacement were performed when the child presented with recurrent aortic valvar and subvalvar stenosis and mitral stenosis. Due to myocardial dysfunction, left ventricular assist was necessary to wean the patient from cardiopulmonary bypass and the child received a cardiac transplant 30 h after his double valve replacement.

Follow up of 54 remaining aortic allograft recipients who were older than 1 year of age at surgery ranges from 4 months to 9.8 years (mean actuarial follow up: 4.4 years) with one child lost to follow up. There have been no late deaths. A child with double outlet left ventricle ultimately required cardiac transplantation. His original repair was a Rastelli-type procedure performed in early childhood. At 11 years of age, he developed severe porcine valved conduit obstruction as well as aortic stenosis and insufficiency. Aortic root replacement was performed and the right ventricular outflow tract was reconstructed with a pulmonary valve allograft. Cardiac transplantation was mandated 4 years later secondary to myocardial dysfunction. Pre-transplant echocardiography, cardiac catheterization, and pathologic examination revealed both allograft valves to be functional. Three of 53 older children (6%) have required aortic valve allograft explantation at 4 months to 8.2 years after their aortic root replacement. Each case is detailed in Table 6. All of the children remain asymptomatic at 1 to 4.4 years following receipt of a replacement allograft.

Mean age of the 16 infants who were 1 year of age or younger at the time of surgery was 3.3 months with a range of 1 day to 12 months. There were four perioperative deaths (25%). Two infants died in the operating room as a result of left ventricular failure; one child was 11 days of age with critical aortic stenosis and endocardial fibroelastosis, and the other was a 5-month-old with truncus arteriosus and distal pulmonary artery stenosis who underwent simultaneous left and right ventricular outflow tract reconstruction with aortic and pulmonary allografts respectively. A 1-day-old male with truncus arteriosus and interrupted aortic arch underwent aortic root replacement. The neonate succumbed to low cardiac output caused by myocardial dysfunction on the operative evening. The fourth death occurred in a 2-week-old boy who previously had undergone repair of interrupted aortic arch. Due to poor postoperative cardiac function, the chest was not reapproximated and the infant became septic and died 19 days postoperatively. Ten operative survivors encountered a variety of early postoperative complications (Table 5). Only two infants (17%) experienced uncomplicated recoveries.

Twelve infants have been followed for 2 months to 7.5 years (mean follow up: 2.2 years). There have been four late deaths (33%) in the infant group. Two of the late deaths occurred in children who had undergone left and right ventricular outflow tract reconstruction with aortic and pulmonary allografts respectively. A girl who was 2 weeks old at operation died of a pulmonary embolus 2.5 months postoperatively and a 12-day-old boy succumbed to sepsis following 3.5 months of multi-organ failure. One sudden death occurred 2 months after reoperative aortic root replacement in a 4-month-old boy and was most likely arrhythmia-related. One reoperative aortic root replacement resulted in late death from infectious cardiomyopathy 8 months after reoperation.

Six of the younger survivors (50%) have undergone allograft explantation. Details of each reoperative case are specified in Table 6. The two youngest infants who underwent reoperative aortic root replacement expired within 1 year of their second surgery; one due to infectious cardiomyopathy and the other due to an arrhythmia that resulted in sudden death as noted previously. Four infants who required allograft replacement are clinically well at 4.4 to 7 years after reoperation.

Table 6. Aortic allograft replacement

Patient	Diagnosis at first allograft repair	Age at first allograft repair	Complication	Reoperation	Months after first allograft repair	Outcome
HG	aortic atresia, atretic proximal ascending aorta	3 days	severe allograft insufficiency	redo ARR	3.5	death 8 mos. after reop
JC	aortic atresia, interrupted aortic arch	8 days	distal allograft stenosis and severe valvar insuff.	redo EARR	4	death 2 mos. after reop
JF	aortic valvar and subvalvar stenosis, aortic insuff.	3 mos.	allograft calcification and insuff. and subvalvar stenosis	mechanical prosthesis	37	well 5.4 yrs. after AVR
LL	dysplastic and stenotic aortic valve, hypoplastic aortic arch	4 mos.	allograft calcification, insuff. and stenosis	pulmonary autograft	45	well 4.4 yrs. after autograft
AB	aortic valvar and subvalvar tunnel stenosis	7 mos.	allograft calcification, insuff. and stenosis	pulmonary autograft	39	well 5.2 yrs after autograft
MA	bicuspid and stenotic aortic valve	12 mos.	allograft calcification, insuff. and stenosis	redo EARR	8	well 7 yrs. after reop
LK	aortic stenosis and insuff.	5.5 yrs.	severe allograft stenosis and moderate insuff.	freesewn allograft AVR and PVR	99	well 1 yr. after AVR and PVR
JD	multilevel aortic stenosis, hypoplastic aortic annulus	6.5 yrs.	allograft stenosis and insuff. (*Staph aureus* endocarditis)	redo EARR	86	well 2 yrs. after reop
CS	stenotic St. Jude aortic prosthesis	14.7 yrs.	*Candida tropicalis* endocarditis	redo EARR	4	well 4.4 yrs. after reop

ARR = aortic root replacement, EARR = extended aortic root replacement, insuff. = insufficiency, AVR = aortic valve replacement, PVR = pulmonary valve replacement.

Discussion

Table 7 compares early and late follow-up between the older and younger patient groups. The proportion of patients who experienced early death was slightly different statistically ($p < 0.10$). Age group differences are not statistically significant when incidence of early postoperative complications is compared. The most dramatic age group differences are exhibited when comparing the proportion of patients who experienced late mortality and allograft explant. The proportion of infants who suffered late death or underwent allograft degeneration that required replacement is significantly greater than the proportion of children older than 1 year old who experienced similar fates. Freedom from hospital death, valve-related death, or valve replacement in the older versus younger children was analyzed actuarially (Fig. 3). Event-free percentages are significantly higher in children older than 1 year of age

Table 7. Comparison of older and younger patient groups in early and late postoperative follow up

Patient age group	Early mortality	Early postoperative complications	Late mortality	Allograft explant
>1 year	3/58 (5%)	36/55 (65%)	0/53	3/53 (6%)
≤1 year	4/16 (25%)	10/12 (83%)	4/12 (33%)	6/12 (50%)
Combined	7/74 (9%)	46/67 (69%)	4/65 (6%)	9/65 (14%)
p value (>1 vs ≤1)	$p < 0.10$*	$p > 0.10$*	$p < 0.001$*	$p < 0.001$*

* chi square for independent samples.

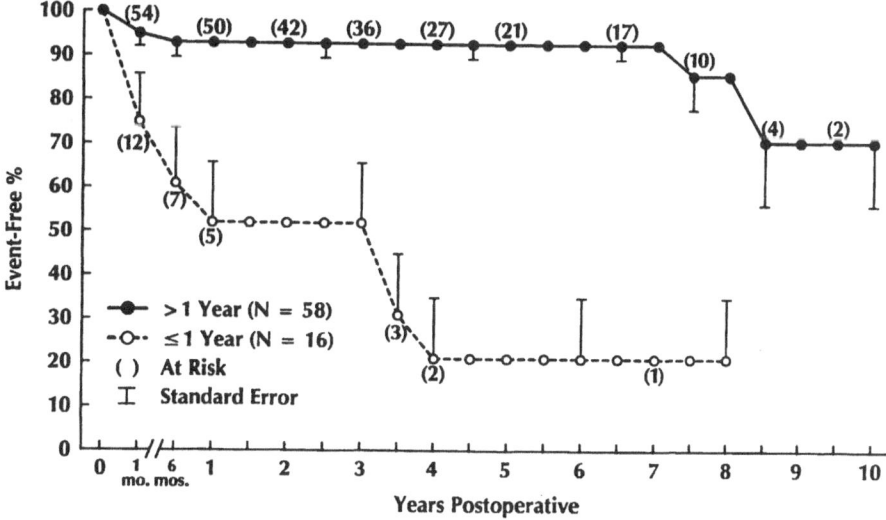

Fig. 3. Actuarial curve showing freedom from hospital death, valve-related death or valve replacement in patients older than 1 year of age at operation compared with children 1 year of age or younger.

between 1 month and 8 years of follow-up. While the mortality differences might be explained by the relative complexity of cardiac disease that requires intervention in infancy, an explanation for the increased incidence of allograft replacement is not so easily derived.

A distinct difference in conduit survival exists between older and younger pediatric aortic allograft recipients. With only 2 years mean follow-up of the infant group, 6 or 50% have had allograft replacements (Tables 6 and 7). Pathologic examination of the explanted allografts demonstrated fibrocalcification and degeneration in every case. In comparison, mean follow up of 4.4 years in the older patients reveals only 3 children or 6% have undergone allograft explantation (Tables 6 and 7) and two of the aortic valve conduits removed were explanted as a result of endocarditis. Therefore, there is only one case of primary allograft tissue failure that can be documented in a patient older than 1 year of age at operation.

There are several theoretical immunologic explanations for the increased incidence of allograft failure in infants. ABO blood type compatibility has been analyzed in the Denver experience with cryopreserved allografts and by others, and reveals no correlation between donor-recipient compatibility or specificity and patient or allograft survival (4).

Cryopreserved allografts are antigenic because the cryopreservation technique retains fibroblast and to a variable degree, endothelial cell viability (11). Small conduit size might contribute to aortic valve allograft failure in younger recipients. Valve conduits of 20 mm internal diameter and larger are more apt to undergo internal manipulation during dissection. The resultant loss of endothelial lining cells might reduce the antigenic stimulus.

One plausible explanation for the increased incidence of allograft fibrocalcification, degeneration and ultimate failure in infants relates to maturation of the immune system. An infant's transition into childhood includes immunologic changes that involve the proportion of circulating CD5 + B (B-1) cells to CD5-B and to T-cells (2). Ninety percent of circulating lymphocytes in an infant are B-1 cells. This proportion decreases to 10 to 20% by age 3 years. The less discriminating infant immune system might mount a more aggressive attack against viable allograft tissue than the more dose-related response of a mature system. Lupinetti and colleagues have demonstrated an association between the immune system and allograft calcification in an animal model (6). In rats, degree of allogenicity did not influence degree of response.

Cryopreserved aortic valve allografts are an appealing alternative for most pediatric patients who require extensive reconstruction of the left ventricular outflow tract. There is an accelerated rate of allograft fibrocalcification and degeneration in children 1 year of age and younger at operation. Because investigation remains in the early stages, explanations for the difference in conduit survival between older and younger aortic allograft recipients are tentative. Until the etiology of allograft failure is further defined, use of non-viable allografts, xenografts, or pulmonary autografts should be considered for infants. Administration of postoperative anti-inflammatory medication or low dose cyclosporine should be considered when of necessity, a viable allograft is implanted in a younger recipient.

References

1. Belcher P, Ross D (1991) Aortic root replacement – 20 years experience of the use of homografts. Thorac Cardiovasc Surgeon 39: 117–122
2. Bhat NM, Kantor AB, Bieber MM, Stall AM, Herzenberg LA, Teng NNH (1992) The ontogeny and functional characteristics of human B-1 (CD5 + B) cells. Int Immunol 4: 243–252

3. Clarke DR (1987) Extended aortic root replacement for treatment of left ventricular outflow tract obstruction. J Cardiac Surg 2(suppl): 121–128
4. Clarke DR, Campbell DN, Hayward AR, Bishop DA (1993) Degeneration of aortic valve allografts in young recipients. J Thorac Cardiovasc Surg 105: 934–942
5. Konno S, Imai Y, Iida Y, Nakajima M, Tatsuno K (1975) A new method for prosthetic valve replacement in congenital aortic stenosis associated with hypoplasia of the aortic valve ring. J Thorac Cardiovasc Surg 70: 909–917
6. Lupinetti FM, Cobb S, Kioschos HC, Thompson SA, Walters KS, Moore KC (1992) Effect of immunological differences on rat aortic valve allograft calcification. J Cardiac Surg 7: 65–70
7. McKowen RL, Campbell DN, Woelfel GF, Wiggins JW Jr, Clarke DR (1987) Extended aortic root replacement with aortic allografts. J Thorac Cardiovasc Surg 93: 366–374
8. Rastan H, Koncz J (1976) Aortoventriculoplasty: a new technique for the treatment of left ventricular outflow tract obstruction. J Thorac Cardiovasc Surg 71: 920–927
9. Somerville J, Ross D (1982) Homograft replacement of aortic root with reimplantation of coronary arteries: results after one to five years. Br Heart J 47: 473–482
10. St. Cyr JA, Campbell DN, Fullerton DA, Grosso M, Bishop DA, Clarke DR (1992) Cryopreserved allograft repair of aortic hypoplasia and interrupted aortic arch. Ann Thoracic Surg 53: 1110–1113
11. Yankah AC, Wottge HU, Muller-Hermelink HK, Feller AC, Lange P, Wessel U, Dreyer H, Bernhard A, Muller-Ruchholtz W (1987) Transplantation of aortic and pulmonary allografts, enhanced viability of endothelial cells by cryopreservation, importance of histocompatibility. J Cardiac Surg 2(suppl): 209–220

Author's address:
D. R. Clarke, MD
The Children's Hospital
Cardiothoracic Surgery, B200
1056 E. 19th Avenue
Denver, CO 80218, USA

Extended aortic root replacement with pulmonary autograft

W. Daenen

Department of Cardiac Surgery, University Hospital Gasthuisberg, Leuven, Belgium

Abstract

The surgical relief of complex multilevel left ventricular outflow tract obstruction remains a challenging surgical problem. We present a new operation which combines the concepts of aortoventriculoplasty, extended aortic root replacement and the use of a pulmonary autograft. Fourteen patients underwent this operation: nine patients after previous attempts to relieve diffuse subvalvular stenosis and five patients who presented excessive gradients over an outgrown aortic valve prosthesis. All patients except one survived the operation. One patient developed complete heart block after a septal infarction.

One patient remained in congestive heart failure and died suddenly after 17 months. All other patients are in NYHA class I after a mean follow-up of 20 ± 12 months. All patients showed excellent function of the autograft and homograft valve at follow-up.

This operation might present a more durable or even a definitive solution in the management of these complex left ventricular outflow tract obstructions.

The surgical relief of complex multilevel left ventricular outflow tract obstruction (LVOTO) remains a challenging problem. Several aggressive surgical procedures have been developed to treat these lesions. Aortoventriculoplasty (AVP) introduced by Konno (9), and aortic root replacement proposed by Ross (6, 16) are certainly more satisfactory than the placement of a left ventricular apico-aortic conduit (1, 4).

Clarke and associates combined the concepts of the AVP and the use of allografts in an operation described as the extended aortic root replacement (EARR) (13).

Convinced by the superiority of the pulmonary autograft in aortic position (7, 11, 15), we therefore combined the concept of the EARR and the use of a pulmonary autograft. This chapter describes our experience of this operation in 14 patients.

Patients and methods

Fourteen patients underwent an EARR: nine after several attempts of resection of a severe tunnel subvalvular aortic stenosis and five patients because of increasing gradients over an outgrown aortic valve prosthesis (Table 1). The ages at operation

Table 1. Patient material

	Redo SUBV-AS	Redo AVR
Patients (n)	9	5
Ages (years)	2.5 26	17 28
Interval previous surgery (years)	2 15	8 18
Mean preop gradient LVOT (mmHg)	112	80
Patients with CHF (n)	2	1

Legend: SUBV-AS: subvalvular aortic stenosis, AVR: aortic valve replacement, LVOT: left ventricle outflow tract, CHF: congestive heart failure.

ranged from 2.5 to 26 years. The mean preoperative gradient was 112 mmHg in the subvalvular stenosis group and 80 mmHg in the group operated for an outgrown aortic prosthesis. Three patients presented signs of congestive heart failure preoperatively.

Operative technique

Cardiopulmonary bypass is instituted using one aortic and one right atrial canula. The patient is cooled to 25 °C. The ascending aorta and the main pulmonary artery (PA) are separated down to the orifice of the left coronary artery. After aortic cross-clamping the aorta is transected 1 cm distal to the aortic commissures. Multidose cristalloid cardioplegia is delivered through two coronary canulas until a septal temperature of 10 °C is reached. Topical cooling with sludged ice is added to avoid myocardial rewarming.

After confirmation of the diagnosis the aortic valve is removed and the LVOTO is sized with Hegar obturators. The two coronary ostia are excised from the aorta with a generous button of 2–3 mm of aortic wall. The coronary arteries are only mobilised to allow proper excision of the buttons. The proximal aorta is then excised, leaving the annulus in place.

The pulmonary artery is transected at the bifurcation with a slight oblique cut into the left pulmonary artery. The main PA is posteriorly completely separated from the left main coronary artery which is probed to allow proper visualisation. The right ventricular infundibulum is incised transversely 5–6 mm from the pulmonary valve anulus. The excision of the pulmonary root is completed by respecting this distance except in the area of the left anterior descending coronary artery and its first septal branch where the transection is kept close to the pulmonary annulus.

After resection of eventual residual subvalvular tissue the interventricular septum is incised starting at the commissure between the right and left aortic cusp. The septal incision is continued into the infundibular septum as far to the left as possible to avoid the conduction mechanism. The length of the incision depends on the severity of the LVOTO and the size of the native pulmonary valve annulus, which is always much larger than the hypoplastic aortic annulus. Sometimes an aberrant left ventricular tendon inserting in the interventricular septum is recognized (two patients). This tendon should be resected as it might be partially responsible for recurrence of the subvalvular stenosis (8). The margins of the septal incision are bevelled on the left ventricular side to further widen the LV outflow tract.

The LV outflow tract is widened with a triangular Dacron (first 10 patients) or a pericardial patch (last four patients), sewn with a monofilament suture placed at the right ventricular side without the use of Teflon pledgets (Fig. 1).

Then the proximal anastomosis of the pulmonary autograft is begun posteriorly in the aortic annulus with a running monofilament suture. Anteriorly, the autograft is sutured to the Dacron patch. The orientation of the autograft is not important since the site of implantation of the coronary arteries can easily be readjusted. The coronary arteries are implanted in the autograft with 6-0 prolene running sutures at a punch hole made with a number 5.5 aortic punch.

An antibiotic-sterilized cryopreserved pulmonary (11 patients) or an aortic homograft (three patients) is anastomosed distally to the pulmonary bifurcation with a running monofilament suture. The proximal anastomosis starts at the most dorsal aspect of the right ventricle. To the left it stays proximal to the first septal coronary artery; to the right it runs over the base of the autograft to the infundibulum to meet the other end of the running monofilament suture. Since the right ventricular outflow tract (RVOT) is also widened by the Dacron patch, an oversized large pulmonary homograft or an aortic homograft with its mitral septal attachment is used to reconstruct the RV outflow tract. Finally, the distal anastomosis between autograft and aorta is made. The distal native aorta is eventually enlarged (four patients) with pieces of aortic wall obtained at the resection of the native aortic root or with autologous or xenopericardium.

All the anastomoses are sealed with fibrin glue (Tissucol Immuno AG, Vienna, Austria). Cardiopulmonary bypass is discontinued in the usual way. The pericardium is closed with a Gore-Tex surgical membrane to facilitate later eventual sternal re-entry.

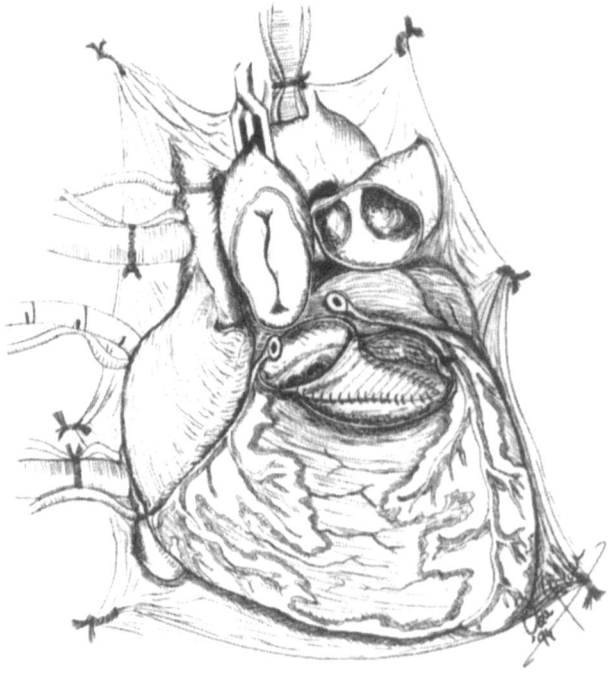

Fig. 1. The aortic and pulmonary roots have been excised. The LVOT is widened with a triangular Dacron patch placed in the infundibular septum.

Results

All patients except one were easily weaned from cardiopulmonary bypass (CPB). This patient was put on a left ventricular assist device (LVAD) because of severe myocardial stunning. Ventricular function did not recover in the next following days. On day five he underwent a heart transplantation. Unfortunately, he suffered from a massive air embolus during the switch from LVAD to CPB. The patient died on day 7 after discontinuation of all supportive treatment. Microscopic examination of the explanted heart revealed an impressive myocardial hypertrophy and fibrosis.

Table 2. Echo-Doppler data in the group with subvalvular aortic stenosis

Patient	Age (years)	ΔP (mmHg)	Minimal LVOT diameter (% of BSA)	
			Preop	Postop
MN	14	170	59	104
CvA	12	98	53	96
LS	11	140	53	98
UG	18	98	73	107
DK	13	56	48	92
BK	5	100	39	123
VS	26	84	39	95
PI	23	90	44	90
SL	2.5	120	45	123

Legend: LVOT: left ventricle outflow tract, BSA: body surface area, ΔP: systolic gradient.

Table 3. Change in minimal LVOT diameter (% of BSA) in group with subvalvular aortic stenosis

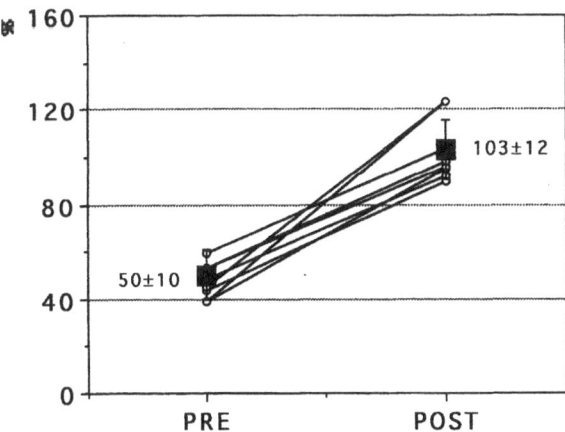

Legend: LVOT: left ventricle outflow tract, BSA: body surface aera.

The mean aortic cross-clamp time was 145 min, reflecting the magnitude of the correction. No anticoagulant therapy was used. Two patients developed surgical heart block: the first patient converted spontaneously to sinus rhyhtm after 2 weeks, the second developed permanent heart block because of a septal infarction and secondary transient tricuspid regurgitation.

One patient remained in congestive heart failure and died suddenly after 17 months. All other patients are in NYHA class I after a mean follow-up of 20 ± 12 months.

Table 2 demonstrates the marked increase of the preoperative minimal LVOT diameter (expressed in percent of body surface area), measured by echocardiogram in the nine patients operated because of redo-subvalvular aortic stenosis. The minimal LVOTO increased from a mean of 50% preoperatively to a mean of 103% postoperatively (Table 3).

In the five patients operated because of an outgrown small aortic valve prosthesis it was possible to increase the annulus by two (three patients) or three sizes (two patients) (Table 4).

All patients presented laminar flow at the level of the reconstruction and complete absence of any LVOT gradient (Table 5). Five patients presented a grade 2/4 aortic regurgitation at their sequential follow-ups. These regurgitations were not evolutive and caused no clinical symptoms. Table 5 also depicts the excellent function of the homograft implanted on the right site.

Table 4. Increase in annular size after redo-valvular replacement

Patient	Indication	Type	Aortic prosth. size (mm)	Pulmonary autograft size (mm)
JP	Δ80 mmHg	BS	19	25
OG	Degeneration	IS	19	23
MP	Δ100 mmHg	BS	19	23
BG	Δ60 mmHg	BS	19	25
SI	Δ120 mmHg	SJM	19	23

Legend: SJM: Saint Jude Medical; BS: Björk-Shiley; IS: Ionescu-Shiley, Δ: systolic gradient.

Table 5. Function auto- and homograft at last follow-up* (Echo-Doppler data)

		Autograft n	Homograft n
Gradient (mmHg)	0	12	5
	1–10	–	3
	10–30	–	3
	Unknown	–	1
Leakage (score 0–4)	0/4	2	1
	1/4	5	10
	2/4	5	–
	Unknown	–	1

* Mean follow-up: 20 ± 12 months.

Discussion

Complex tunnel subvalvular aortic stenosis remains a challenging surgical problem, especially in reoperative surgery. The nine cases with important residual post-operative gradients reported here, prove that the classical membrane resection with or without myectomy is not always sufficient.

Myectomy with or without patch enlargement of the interventricular septum with or without reconstruction of the aortic annulus (2, 19) is only possible in those rare cases where the aortic valve and aortic annulus are morphologically normal.

More radical procedures with aortic valve replacements (3, 9, 10, 14) appear to be more appropriate but have the disadvantages of tissue degeneration (bioprostheses), thrombo-embolic phenomena (mechanical valve prostheses) and lack of growth capacity in small children (5, 12, 17, 18). Aortic root replacement (ARR) with an aortic homograft (6, 16) partially solves the problem of degeneration but cannot relieve the long tunnel-like obstructions. The extended aortic root replacement (13) makes a complete relief of obstructions extending deep into the LVOTO possible. However, it remains questionable whether these homografts will offer a final solution to children, despite the excellent intermediate term results of cryopreserved aortic homografts used as root replacements in adults and older children (6, 7, 15, 20).

Autograft pulmonary valves for aortic valve replacement have proved to be superior to aortic homografts (7). Therefore, we combined the concepts of extended aortic root replacement and the use of pulmonary autografts. This might be a more durable solution in children. The application of this concept in very young children and babies is also attractive since it has been shown that these autografts have growth capacity (6, 21–23).

Extended root replacement is the procedure of choice in those reoperations where the tunnel LVOTO is due to long-standing turbulence caused by an aberrant tendon or fibrous bands inserting low in the interventricular septum (8). If this concept is valid it might be possible to obviate recurrences observed after more classical operations as long as this cause of turbulence is also resected during the primary correction. We feel that streamlining the LVOTO is important, as turbulence may not only cause recurrence of the subvalvular aortic stenosis, but also jeopardise the longevity of the autograft. In every patient where a tendon or a ridge was identified as a cause of subaoritc turbulence, we attempted to visualise this lesion. This would not have been possible after a classical resection of the subvalvular stenosis; only after incising the interventricular septum could these structures be identified and resected.

One patient in this series developed a septal infarction and temporary secondary tricuspid regurgitation. An important first septal artery was identified at operation. We felt however that it was necessary to divide this coronary artery in order to be able to make a sufficiently wide enlargement of the interventricular septum. Fortunately, this patient survived the operation and has normal documented right and left ventricular contractility on echocardiography. Nevertheless, we recommend a coronarography preoperatively to assess the importance of the first septal coronary branches.

The concept of this operation can also be applied to replacement of a too small, outgrown aortic valve prosthesis. A classical root replacement is often not effective because of the marked septal hypertrophy and secondary dynamic obstruction.

The short-term results of this EARR with pulmonary autografts seem to be very gratifying. The use of autografts in the subcoronary position is obviously technically more demanding in children and more prone to regurgitation. Therefore, we abandoned this technique and currently exclusively use aortic root replacement as well with aortic homografts as with autografts. It has been shown that tissue failure following ARR with aortic homografts is less likely than when homografts are implanted in the subcoronary position (20). It might, however, be erroneous to conclude that this will also be the case for ARR with pulmonary autografts. Long-standing pulmonary hypertension at systemic pressure level can cause pulmonary regurgitation of the native pulmonary valve. Therefore, longer follow-up than reported here is needed to ascertain whether late aortic regurgitation will occur. Several authors have published excellent results in this respect (21–23). The excellent long-term performance of the neo-aortic valve after the switch operation for transposition of the great arteries is also very promising.

Other drawbacks of EARR with pulmonary autograft are the technical difficulties encountered at primary repair and certainly at eventual reoperation. Only centers familiar with the use of homo- and/or autografts in correction of congenital heart disease in children should undertake this type of correction. Reoperation for autograft failure might be a problem but has been performed with low morbidity and mortality (11). Endocarditis prophylaxis should be maintained after autograft replacements since a certain risk of endocarditis persists (7). Excellent results however have been reported after pulmonary autograft replacement for native and/or prosthetic valve endocarditis (24).

Finally, one should realize that this operation is a double valve replacement with two valves (one autograft and one homograft) at risk during follow-up.

Conclusions

1) EARR with pulmonary autograft might be a more durable (definitive?) solution for the correction of complex tunnel subvalvular aortic stenosis than the classical Konno operation or even the EARR with cryopreserved aortic homografts.

2) This operation is very attractive for the correction of this lesion in the very young, since growth capacity of the autograft has been documented.

3) Aortic incompetence might become a problem if the neo-aortic root dilates. The short-term results however are very encouraging.

4) The surgical complexity of this operation should not discourage its use in the management of this difficult lesion.

References

1. Brown JW, Girod DA, Hurwitz RA, Caldwell RL, Rocchini AP, Behrendt DM, Kirsch MM (1984) Apicoaortic valved conduits for complex left ventricular outflow obstruction: technical considerations and current status. Ann Thorac Surg 38: 162–168
2. DeLeon SY, Ilbawi MN, Roberson DA, Arcilla RA, Thilenius OG, Wilson WR, Duffy EC, Quinones JA (1991) Conal enlargement for diffuse subaortic stenosis. J Thorac Cardiovasc Surg 102: 814–820
3. de Vivie ER, Koncz J, Rupprath G, Vogt J, Beuren AJ (1982) Aortoventriculoplasty for different types of left ventricular outflow obstructions. J Cardiovasc Surg 23: 6–11
4. DiDonato RM, Danielson GK, McGoon DC, Driscoll DJ, Julsrud PR, Edwards WD (1984) Left ventricular-aortic conduits in pediatric patients. J Thorac Cardiovasc Surg 88: 82–91

5. Fleming WH, Sarafian LB (1987) Aortic valve replacement with concomitant aortoventriculo-plasty in children and young adults. Ann Thorac Surg 43: 575–578
6. Gerosa G, McKay R, Ross DN (1951) Replacement of the aortic valve or root with a pulmonary autograft in children. Ann Thorac Surg 51: 424–429
7. Gerosa G, McKay R, Davies, J, Ross DN (1991) Comparison of the aortic homograft and the pulmonary autograft for aortic valve or root replacement in children. J Thorac Cardiovasc Surg 02: 51–61
8. Gewillig M, Daenen W, Dumoulin M, Van der Hauwaert L (1992) Rheologic genesis of discrete subvalvular aortic stenosis: A Doppler Echocardiographic study. J Am Col Cardiol 19: 818–824
9. Konno S, Imai Y, Iida Y, Nakajima M, Tatsuno K (1975) A new method for prosthetic valve replacement in congenital aortic stenosis associated with hypoplasia of the aortic valve ring. J Thorac Cardiovasc Surg 70: 909–917
10. Koul BL, Henze A, Björk VO (1984) Aortoventriculoplasty ad modum Konno. Experience with five cases. Scand J Thorac Cardiovasc Surg 18: 239–242
11. Matsuki O, Okita Y, Almeida RS, McGoldrick JP, Hooper TL, Robles A, Ross DN (1988) Two decades' experience with aortic valve replacement with pulmonary autograft. J Thorac Cardiovasc Surg 95: 705–711
12. McIntyre B, Guyton RA, Jones EL, Graver JM, Williams WH, Hatcher CR Jr (1986) Reoperation for prosthetic valve degeneration after Konno aortoventriculoplasty. J Thorac Cardiovasc Surg 91: 934–936
13. McKowen RL, Campbell DN, Woelfel GF, Wiggins JW, Clarke DR (1987) Extended aortic root replacement with aortic allografts. J Thorac Cardiovasc Surg 93: 366–374
14. Misbach GA, Turley K, Ullyot DJ, Ebert PA (1982) Left ventricular outflow enlargement by the Konno procedure. J Thorac Cardiovasc Surg 84: 696–703
15. Randolph JD, Toal K, Stelzer P, Elkins RC (1989) Aortic valve and left ventricular outflow tract replacement using allograft and autograft valves: a preliminary report. Ann Thorac Surg 48: 345–349
16. Ross DN (1967) Replacement of aortic and mitral valves with a pulmonary autograft. Lancet 2(523): 956–958
17. Terada M, Imai Y, Kurosawa H, Kawada M, Nakazawa M, Satomi G (1990) Left ventricular function after Konno procedure for congenital aortic stenosis. Nippon Kyobu Geka Gakkai Zasshi 38: 201–206
18. Vogt J, de Vivie ER, Koncz J, Beuren AJ (1986) Haemodynamic and echocardiographic findings after aortoventriculoplasty. Eur Heart J 7: 501–508
19. Vouhe PR, Poulain H, Bloch G, Loisance DY, Gamain J, Lombaert M, Quiret JC, Lesbre JP, Bernasconi P, Pietri J (1984) Aortoseptal approach for optimal resection of diffuse subvalvular aortic stenosis. J Thorac Cardiovasc Surg 87: 887–893
20. Yacoub M, Personal communication. 2nd International Live Teleconference on homograft and autograft implantation. London-Harefield, UK, October 26–28, 1991
21. Elkins CE, Knott-Craig CJ, Ward KE, McCue C, Lane MM (1994) Pulmonary autograft in children: realized growth potential. Ann Thorac Surg 57: 1387–94
22. Schoof PH, Cromme-Dijkhuis AH, Bogers JJ, Thijssen EJ, Witsenburg M, Hess J, Bos E (1994) Aortic root replacement with pulmonary autograft in children. J Thorac Cardiovasc Surg 107: 367–73
23. Quaegebeur JM, Solowiejczyk D, Hus D, Bourlon F, Hess J, Gersony W, Personal communication. 73rd Annual Meeting AATS, New York, April 25–27, 1994
24. Oswalt JD, Dewan SJ (1993) Aortic infective endocarditis managed by the Ross procedure. J Heart Valve Dis 2: 380–4

Author's address:
W. Daenen, MD, PhD
Department of Cardiac Surgery
University Hospital Gasthusberg
3000 Leuven, Belgium

Pulmonary autograft: "Valve of choice" for aortic infective endocarditis?

J. D. Oswalt

Cardiothoracic and Vascular Surgeons, Austin, Texas, USA

Introduction

Current literature recommends the use of an aortic homograft for replacement of the aortic valve when involved with an infective process (12, 2). Some attributes of the aortic homograft include its pliable annulus, allowing for molding to an irregular annulus destroyed by abscess. With increased resistance to infection, as suggested by Kirklin and Barratt-Boyes (8), the homograft has a relative "safe" post-implantation period against re-infection. The anterior mitral leaflet which accompanies the valve can be used as patch material when repairing annular discrepancies caused by annular abscesses.

The pulmonary autograft has similar attributes and more. It is completely viable which should allow growth if needed in a pediatric-age patient. It is more supple and easier to handle than the homograft, and by harvesting more of the muscular pulmonary outflow tract beneath the annulus of the autograft, one can use the added length to fill annular discrepancies or patch fistulae. It also is resistant to infection since the valve can be permeated by systemic antibiotics administered preoperatively. The living tissue or leaflets continue to absorb antibiotics provided via the blood stream through the normal pathways.

Recognizing the attributes of the pulmonary autograft plus knowing that all infected areas heal best following complete debridement and replacement or supplement with viable tissue, we chose the autograft as our valve of choice in the management of aortic infective endocarditis.

Materials and methods

Since April 1990, 31 consecutive patients with aortic endocarditis have been managed by root replacement of the aortic valve using the pulmonary autograft (Ross Procedure). There were 26 (84%) males and five (16%) females ranging in ages from 19 to 62, mean 39 years. Six percent (two patients) were in New York Heart Association Class II, sixty-eight percent (21 patients) were in NYHA Class III, and 21% (six patients) in Class IV. All patients except one had severe aortic regurgitation at the time of surgery; that patient had severe aortic stenosis. Seventy-one percent had active vegetations with continuing positive blood cultures at the time of surgery. Six (21%) patients had annular abscesses. One had a ventriculoaortic disconnection

Table 1. Clinical summary of patients

Age	Sex	Organism	Infection	Pre-op complication
29	M	Enterococcus	Active	–
53	M	S. viridans	Active	–
34	F	S. viridans	Inactive	–
32	M	Unknown	Inactive	–
58	M	S. viridans	Active	–
23	M	S. viridans	Active	–
32	M	S. aureus Enterococcus	Active	–
39	M	S. viridans	Active	–
50	M	Enterococcus	Active	
39	M	S. viridans	Inactive	Stroke/Speech
61	M	S. bovis	Active	> P-R Interval
59	M	S. viridans	Active	–
31	M	S. viridans	Active	Previous free hand homograft
53	M	Unknown	Inactive	–
46	M	S. aureus	Active	Peripheral emboli
37	M	S. aureus C. albicans	Active	–
34	F	Unknown	Inactive	–
31	F	Grp B Strep galactica	Active	Hypotensive Pulm Edema Sepsis
38	M	S. aureus	Active	Sepsis
32	M	H. influenzae	Active	–
33	F	Brucellosis	Active	CHF
28	M	S. viridans	Inactive	Cerebral emboli with seizures
27	M	S. aureus	Active	–
38	M	S. viridans	Active	–
19	M	S. viridans	Inactive	–
27	M	S. aureus S. viridans	Inactive	–
39	M	S. viridans	Active	–
31	M	Enterococcus	Active	–
39	M	S. viridans	Active	–
54	M	Alpha strep	Inactive	–
50	F	Enterococcus	Active	End Stage Renal Dialysis

secondary to the abscesses. One patient had an aorto-right atrial fistula which caused florid pulmonary edema and shock, and one had infection and abscess in a previously placed aortic homograft. Four patients suffered emboli pre-operatively, three with neurological injury and one with a peripheral embolus requiring embolectomy of the brachial artery the night prior to his root replacement (Table 1).

The diagnosis was based on clinical and laboratory data including cardiac murmur, systemic embolization, blood cultures, Doppler echocardiography and in two cases cardiac catheterization with angiography. All patients were on appropriate intravenous antibiotics prior to surgery.

Surgical technique

All operations performed used transesophageal echocardiography for initial evaluation and postoperative evaluation of the valve. Systemic cooling to 30 °C was achieved via single two-staged venous cannula and ascending aortic return. Cardiac protection was achieved in early years with cold-oxygenated crystalloid cardioplegia and more recently with antegrade and retrograde cold blood cardioplegia. The Ross procedure has been previously described (14, 15), but we include our modifications which we feel have shortened our cross-clamp times and added to our success. Initially, the autograft is harvested as a root with a cuff of ventricular myocardium. More muscle can be harvested if the TEE shows an extensive annular abscess. The autograft is preserved in fresh blood, usually in the pericardial cavity, and the pulmonary outflow tract is then reconstructed using a freshly-thawed pulmonary homograft. No aortic homografts have been used. This early reconstruction allows for two things: avoidance of air-locks in the venous drainage system of CPB, and protection of the RVOT from exposure to the infected area of the aortic root. A running polypropylene suture is used both proximally and distally.

The aortotomy is then performed in a transverse fashion just above the sino-tubular junction and complete resection of the valve and root is accomplished. The coronary ostia are left as buttons or the left coronary ostia can remain attached to the ascending aorta as a tongue. All infected material is debrided to viable tissue and the area is irrigated clean. Reconstruction is accomplished using a triangulated running polypropylene suture. The autograft root is sewn intra-annular or below to left ventricular muscle if abscesses are present. It is important to sew to viable non-infected tissue. This suture-line is bolstered with a strip of autologous pericardium placed as a ring within the initial triangulating sutures. Also important is maintaining a plane for the insertion of this new annulus to allow for maximum coaptation of leaflets. The left coronary ostial button can then be inserted or if left on a tongue of aorta, the new left coronary sinus is excised to match the tongue so as not to enlarge the sino-tubular junction. The distal anastomosis is then performed with running polypropylene suture. Prior to completion of this anastamosis, the two commissural posts of the right sinus are identified externally on the autograft so as not to injure them with re-implantation of the right coronary button. The right coronary ostium is then anastamosed again with polypropylene suture. Cross-clamp times ranged from 65 to 151 min (average cross-clamp 84 min). Post cross-clamp TEE examination of the valves can be performed. No patient has been anticoagulated postoperatively.

Results

All 31 patients initially were cured of their infections by the end of their antibiotic therapy. Antibiotics were administered for 3 to 6 weeks, depending on culture results at the time of surgery. If the culture was negative on tissue submitted at surgery, the shorter course was chosen. Subsequent to cessation of antibiotics, follow-up has been 71% from 1 month to 5 years (mean 24 months). There was no operative mortality (30 days). There has been one recurrence of endocarditis and this occurred 5 years postoperatively. It should be noted that this patient was HIV positive and was an IV

OPERATIVE MORBIDITY

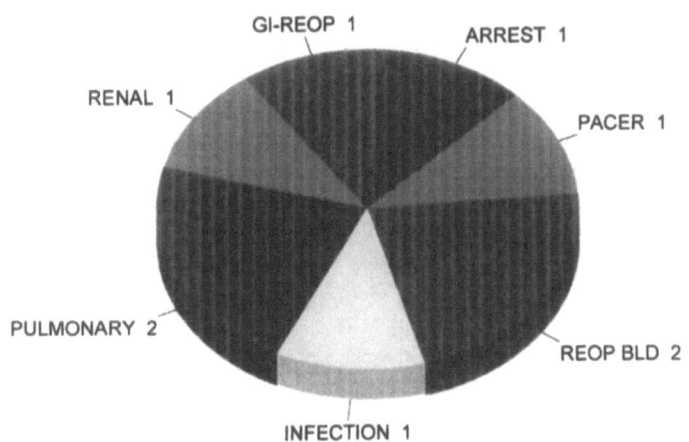

Fig. 1.

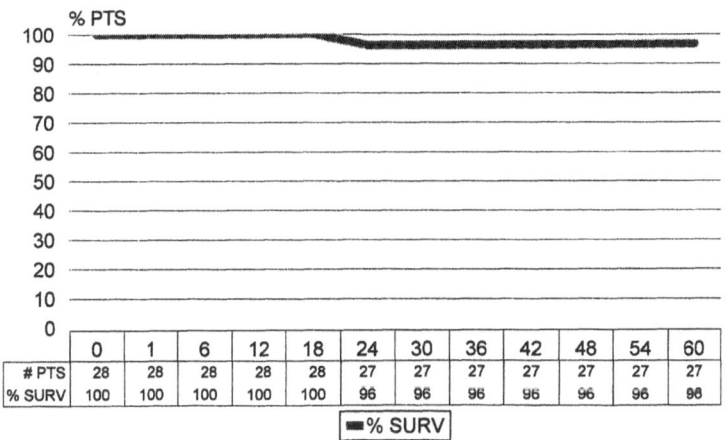

Fig. 2.

drug abuser at the time of his first endocarditis. He now has clinical AIDS and continues his IV drug use. All patients are in NYHA Class I. Doppler echocardiography shows 13 patients (42%) with trivial to no aortic regurgitation, four patients (13%) have mild regurgitation, two patients (6%) have moderate regurgitation, and one patient (3%) had severe aortic regurgitation.

Post-operative complications have occurred in 17% (Fig. 1), one of which was complete heart block (patient with the ventriculo-aortic disconnection) requiring a permanent pacemaker. Post-operative bleeding occurred in two patients. One patient also required later re-operation for a false aneurysm at the proximal aortic anastamosis. Tissue from this area grew Candida. The patient was placed on anti-fungal agents and his autograft continues to function well at 21 months post-op.

The other patient had bleeding from the aortic distal anastomosis and this was repaired with no complications. The fourth patient had post-op cardiac arrest due to hyperkalemia with subsequent renal failure requiring dialysis, small bowel infarction requiring resection, respiratory failure requiring intubation, and Candida septicemia without re-infection of his new valves. There has been one late death from pulmonary complications. Actuarial survival at 5 years by Kaplan–Meier is 93.7% (Fig. 2). Freedom from endocarditis is 97%. Thromboembolic events have not been seen in late follow-up and no patient is on anticoagulation with the exception of the 2 patients with mechanical prostheses. The mean length of stay postoperatively was 8.8 days, range 3 days to 36 days. Of note, one patient left the hospital against medical advice on the fifth postoperative day without antibiotics. He has since returned to follow-up without recurrence of his infection.

Discussion

Since the 1964 and 1965 reports of Dr Yeh and Dr. Wallace (19, 16), aortic infective endocarditis is most commonly managed surgically by valve replacement. For approximately 20 years, the valve of choice was a mechanical valve. Kirklin and Barratt-Boyes (8) in 1986 suggested that the aortic homograft may be the valve of choice for infective endocarditis. Support for this is seen in articles by Tuna and Okita (11, 15) separately reporting the use of the aortic homograft for endocarditis. Donaldson, Lau and Farnsworth (2, 3, 10) likewise report on homograft use for prosthetic valve endocarditis. Recently, Petrou (12) reported on 48 patients with prosthetic endocarditis – all replaced with a homograft, 19 root, 29 free-hand, with an 8.3% early death rate, 20% complication rate and a mean length of stay of 23 days. James Kirklin (9) in his support of the homograft had 22 patients with native or prosthetic valve endocarditis with good results in the 11 surviving patients. He believes that subcoronary, inclusion technique, or root replacement with the homograft are all acceptable. In two large series, multiple valves were used and reported. Haydock (5) had 108 patients, sixty-six native and 42 prosthetic. Seventy-eight were replaced with a homograft (free-hand and root) and 30 replaced with a mechanical or xenograft valve. Operative mortality was 16% and 20% with the homograft and mechanical/xenograft respectively. Recurrent endocarditis occurred in 13%, all free-hand homografts. The other report by Aranki (1), a 20-year review with a predominance of porcine valves, showed a 7.5% mortality in the native valve endocarditis.

Considering the recommendations to use the aortic homograft and the pulmonary autograft having similar attributes, we chose the autograft as our valve of choice to manage active endocarditis.

A major factor influencing this decision was the fact that we would be implanting a truly viable heart valve. Not only would it be viable, but it would be totally permeated with antibiotic solution from the systemic administration of antibiotics preoperatively. Its use would be consistent with the surgical practice of placing viable tissue perfused with antibiotics in the area of infection to achieve improved healing.

In keeping with the homograft, the autograft's pliability is beneficial in the proximal anastomosis. A rigid ring creates more stress for potential dehiscence in the less than ideal tissue seen with endocarditis. This was particularly useful in the patient with ventriculo-aortic disconnection where the autograft muscular ring was anastamosed directly to the left ventricular muscle and edge of mitral leaflet. The flexibility still allowed for coaptation of the leaflets and a competent valve.

A comparison of our series with that of other institutions would not be scientific. But without a prospective single institute study, some inferences can be made. The autograft has excellent results not only in curing the infection but in survivability. The complications appear to be as low or lower and the length of stay is improved. This last observation may not be totally comparable as this series occurred when LOS is a more important issue in today's healthcare picture. Nonetheless, the LOS remains quite short and acceptable. We believe a strong factor in our short LOS and diminished pre- and post-op complications is that the decision to perform surgery is made early. Long-term antibiotics or sterilization are not necessary and delays may only allow for further destruction of the aortic annulus or embolization. The key factor in the decision process is not the infection but the valve. If the valve will require replacement, then all that is necessary is adequate antibiotic coverage to achieve tissue levels. Surgery should then be performed. If the valve is not insufficient or diseased enough to warrant replacement, then, medical therapy should be continued.

Some technical features should be mentioned in relation to this valve and the operative technique involving endocarditis. The excellent results shown in Ralph-Edwards (13) paper presenting extremely difficult cases of infected, previously-replaced aortic roots, were based on meticulous debridement and accurate repair of all tissues in the surrounding outflow tract. Also, the type of prosthesis used in repair was found not to be significant. All patients did require surgical management. In our experience, we also believe the first technical principle is debridement. In addition, we believe the autograft is superior because many of the defects can be repaired or excluded while replacing the root. This allows for no foreign material in the infected area. Likewise, we feel the replacement should be a root replacement, not as an inclusion or free-hand sub-coronary valve. Aortic endocarditis is an infection of the leaflets with or without extension into the annulus and surrounding structures. To replace the leaflets with a sub-coronary or inclusion root autograft does not allow for complete debridement or exteriorization of the infection. Thus, they may form a closed area between inclusion wall and the aorta or the non-coronary sinus and aorta in the sub-coronary technique.

Concern about this technique being a double valve replacement has been raised on two accounts. One, that increased length of operative time is required. We have found that with standardization of technique these times have not been excessive. With the myocardial protection techniques now available the ischemic times are certainly acceptable. Two, this procedure places the pulmonary homograft and RVOT at risk of infection. We have not experienced any difficulty with new infection. Perhaps this area remains protected since we totally reconstruct the RVOT prior to opening the aorta. Certainly, the pulmonary homograft *not* implanted in the infected area has less chance of new infection than an aortic homograft placed *in* the infected area. (*Vis-a-vis* the recommendation to use an aortic homograft as the valve of choice).

Other authors find agreement with our ideology and technique. Joyce (7) has reported a series, initially of six patients, but larger now, managing them with auto-graft root replacement. They also show no mortality, no re-infection, and no late deaths. Yankah (17) has found little difference between homograft or autograft but points out increased availability of the pulmonary homograft. One last favorable point for the autograft is that it is likely a permanent valve as supported by Mr. Ross' data (4).

In summary, we believe from our data and by inferring comparison with other valves in similar clinical settings, the pulmonary autograft may be the valve of choice for the treatment of aortic infective endocarditis. We are convinced that it is the solution to the dilemma described by Dr. Hufnagel (6) in *Surgical Techniques in the Treatment of Infected Valvular Prostheses.*

"One of the first recognized principles in the surgical approach to infections is that they must be adequately drained and that no foreign materials may be left in the infected areas. However, within the heart and aortic root the problems of drainage in unhealed and unsterilized abscess areas are quite different; the methods required for valvular implantation require the insertion of some foreign material, whether it be a prosthesis, homograft or xenograft".

References

1. Aranki S, Santini F, Adams DH, Rizzo RJ, Couper GS, Kinchla NM, Gildea JS, Collins JJ, Cohn LH (1994) Aortic valve endocarditis: determinants of early survival and late morbidity. Circulation 90 [part 2]: II-175–II-182
2. Donaldson RM, Ross DN (1982) Homograft replacement of the aortic root replacement for complicated prosthetic valve endocarditis. Circulation 70 [part 2]: IL 78–82
3. Farnsworth AE (1993) Homograft aortic root replacement for destructive prosthetic endocarditis. Annals of Thoracic Surgery 55: 386–388
4. Gerosa G, McKay R, Davies J, Ross DN (1991) Comparison of the aortic homograft and the pulmonary autograft for aortic valve or aortic root replacement in children. J Thorac Cardiovasc Surg 102: 51–61
5. Haydock D, Barratt-Boyes B, Macedo T, Kirklin JW, Blackstone E (1992) Aortic valve replacement for active infectious endocarditis in 108 patients. J Thorac Cardiovasc Surg 103: 130–139
6. Hufnagel CA (1977) Surgical techniques in the treatment of infected valvular prosthesis. University Park Press, Baltimore, pp 143–160
7. Joyce F, Tingleff J, Aagaard J, Pettersson G (1994) The Ross operation in the treatment of native and prosthetic aortic valve endocarditis. Journal of Heart Valve Disease 3: 371–376
8. Kirklin JW, Barratt-Boyes BG (1986) Aortic valve disease. In: Kirklin JW, Barratt-Boyes BG (eds) Cardiac Surgery. John Wiley and Sons, New York pp 373–429
9. Kirklin JK, Pacifico AD, Kirklin JW (1989) Surgical treatment of prosthetic valve endocarditis with homograft aortic valve replacement. Journal of Cardiac Surgery Vol. 4, No. 4
10. Lau JKH, Robles A, Cherian A, Ross DN (1984) Surgical treatment of prosthetic endocarditis: aortic root replacement using a homograft. J Thorac Cardiovasc Surg 87: 712–716
11. Okita Y, Franciosi G, Matsuki O, Robles A, Ross DN (1988) Early and late results of aortic root replacement with antibiotic-sterilized aortic homografts. J Thorac Cardiovasc Surg 95: 696–704
12. Petrou M, Wong K, Albertucci M, Brecker SJ, Yacoub MH (1994) Evaluation of unstented aortic homografts for the treatment of prosthetic aortic valve endocarditis. Circulation 90 [part 2]: II-198–II-204
13. Ralph-Edwards A, Tirone DE, Bos J (1994) Infective endocarditis in patients who had replacement of the aortic root. Annals of Thoracic Surgery 58: 429–433
14. Stelzer P, Jones DJ, Elkins RC (1989) Aortic root replacement for pulmonary autograft. circulation 80 [part 2]: III-209–213
15. Tuna IC, Orszulak TA, Schaff HV, Danielson GK (1990) Results of homograft aortic valve replacement for active endocarditis. Annals of Thoracic Surgery 49: 619–624
16. Wallace AG, Young WG, Osterhout S (1965) Treatment of acute bacterial endocarditis by valve excision and replacement. Circulation 31: 450–453
17. Yankah AC (1994) Surgical management of infective endocarditis: pulmonary autograft or allograft? Journal of Heart Valve Disease 3: 380–383
18. Yeh TJ, Hall D, Ellison RG (1964) Surgical treatment of aortic valve perforation due to bacterial endocarditis. Annals of Thoracic Surgery 30: 766–769
19. Zwischenbrewer JB, Tarec ZS, Conti VR (1989) Viable cryopreserved aortic homograft for aortic valve endocarditis and annular abscess. Annals of Thoracic Surgery 48: 365–370

Author's address:
J. D. Oswalt, MD
Cardiothoracic and Vascular Surgeons,
1010 W. 40th Street,
Austin, Texas 78756, USA

Treatment of aortic valve endocarditis with the Ross operation

F. Joyce, J. Tingleff, G. Pettersson

The Department of Cardiothoracic Surgery, The National University Hospital –
Rigshospitalet, Copenhagen, Denmark

Introduction

Eradication of advanced endocarditis requires complete debridement of all infected
and non-viable tissue and successful reconstruction of the heart. Many treatment
strategies have been proposed, but because of the relatively small number of patients
in each series and the large number of variables, it is virtually impossible to make
a strict scientific evaluation of the alternatives, nor can help be expected from
prospective, randomized trials in the future. Deciding on a treatment strategy can, in
and of itself, be difficult, but thought must be followed by action, and the surgical
challenge in these patients is often extreme.

Homograft root replacement has become an increasingly popular treatment modal-
ity for these patients and is considered treatment-of-choice by many (8, 14, 17, 25).
Good results have been obtained, but the homograft has limited durability and other
drawbacks, and is, therefore, a less-than-perfect solution. Good results have also been
reported with the composite graft (4), but it, too, has a number of drawbacks. Our
view on the strengths and weaknesses of the different treatment alternatives are
summarized in Table 1.

The Copenhagen experience with the Ross operation for aortic valve endocarditis
began in December, 1992 and was motivated by a number of theoretical considerations which will be elaborated on below. So far, our hopes and expectations have
been fulfilled, and as our experience grows, we are becoming more and more confident
that the Ross operation will play an increasing role in the treatment of these patients
and possibly emerge as treatment-of-choice (10, 11, 12, 19, 26).

Patient population

Since December, 1992, 67 patients have undergone a Ross operation. Eighteen of
these had aortic valve endocarditis. Twelve patients had active endocarditis with an
isolated bacteria at the time of, or just prior to, their operation. Six patients were
operated because of sequelae to an earlier endocarditis (culture positive) (four patients) or a suspected earlier endocarditis (culture negative) (two patients). Seventeen
patients had advanced pathology, defined as pathology secondary to proven or
suspected endocarditis with extension beyond the aortic valve cusps. Ten patients
(56%) had undergone from one to four previous heart operations. Eight of these had

Table 1. Strengths and weaknesses of the alternatives for treatment of advanced aortic valve endocarditis.

Treatment modality	Strengths	Weaknesses
Composite graft (mechanical valve and vascular prosthesis)	• Unlimited availability • More familiar procedure for most surgeons • Favorable long-term durability	• Stiff sewing ring may have difficulty seating in abnormal outflow tract tissue and lead to the development of pseudoaneurysms • Higher reinfection frequency, possibly due to harboring of bacteria by sutures, sewing ring, and vascular prosthesis • Requires life-long anticoagulation • Thromboembolic risk • Valve noise • Non-physiologic hemodynamics
Homograft root replacement	• Resistant to early and late infection • Possible advantage of antibiotics used in homograft preparation • Exteriorizes root pathology • Physiologic hemodynamics • Negligible thrombogenicity without anticoagulation • No valve noise	• Limited availability • Not familiar procedure for most surgeons • More difficult procedure than composite graft • Limited durability • Less pliable than the autograft
Aortograft root replacement	• Living tissue • Exteriorizes root pathology • Resistant to early and late infection • Possible advantage of preoperative systemic antibiotics • Delicate, pliable tissue which seats well in abnormal outflow tract tissue and allows safe implantation of pathologic coronary arteries • Improved exposure after aortic root and autograft excision • Favorable long-term durability of autograft • Physiologic hemodynamics • Negligible thrombogenicity without anticoagulation • Growth potential • No valve noise • Makes use of surplus of pulmonary homografts	• Exposes the right side of the heart to infection? • Two-valve instead of one-valve procedure • Performed by a minority of surgeons • More difficult procedure than composite graft or homograft • Limited pulmonary homograft durability, but expected better durability than homograft in aortic position • Limited homograft availability

Table 2. Surgical findings

Pathology	Number of patients
Aortic root pseudoaneurysm	12
Pathology of or around coronary arteries	4
Cusp pathology (vegetations, perforations, calcification)	10
Valve prosthesis	8
Paravalvular leakage	7
Valve leaflet dysfunction	1
Fistula from aortic root to right ventricle and left atrium	1
Perforation of anterior mitral leaflet (jet lesion)	2
Tricuspid valve endocarditis	1

undergone one or more prior aortic valve replacements (one composite graft, one bioprothesis, and six mechanical valve prostheses). Two patients had previously undergone balloon valvuloplasty for congenital aortic stenosis. There were three females and 15 males, median age 29 years, range 10–71 years. Of the 12 patients with active endocarditis, eight had *Streptococcus* and four had *Staphylococcus* endocarditis. *Streptococcus* was isolated from three and *Staphylococcus epidermidis* from one of the six patients with previous confirmed- or suspected endocarditis, while in the remaining two, it was not possible to isolate the causative microorganism. Two patients were intravenous drug abusers.

The pathology observed at operation is presented in Table 2. The most commonly observed pathology was pseudoaneurysm formation, ventriculo-aortic separation, and paravalvular leakage in patients with valve prostheses. One patient had a circular pseudoaneurysm at the orifice of the left coronary artery, and one patient had a fistula between his right coronary artery and a vascular prosthesis after earlier composite graft insertion according to the method of Cabrol (3). Two patients had pseudoaneurysms that partially encircled the left coronary artery. Three patients underwent concomitant procedures (patch repairs of a mitral valve perforations and intracardiac fistulas).

Surgical principles and technique

The following general surgical principles in the management of endocarditis were observed.

1) Aggressive and complete debridement of infected or necrotic tissue;
2) Irrigation with large amounts of saline;
3) Subannular autograft insertion in healthy tissue along the proximal border of debrided cavities (Fig. 1);
4) Strict avoidance of foreign material except for monofilament polypropylene suture material;
5) Culture- and sensitivity-relevant intravenous antibiotics for six weeks after operation, in cases of suspected or verified active endocarditis (but we are considering shortening the length of postoperative antibiotic treatment to 2 weeks).

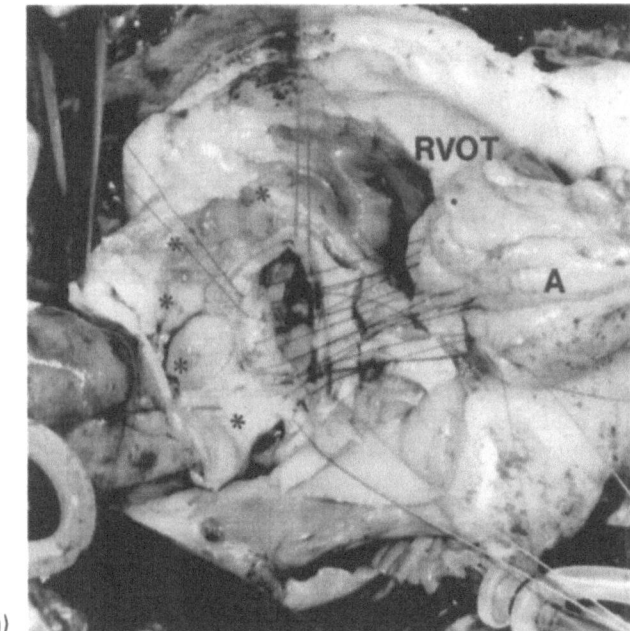

(a)

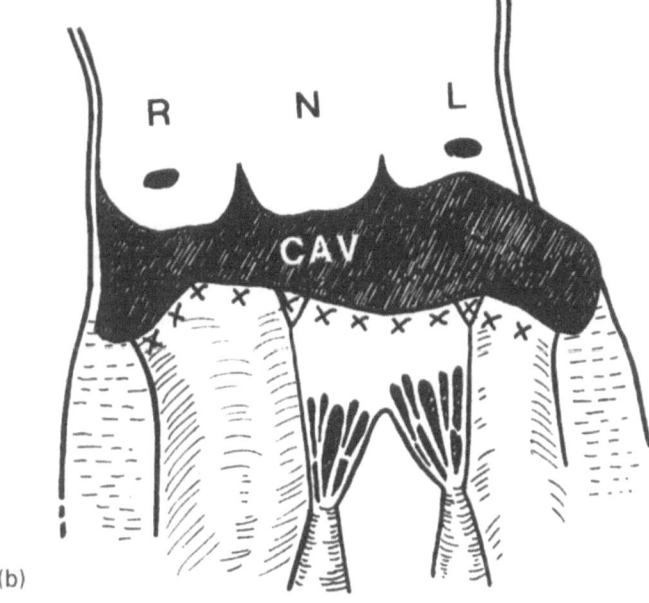

(b)

Fig. 1. After preparation of the aortic root, autograft excision, and debridement of infected tissue, the autograft is inserted deep in the annulus or proximal to the border of debrided cavities. **a)** Here one-third of the suture line between the annulus and the autograft is seen. Notice that the suture line is below the pseudoaneurysm (∗) so that it will exteriorize the pathology when lowered into position. Notice also the lack of substance loss of the outflow tract. RVOT = right ventricular outflow tract. A = autograft. **b)** Schematic drawing of level of proximal suture line (XXX). The fibrous trigones are used as landmarks in autograft orientation. CAV = pseudoaneurysmal cavity which has resulted in ventriculo-aortic separation.

Particularly points 1, 3, and 4 are considered essential, and point 1 most of all. Complete debridement of infected tissue removes the source of reinfection, unless, of course, another focus exists. If residual bacteria contaminate the field, they will be diluted by irrigation and fought off by antibiotics and the patient's immune defense. The logic behind using infection-resistant valve replacements, i.e. the homograft or autograft, is to provide a maximal barrier to reinfection.

All operations were performed through a median sternotomy and on cardiopulmonary bypass (CPB) with systemic temperatures below 30 °C. Two-stage atrial cannulation was standard unless access to the tricuspid or mitral valve was necessary, in which case bi-caval cannulation was performed. Aortic cannulation for arterial return was standard, but in one patient, the femoral artery was used. Myocardial protection was provided by antegrade and retrograde intermittent cold crystalloid cardioplegia. Aorta cross-clamp times ranged from 102–224 min (median 161) and CPB times from 134–302 min (median 209).

All operations were performed as total root replacements with reimplantation of the coronary arteries. The pulmonary valve and artery were reconstructed with a cryopreserved pulmonary homograft in 17 cases and an aortic homograft in one case. The technique of autograft root replacement is well-described elsewhere (11, 12), however, the following principles should be emphasized. The size of the pulmonary valve sinotubular junction is measured before going on CPB. Before autograft harvesting, the aortic root pathology is evaluated and the annulus is sized. A significant size discrepancy exists if the aortic annulus is more than 15–20% larger than the pulmonary artery sino-tubular junction diameter, and the Ross operation is aborted. We evaluate the size of the autograft by the pulmonary artery sino-tubular junction diameter because we have found that this is a more reliable measurement than the diameter of the pulmonary valve at the base of the cusps, the pulmonary equivalent of the aortic annulus. In case of advanced pathology with destruction, abscess, and pseudoaneurysm formation close to the pulmonary artery and valve, it is important to perform the autograft dissection in a very careful and controlled fashion. Although in our experience autograft quality has been good in all cases, infectious or iatrogenic damage of the autograft precluding a Ross operation must be looked for. Autograft removal will further expose the pathology and the left ventricular outflow tract. The surgeon should at this time finalize the debridement and the planning of the reconstruction. The autograft is positioned with 3 mid-cusp stay sutures, one in each fibrous trigone and the third anteriorly. The symmetry of the positioning sutures is controlled with a Plexiglas disk with marks that trisect the circumference of the disk (Toronto SPV sizer). The autograft is usually rotated so that the septal third (the thinnest part) of the valve is positioned anteriorly and to the left, where it is supported by the septal third of the aortic annulus. The autograft is inserted in vital tissue below debrided root pathology, even when it is necessary to insert the valve deep in the left ventricular outflow tract (Fig. 1). Autograft anastomoses are performed with continuous suture technique with monofilament polypropylene interrupted directly below the middle of each cusp. The sutures are placed under direct vision in parachute fashion from mid-cusp to mid-cusp. No felt is used. Finally, the graft is lowered into place and the sutures tightened with gentle traction on each individual throw with a nerve hook. Coronary arteries are implanted into the autograft with continuous 5-0 monofilament polypropylene suture. Both coronary arteries are now inserted as buttons. Early in the series, the left coronary artery was inserted on a tongue attached to the aorta in some cases, but this technique has been abandoned following the experience of early autograft insufficiency in one non-endocarditis case. Homograft reconstruction of the pulmonary artery is performed with running 4-0 monofilament polypropylene suture at each anastomosis. The homograft is aligned in its natural position using the duct

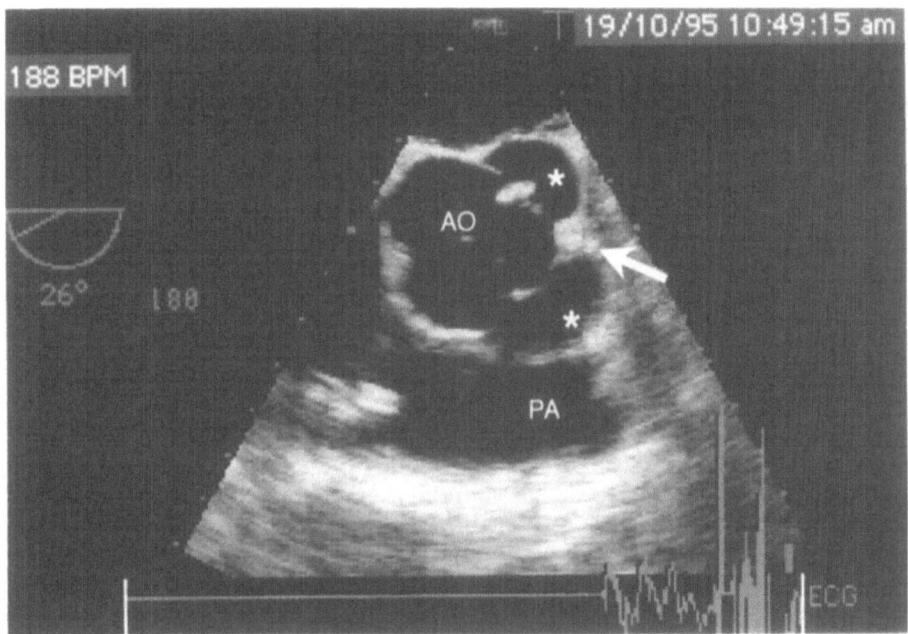

Fig. 2. Transesophageal multiplane echocardiogram demonstrating pseudoaneursym (∗) which involves 2/3 of the circumference of the aortic root. The pseudoaneurysm is divided into two cavities by the left main coronary artery (arrow). AO = aortic valve, PA = pulmonary artery.

ligament as a landmark. For the greater part of the series, fibrin glue was placed on suture lines and on the dissection plane of the right ventricular outflow tract/septum, but this practice has recently been abandoned.

Intraoperative transesophageal echocardiography (TEE) is performed in all patients. The pre-pump study is used to evaluate the pathology and the pulmonary valve, and it can guide the surgeon in the search for abscesses, cavities, pseudoaneurysms, fistulas, and septum defects (24) (Fig. 2). The post-pump study is useful in the evaluation of thoroughness of intracardiac air evacuation, success of repair of defects, ventricular function, and autograft and homograft valve function.

Results

There was one operative death and no late deaths. The patient who died was a 240 kg 55-year-old man with advanced endocarditis, sepsis, severe AI and fistulas to the left atrium and right ventricle. One patient was reoperated for bleeding. There have been no new cases of complete heart block and no cases of recurrent endocarditis. One patient who had been operated three times previously developed a sternal pseudo-arthrosis. She also developed a deep vein thrombosis and a transient neurologic deficit.

All patients had < grade 1 autograft insufficiency immediately postoperatively. At follow-up, which is 100% complete, no deterioration in autograft function has been seen on echocardiography. One patient has, however, required reoperation for pulmonary homograft stenosis. At reoperation, fibrosis of the homograft was seen, and immunologic mechanisms are suspected. The patients are doing well clinically, except the woman with the sternal problems. She continues to have debilitating chest pain.

Advantages and disadvantages of the Ross operation

Oswalt was the first to take the courageous jump from homograft to autograft in patients with endocarditis in 1990 (19). In his series, presently of 27 patients (personal communication), there has been no mortality or endocarditis recurrence. These excellent results support our belief that the Ross operation is a good and probably even better alternative than the homograft, mechanical valve prosthesis, and bioprosthesis for many patients with endocarditis. There are, however, a number of important issues that concern us which only further studies will resolve.

Exposure

In the treatment of advanced endocarditis, excision of most of the aortic root is common to all three major treatment modalities; the composite graft, the homograft root, and the autograft root, but removal of the autograft provides even greater exposure of the left ventricular outflow tract, the interventricular septum, and the root pathology. If access to the atrio-ventricular valves is necessary, exposure can be enhanced even more by a transatrial/transseptal incision (Fig. 3). It is our firm belief that optimal exposure is a key element in the successful treatment of advanced aortic endocarditis. After the aortic root, coronary arteries, and autograft are prepared, surgical exposure is optimal, and the safe and complete debridement of pathologic tissue is facilitated. After this has been accomplished, it has been our experience that reconstruction of the heart is remarkably straightforward and comparable to a standard Ross operation in most cases.

Tissue quality

The autograft has a delicate pliability which makes it uniquely well-suited for insertion in the edematous, friable tissue that is often present in patients with active endocarditis. The autograft adapts easily to these surfaces and the risk of bleeding and pseudoaneurysm development is minimized. The only limitation is the degree of distortion that the autograft can tolerate and still remain competent. In our experience, homograft tissue pliability is inferior to the autograft's. Indeed, occasionally the homograft is stiff and friable. The composite graft with its rigid design forces the tissue to adapt to it, rather than the reverse. The coronary arteries of these patients are occasionally damaged by the infective process or are atherosclerotic, or both, and the autograft is particularly well-suited for the safe insertion of even severely diseased or

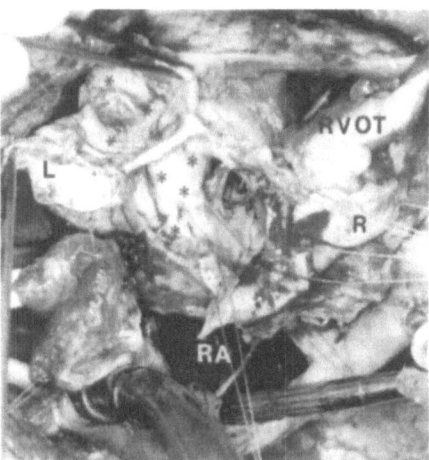

Fig. 3. Unparalleled exposure to the left ventricular outflow tract and the pathology is one of the important strengths of the Ross operation. Exposure can be improved even more, if access to the atrio-ventricular valves is necessary, with a transatrial/transseptal incision, as seen in this photograph of a patient with tricuspid and aortic valve endocarditis. ∗ = pseudoaneurysm, RVOT = right ventricular outflow tract, L = left coronary artery, R = right coronary artery, RA = right atrium.

naked coronary arteries devoid of an aortic wall cuff. This point is well-illustrated by our second Ross patient, a 19-year-old boy who had previously undergone four aortic valve operations, the most recent a Cabrol procedure. A fistula developed between his right coronary artery and the vascular prosthesis which communicated with a large cavity and ultimately to the left ventricular outflow tract (Fig. 4). Because of the favorable tissue quality of the autograft, it was possible to establish successful anastomoses between the autograft and the naked ends of his coronary arteries that remained after removal of the vascular prosthesis. The autograft's tissue quality is a strong argument in favor of the Ross operation in the treatment of advanced endocarditis.

Other autograft strengths

Treatment of endocarditis patients with a homograft is appealing in many ways. It is a simpler, shorter operation in a situation where the surgeon may feel threatened by the complexity of the problem, and it is a universally accepted surgical truth that there can be no long-term follow-up, unless there is short-term survival. However, it may be possible to afford oneself the luxury of short- *and* long-range thinking, and if that is the case, the limited durability of the homograft detracts from the appeal of that solution. Homograft deterioration is inevitable and the later reoperation of an aortic homograft root in this patient category is not without difficulty or risk. The autograft's and homograft's negligible thromboembolic potential without anticoagulation is well-established (9, 15, 21, 23), and both valves' hemodynamics are physiologic. However, if our expectations to autograft durability are upheld, it can be assumed that these attractive qualities will continue to characterize the autograft, whereas they will probably diminish in the homograft. It can also be speculated how well the homograft's endocarditis-resistance will be maintained as valve function and surface

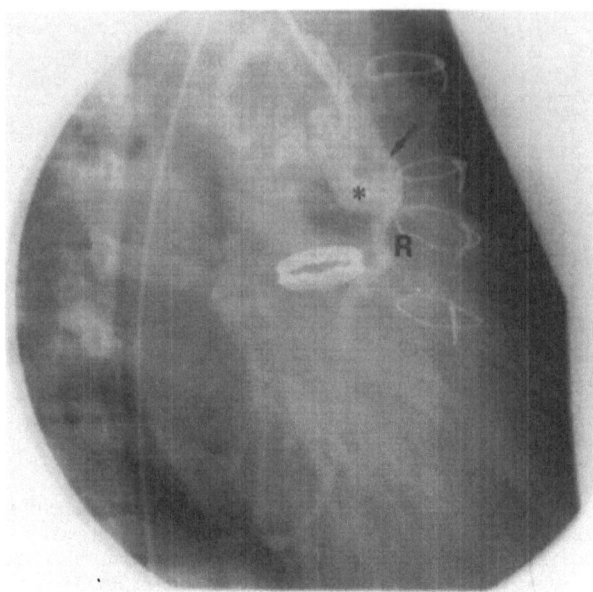

Fig. 4. Selective angiogram with catheter in Cabrol graft (∗) with fistula (arrow) at anastomosis to the right coronary artery (R).

integrity deteriorates with time. These arguments are based on the presumption that the pulmonary homograft used to reconstruct the right ventricular outflow tract will have a better durability or be easier to replace than a homograft in the aortic position.

The growth potential of the autograft makes its use in neonates and children attractive (5,6,16,22). Our first Ross patient was a 10-year-old boy from Greenland with aortic valve endocarditis secondary to a ventricular septum defect. The autograft's growth capabilities and the fact that anticoagulation could be avoided in a young Eskimo made the Ross operation particularly attractive in that case. Additional advantages with the Ross operation are the lack of valve prosthesis noise and the fact that surplus pulmonary homografts can be put to use.

Infection resistance

The autograft is living tissue and maintains its vitality after translocation to the aortic position. Although the homograft may contain living cells at insertion, the inevitable immune reaction will quickly damage or kill these cells, although there are opposing views on this issue (1, 2, 18). It is expected that living tissue is more resistant to bacterial invasion. The autograft is "pre-treated" with pre-operative systemic antibiotics and the homograft is treated with antibiotics before cryopreservation, and these treatments may contribute to infection resistance. In the early Ross material, there was a disturbing frequency of autograft endocarditis (7), but in later series this does not appear to be a problem (5, 13, 15, 19, 23).

One of our non-endocarditis cases illustrates a rather remarkable degree of autograft (and homograft) resistance to infection. A 3-month-old baby had undergone open aortic valvuloplasty and atrial septal defect and patent ductus closure 2 days after delivery. The mitral valve was insufficient, but no attempt was made to repair it during this initial operation. There was a residual aortic stenosis, persistent grade 4 mitral insufficiency, and pulmonary hypertension. The child's condition deteriorated and at 3 months, a Ross operation and mitral valve repair (annuloplasty) were performed. The mitral repair was unsuccessful and 3 weeks later, a mechanical valve prosthesis was inserted. Postoperative *Staphylococcus aureus* sepsis resulted in prosthetic valve endocarditis with annular destruction, pseudoaneurysm formation, and paravalvular leakage which required re-replacement of the mitral valve prosthesis after an additional 6 weeks. The baby has recovered and neither the autograft nor the pulmonary homograft were affected by the infection.

Nevertheless, the homograft has proven to be infection-resistant in this setting in many reports (8, 14, 17, 25), and our view on the autograft's potentially superior qualities in this respect must be relegated to the realm of speculation.

Autograft drawbacks

A possible drawback to the Ross operation in the case of endocarditis is the fact that the right side of the heart is opened and exposed to infection. This fear has been a major factor in Donald Ross' reluctance to use the autograft in endocarditis, but Oswalt's and our data suggest that this fear may be ungrounded (10–13, 19). The Ross operation is a 2-valve operation for a one-valve disease, and is more difficult and time-consuming than alternative procedures. However, modern strategies for myocardial protection allow us ample time and more and more surgeons are performing the operation with success (20).

Primary autograft function is always a concern with this operation. If the pulmonary valve is normal, early autograft dysfunction must be related to surgical technique and judgement, a particular concern in patients with endocarditis who have required extensive debridement. In our experience, most patients, even those with very large cavities and pseudoaneurysms have not suffered significant substance loss. Therefore, the autograft can be inserted after debridement in the left ventricular outflow tract with correct size match, without severe distortion, and with acceptable support from the surrounding heart (Fig. 1).

Another concern with the autograft is whether it will dilate and become insufficient with time. We do not believe that the risk of late autograft dilatation and insufficiency should be greater following operation for endocarditis than after any Ross operation. There are, however, no really long-term autograft root replacement results available yet, since the early Ross material was with subcoronary autograft implantation.

We are also concerned with the fate of the pulmonary homograft, and the potential problems attendant to its later replacement. We assume that replacement of a homograft in the pulmonary position would be safer and easier than replacement of an aortic homograft root, which would involve operating in a previously infected area and dealing with the coronary arteries. However, we do not believe that the difficulties involved in replacing a pulmonary homograft should be underestimated. The left main, the septal, and the left anterior descending coronary arteries are often exposed during autograft harvesting and will lie in direct contact with the homograft proximally posteriorly (Fig. 5).

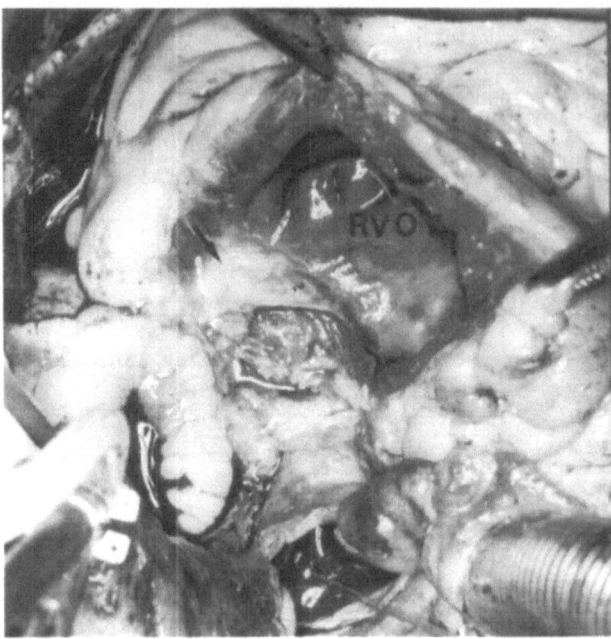

Fig. 5. The septal artery is often exposed in the septal dissection plane during autograft harvesting (arrow). The myocardium above the septal artery is extremely thin, just a few millemeters in many cases, and care must be taken during autograft harvesting and homograft insertion not to damage this artery. RVOT = right ventricular outflow tract.

Conclusion

The Ross operation is an exciting and promising alternative to available treatment modalities for endocarditis. This series demonstrates that the Ross operation can be performed successfully, even in patients with advanced endocarditis. It is especially in these patients that the autograft may provide substantial advantages over alternative treatment modalities. Although we have a number of concerns with the Ross operation, foremost among these being the long-term durability of the autograft when inserted as a root, and the fate of the pulmonary homograft used for right ventricular outflow tract reconstruction, our results with the Ross operation in endocarditis are encouraging. In Copenhagen, the following therapeutic guidelines have evolved and are now adhered to. Patients with non-advanced endocarditis are given a Ross operation if standard criteria for this operation are fulfilled, such as contraindication for anticoagulation, children, potential mothers, other patients under 65 years of age who wish to avoid anticoagulation, and some special indications (13). Advanced endocarditis is treated with a Ross operation if the patient's life expectancy is greater than the expected life of a homograft, or other factors such as autograft tissue quality, improved exposure with the Ross operation, or autograft growth potential tip the scales in favor of the autograft.

References

1. Angell WW, Oury JH, Koziol JA, Dussault MH (1988) Survival of aortic allograft containing living cells. In: Yankah AC, Hetzer R, Miller DC, Ross DN, Somerville J, Yacoub MH (eds) Cardiac Valve Allografts 1962–1987. Springer-Verlag New York, pp 273–280
2. Barrett-Boyes BG, Roche AH, Subramanyan R, Pemberton JR, Whitlock RM (1987) Long-term follow-up of patients with the antibiotic-sterilized aortic homograft valve inserted freehand in the aortic position. Circulation 75: 768–777
3. Cabrol C, Pavie A, Mesnildrey P, Gandjbakhch I, Laughlin L, Bors V, Corcos T (1986) Long-term results with total replacement of the ascending aorta and reimplantation of the coronary arteries. J Thorac Cardiovasc Surg 91: 17–25
4. David TE, Komeda M, Brofman PR (1989) Surgical treatment of aortic root abscess. Circulation 80 (suppl I): I-269–274
5. Elkins RC, Knott-Craig CJ, Randolph JD, Razook JR, Ward KE, Overholt ED, Lane MM (1994) Medium-term follow-up of pulmonary autograft replacement of aortic valves in children. Eur J Cardiothorac Surg 8: 379–383
6. Gerosa G, McKay R, Ross DN (1991) Replacement of the aortic valve or root with a pulmonary autograft in children. Ann Thorac Surg 51: 424–429
7. Gerosa G, McKay R, Ross DN (1991) Replacement of the aortic valve or root with a pulmonary autograft in children. Ann Thorac Surg 51: 424–429
8. Glazier JJ, Verwilghen J, Donaldson RM, Ross DN (1991) Treatment of complicated prosthetic valve endocarditis with annular abscess formation by homograft aortic root replacement. J Am Coll Cardiol 17: 1177–1182
9. Gonzalez Lavin L, Robles A, Graf D (1988) The Ross operation: the autologous pulmonary valve in the aortic position. J Card Surg 3: 29–43
10. Joyce F, Tingleff J, Aagaard J, Pettersson G (1994) The Ross operation in the treatment of native and prosthetic aortic valve endocarditis. J Heart Valve Dis 3: 371–376
11. Joyce F, Tingleff J, Pettersson G (1995) The Ross operation in the treatment of prosthetic valve endocarditis. Sem Thorac Cardiovasc Surg 7: 38–46
12. Joyce F, Tingleff J, Pettersson G (1995) The Ross operation: results of early experience including treatment for endocarditis. Eur J Cardio-thorac Surg 9: 384–392
13. Joyce F, Tingleff J, Pettersson G (1995) Expanding indications for the Ross operation. J Heart Valve Dis 4: 352–363
14. Kirklin JK, Kirklin JW, Pacifico AD (1988) Aortic valve endocarditis with aortic root abscess cavity: surgical treatment with aortic valve homograft. Ann Thorac Surg 45: 674–677
15. Kouchoukos NT, Davila Roman VG, Spray TL, Murphy SF, Perrillo JB (1994) Replacement of the aortic root with a pulmonary autograft in children and young adults with aortic-valve disease. N Engl J Med 330: 1–6
16. Matsuki O, Yagihara T, Yamamoto F, Nishigaki K, Uemura H, Kagisaki K, Kawashima Y (1993) Growth potential after root replacement of the right and left ventricular outflow tracts. J Heart Valve Dis 2: 308–310
17. McGiffin DC, Galbraith AJ, McLachlan GJ, Stower RE, Wong ML, Stafford EG, Gardner MAH, Pohlner PG, O'Brien MF (1992) Aortic valve infection. Risk factors for death and recurrent endocarditis after aortic valve replacement. J Thorac Cardiovasc Surg 104: 511–520
18. O'Brien MF, Stafford EG, Gardner MAH, Pohlner P, McGiffin DC, Johnston N, Tesar P, Brosnan A, Duffy P (1988) Cryopreserved viable allograft aortic valves. In: Yankah AC, Hetzer R, Miller DC, Ross DN, Somerville J, Yacoub MH (eds) Cardiac Valve Allografts 1962–1987. Springer-Verlag New York, pp 311-321
19. Oswalt JD, Dewan SJ (1993) Aortic infective endocarditis managed by the Ross procedure. J Heart Valve Dis 2: 380–384
20. Oury JH (1995) Editorial: an appraisal of the Ross procedure. J Heart Valve Dis 4: 350–351
21. Ross DN, Jackson M, Davies J (1992) The pulmonary autograft – a permanent aortic valve. Eur J Cardio-thorac Surg 6: 113–117
22. Schoof PH, Cromme Dijkhuis AH, Bogers JJ, Thijssen EJ, Witsenburg M, Hess J, Bos E (1994) Aortic root replacement with pulmonary autograft in children. J Thorac Cardiovasc Surg 107: 367–373
23. Stelzer P, Jones DJ, Elkins RC (1989) Aortic root replacement with pulmonary autograft. Circulation 80: III-209–III-213 (suppl)

24. Tingleff J, Egeblad H, Gøtzsche CO, Baandrup U, Kristensen BØ, Pilegaard H, Pettersson G (1995) Perivalvular cavities in endocarditis: abscesses versus pseudoaneurysms? A transesophageal Doppler echocardiographic study in 118 patients with endocarditis. Am Heart J 130: 93–100
25. Tuna IC, Orszulak TA, Schaff HV, Danielson GK (1990) Results of homograft aortic valve replacement for active endocarditis. Ann Thorac Surg 49: 619–624
26. Yankah AC (1994) Surgical management of infective endocarditis: pulmonary autograft or allograft? J Heart Valve Dis 3: 380–383.

Author's address:
G. Pettersson, MD
Department of Cardiothoracic Surgery
The National University Hospital Rigshospitalet
2100 Copenhagen, Denmark

Techniques of reconstruction of the right ventricular outflow tract at Ross operation

D. Metras

University Hospital Marseille, Dept. Thoracic and Cardiovascular Surgery

Introduction

Although it is done after the two main steps of the Ross operation (i.e., pulmonary autograft harvesting, insertion of the autograft in the aortic position with coronary reimplantations), and sometimes considered as the easy part of the operation, the right ventricular outflow tract (RVOT) reconstruction is a critical step of this procedure.

The RV septal muscle bed is at risk of two major complications: hemorrhage and first septal coronary artery lesion, both being reported as the main reason for early reoperation and the main reason for peri-operative mortality (1, 2).

In addition, the RVOT is the main area at risk of late reoperations, due to the inevitable deterioration of the substitute.

Therefore, a lot of care must be given to this step of the operation and some discussion is deserved for the type and fate of the RVOT substitute.

Technique

Standard present technique: the RVOT reconstruction with a cryopreserved homograft

Presently, in the majority of the cases, the RVOT reconstruction is done with a cryopreserved homograft, preferably a pulmonary homograft.

There are different steps in the RV outflow tract repair after a Ross procedure, we will briefly comment on all of them.

Preparation of the RV septal muscle bed

After harvesting of the pulmonary autograft, there is a "bed" of RV septal muscle, cut obliquely. There are a number of very small coronaries cut during this harvesting. In view of the hazard of intra and peri-operative bleeding of this area, it is absolutely essential to insure an excellent hemostasis of this area, since the main reason for early reoperation for bleeding comes from this area (2).

A direct injection of cardioplegic solution in the left coronary helps to show the small bleeders. They have to be occluded by cautery or if more important by a fine 6/0 suture. Care must be taken to avoid the first septal artery if it is seen. If it is not seen, the sutures must remain very superficial.

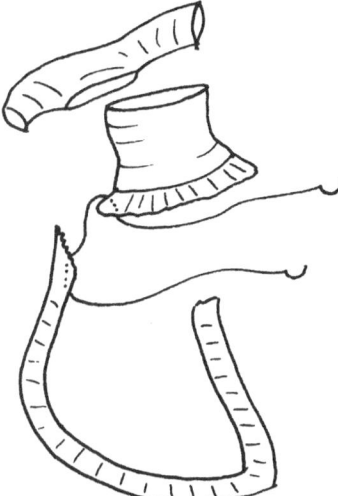

Fig. 1. The proximal anastomosis is done first. The posterior septal suture is done taking bites low in the RV septum, including the endocardial layer, avoiding the oblique thin part with the first septal artery.

When it is sure that no obvious bleeder exists, we favor application of fibrin glue, although the placement of an absorbable hemostatic gauze layer is also used (1).

Proximal suture of the pulmonary homograft

The proximal suture is an end-to-end anastomosis between the recipient's RV muscle and the homograft RV muscle. A simple 4 or 5/0 circumferencial polypropylene continuous suture is adequate.

The only particular aspect is the way the recipient RV septum is handled. As seen on Fig. 1, with the oblique cutting of this muscle, the thickest layer with endocardium is rather low. The suture should take bites only in this area, since the muscle bite including the endocardial layer is the most solid one, and since in the oblique thin part there is a danger of first septal artery wound.

The distal anastomosis

It is also done with a running suture of 4 or 5/0 polypropylene suture. Prior to the suture an adequate trimming of the HG is necessary to obtain a geometrically perfect alignment of the RVOT reconstruction. This is why the distal anastomosis should be done after the proximal one.

The essential feature of this anastomosis being avoidance of a stenosis, this anastomosis can be done after trimming of the HG at the level of the pulmonary artery bifurcation. To avoid the purse string effect of the continuous running suture, one can use a loose suture, several running sutures, or interrupted sutures on the anterior aspect of the anastomosis.

Strategy and timing of the RVOT reconstruction

A compromise must be found between a safe and easy HG implantation and a shorter aortic cross-clamping time (3).

Most surgeons perform the RVOT repair after the aortic replacement but some still perform it before (1, 3). The part needing most care with the technique of suture is the posterior septal proximal suture; we do this part with a quiet and flaccid heart under cross-clamping and cardioplegia. The rest of the HG implantation (anterior proximal suture, distal anastomosis) is performed with the aortic cross-clamp released.

Choice of the substitute and alternatives

Pulmonary cryopreserved homograft

This is presently the preferred substitute in most teams, since it is thinner, has a bifurcation, and has less content of elastin and calcium, and is less prone to degeneration than the aortic homograft.

The size of the graft has to be an adult size in most cases over 18–20 mm of annular diameter. The goal is to avoid any reoperation for outgrowing of the HG by the recipient, and to delay as much as possible the reoperations.

In children, one can use down-sizing of a pulmonary homograft transformed in a bicuspid conduit (4, 5), but in most cases, due to the compliance of the RV after harvesting of the autograft, a larger HG can be used (6). In our experience, a 6 kg 4 month-old child could receive an adult size HG of 20 mm diameter, without particular difficulties.

Aortic homograft

In the past, it was used before it was evidenced that the pulmonary HG was superior in terms of degeneration, calcifications and actuarial freedom from reoperation (7).

Presently, it is used only if no pulmonary HG is available.

In children, neo-aortic growth has been demonstrated experimentally (8) and clinically (9). It is not the case for the RVOT and one has to find a compromise between using a larger homograft and avoid the inconvenience of the possible compressions by a large conduit. Still, as we had the experience and some authors have reported (6) a quite large homograft can be used without inconvenience.

Other substitute

A pulmonary porcine xenograft stored in glutaraldehyde, is an option, although its use has not yet been reported. It is possible that the pulmonary nature of the xenograft procures less tendency to structural deterioration and calcified deposit, compared to aortic xenograft, like the pulmonary HG compared to aortic HG, but this remains to be demonstrated. Aortic porcine xenograft has been used in some patients (10) and only early results are available.

If this is evidenced, it will be possible to safely perform a pulmonary autograft with an acceptable late result even in the absence of homografts, using a porcine pulmonary conduit.

Use of aortic native valve

In the hope to reduce the use of a foreign material, it has been proposed to use the patient's own moderately diseased aortic valve (11), mainly in aortic insufficiency, to replace the pulmonary valve during a Ross procedure. The reconstruction of the native PA wall is done using part of the PA wall, part of the aortic wall, and a prosthetic patch.

Experimentally, a direct anastomosis

(12) has been performed between the pulmonary bifurcation, after extensive dissection of the branches and lowering to the level of the RV outflow. Therefore, no foreign or prosthetic tissue was used. In addition, the authors found enough pulmonary arterial wall tissue to construct a valve-like structure. This remains to be attempted and evaluated in clinical practice to gain acceptance.

Discussion

Although thought to be the easy part of the operation, the RVOT reconstruction must however be done very carefully. Early reoperations for bleeding were practically always due to bleeding of the proximal area of the RVOT repair (2), although most cases are unreported.

Late reoperations have been in part due to HG replacement for late failure. It is interesting to notice that an early mild dysfunction with pulmonary valve insufficiency and distal anastomotic site mild stenosis have been reported (13). This emphasizes the importance of the care in the anastomosis constructions.

The RV outflow reconstruction with a cryopreserved pulmonary homograft remains, at present, the preferred option in most series.

As recently demonstrated for the RVOT reconstruction in other types of operations for congenital heart defects, the pulmonary HG is much superior to the aortic HG in terms of degeneration, calcification, dysfunction, freedom from reoperation (7).

The clinical results with the other types of substitutes and even without substitute are expected with great interest, but at present, the safe future of the neo-aortic valve is still the essential point to be demonstrated in the procedure (14). An interesting point of debate concerns small children.

Conclusion

Although considered as one of the minor steps of the Ross pulmonary autograft procedure, the RVOT reconstruction deserves great care to insure the best early and late results. Also, the various modalities in repairing the RVOT show that, as opposed to the aortic part of the operation, the optimal solution is not yet standardized. If one considers the aortic replacement with an autograft as the ideal and permanent substitute, this goal has not yet been achieved for the RVOT repair.

References

1. Ross DN (1991) Replacement of the aortic valve with a pulmonary autograft: the "Switch" operation. Ann Thorac Surg 52: 1346–1350
2. Gonzalez-Lavin L, Robles A, Graf D (1988) Morbidity following the Ross operation. J Cardiac Surg 3 (Suppl): 305–308
3. Ross DN (1994) in: Metras D (ed) Allogreffes et autogreffes valvulaires cardiaques: conservation et chirurgie. 1st Ed. Paris, Masson
4. Hiramatsu T, Miura T, Forbess JM et al. (1994) Downsizing of valve allografts for use as right heart conduits. Ann Thorac Surg 58: 339–343
5. Monro JL, Tolan MJ, Slavek Z et al. (1995) Bicuspidisation of homografts used in reconstruction of the right heart. Ann Thorac Surg 59: 789
6. Sardari F, Gundry R, Razzouk J, Shilari S, Bailey L (1996) The use of larger size pulmonary homografts for the Ross operation in children. J Heart Valve Dis 5: 410–413
7. Bando K, Danielson GK, Schaff HV, Mair DD, Julsrud PR, Puga FJ (1995) Outcome of pulmonary and aortic homografts for right ventricular outflow tract reconstruction. J Thorac Cardiovasc Surg 109: 509–518
8. Kreitmann B, Riberi A, Jimeno MT, Metras D (1995) Experimental basis for autograft growth and viability. J Heart Valve Dis 4: 379–383
9. Elkins RC, Knott-Craig CJ, Ward KE (1994) Pulmonary autograft in children: realized growth potential. Ann Thorac Surg 57: 1387–94
10. Konertz W, Sidiropoulos A, Hotz H, Borges A, Baumann G (1996) Ross operation and right ventricular outflow tract reconstruction with stentless xenografts. J Heart Valve Dis 5: 418–420
11. DeLeon SY, Quinones JA, Miles RH et al. (1995) Use of the native aortic valve as the pulmonary valve in the Ross procedure. Ann Thorac Surg 59: 1007–1010
12. Couetil JP, Pellerin M, Tolan M, Berrebi A, Pelissier J, Carpentier A (1996) Reconstruction of a pulmonary outflow tract after Ross procedure using the pulmonary artery wall to fashion a monocusp valve. Eur J Cardio Thorac Surg 10: in press
13. Pieters AA, Al-Halees Z, Zwaan E, Hatle L (1996) Autograft failure after the Ross operation in a rheumatic population: pre- and postoperative echocardiographic observations. J Heart Valve Dis 5: 404–409
14. Ross DN, Jackson M, Davies J (1991) Pulmonary autograft aortic valve replacement: long-term results. J Cardiac Surg 6: 529–533

Author's address:
Prof. Dominique Metras
Hopital d'Enfants de la Timone
Service de Chirurgie Thoracique
et Cardio-Vasculaire
13385 Marseille
France

Allograft vs. prosthetic aortic valve replacement for active infective endocarditis

D.-A. Haydock

Green Lane Hospital, Auckland, New Zealand

The allograft valve in infective endocarditis

Endocarditis is a lethal problem and despite advances in diagnostic methods, improvements in antibiotic treatment, surgery with its attendant risks is often required. Ever since the first replacement of a heart valve for treatment of an infected valve (11) endocarditis has remained a major challenge for the cardiac surgeon. In endocarditis, as opposed to standard valve replacement for non-infective reasons, the surgeon must be concerned about eradication of infection as well as correction of the haemodynamic lesion. This has led to debate in the literature about which valve operation is the best in the infected field. The purpose of this chapter is to review the reported performance of the allograft valve in this situation. Clearly almost all information relates to endocarditis of the aortic valve for obvious reasons. Patients with endocarditis are usually treated by a cardiologist until it is clear that there are indications to proceed to surgery. The standard surgical indications often quoted are uncontrolled sepsis, uncontrolled heart failure and septic embolic events. Along with this many would add in such reasons as *Staphylococcus aureus* or fungal infection, presence of large vegetations, onset of heart block or increasing delay in AV conduction associated with a paravalvular abscess.

Native valve endocarditis (NVE) can often be treated successfully with antibiotics and if not is reasonably straightforward to deal with as long as surgery is not too delayed. With prosthetic valve endocarditis (PVE) the valve itself serves as a focus of infection and as a result tissue destruction is often extensive and makes surgical treatment quite a challenge (1). These operations are often the most difficult to perform as there is sometimes extreme distortion of the anatomy even leading to aorto-ventricular discontinuity and false passages into other cardiac chambers. To obtain a survivor that is completely cured of recurrent infection is each surgeon's aim but unfortunately not always achieved.

The survival difference between those undergoing surgery for native valve versus prosthetic valve endocarditis is demonstrated in Table 1 from the Green Lane Hospital data (2). There was significantly better survival in those patients with endocarditis of their native valve. The majority of the difference between the two groups had occurred by the 1-year mark.

Clearly the most difficult test of a valves' ability to resist infection and for the surgeon to obtain a survivor is in the setting of prosthetic endocarditis or in those with gross infection in the destroyed aortic annulus. Reports of patients undergoing allograft root replacement for endocarditis generally contain small numbers (4, 8, 13). These reports are interesting and often contain excellent results in patients with marked anatomical destruction of the aortoannular area. Unfortunately because of the small numbers of patients conclusions are difficult to make with any statistical

Table 1. Survival results following surgery for native versus prosthetic valve infection

Survival	NVE $n = 66$	PVE $n = 42$
1 month	86%	74%
1 year	80%	59%
5 years	72%	57%
10 years	50%	41%
15 years	50%	16%

conviction. Our own experience with this technique when there is gross destruction of structures in the surgical field has been favourable (19/19 survivors with no recurrent endocarditis).

The aims of all endocarditis surgery must include the following:

1) Eradication of the infection;
2) Correction of the valvular incompetence;
3) Prevention of further embolization;
4) Patient survival.

The ideal valve replacement would be one that resists reinfection both early and late, that is completely durable and has a low thromboembolic rate. Apart from the possible potential with valve repair most of the options listed below fall short of the ideal.

Surgical options.

1) Homografts as a subcoronary placement or a root replacement (3);
2) Pulmonary autografts (7, 12);
3) Porcine and other non-allograft tissue valves (9);
4) Mechanical valves (9).

The following discussion is limited to the use of allograft valves in the treatment of endocarditis and the other options will not be discussed apart from their use as a comparison group. The technical aspects of insertion of the allograft will not be discussed as these have been well described in other documents (3).

The problem presenting the surgeon when he tries to find out how the use of an allograft for aortic endocarditis will benefit his patient is that there is no randomized study that can truly answer this question. Allograft enthusiasts have attempted to indoctrinate the remainder of the surgical community with the belief that it is best to use an allograft for those patients with important aortic valve infection. This information has not been derived from a randomized trial but by retrospective reports. These reports are scattered through the literature and on the whole involve small numbers of patients and show that allografts can be used with satisfactory results in most situations involving aortic valve endocarditis (2, 4, 5, 8, 10, 12, 13). Unfortunately it is difficult to directly compare many of these studies as the patients they report on tend to belong to different clinical subgroups. Some authors have included those patients with remote healed endocarditis which tends to dilute down the data with a group of less seriously ill patients. Some series have a group of patients who are intravenous drug abusers which is probably the biggest risk factor for recurrent endocarditis. The overall risk of complications, including reinfection, is greatest for those patients that have active endocarditis leading to emergency or semi-urgent surgery.

To illustrate the information that can get us close to current understanding of the performance of the allograft two papers have been chosen in which a significant number of allograft valves have been used in the treatment of endocarditis (2, 6).

The two chosen studies arise from two hospitals with a very large allograft experience. They are our group at Green Lane Hospital in Auckland, New Zealand and the Prince Charles Hospital group in Brisbane, Australia. There are many similarities between the two studies and some important differences. The combination of the two studies covers over 300 patients with over two-thirds of them having active endocarditis. The details of each centers patient groups are listed separately below in detail as it is only with this information that the overall performance of the allograft can be assessed. A comparison of the results from the two centers follows these important patient details. Both groups have had a similar aim and that was to compare how different valve types had performed in resisting infection that was present in the surgical field. In particular both groups looked to determine whether the allograft performed better than other valves.

Green Lane Hospital study group

The Green Lane group (2) looked at aortic valve replacement in the most provocative setting of active infectious endocarditis in 108 patients.

Between 1965 and 1985 a total of 348 surgical patients had had endocarditis as the cause of their aortic valve lesion. Only 108 had acute endocarditis at the time of their operation. This was defined as the need to proceed with valve replacement during the hospital admission for acute endocarditis because of the severity of the patient's illness. There were 87 males and 21 females. Ages ranged from 9 up to 76 (mean 44 years). As can be seen from the NYHA class in Table 2, the patients were very ill in the majority of cases.

Overall at the time of surgery 90% had deterioration in valve function, 44% had uncontrolled infection, 31% had had embolization. All patients had been on antibiotics (mean 26 days) and these were continued for 4 weeks postoperatively if the culture of tissue removed was negative and for 6 weeks if they were positive and longer if infection persisted.

No operation was elective. Around 95% had blood cultures that were positive and 31% of the cultures taken at the time of surgery were positive. Gram stain was positive in 64%. The surgeon considered the disease process to be active in 88% and extensive in 34%. Vegetations were present in 77%. In only four instances was the diagnosis of active infection based solely on the appearance of the valve at operation.

Table 2. NYHA class for the 108 patients operated on for active endocarditis

NYHA		
	Class 1	0
	Class 2	11
	Class 3	16
	Class 4	40
	Class 5	41

At the time of the operation the infection was felt to have spread beyond the confines of the annulus in 35%. Eighteen had involvement of the anterior mitral leaflet often with spread to the adjacent membranous septum, four had frank abscesses and 17 had false aneurysms. One of the false aneurysms was associated with a fistulous connection to the left atrium and another with an infection generated VSD. Two had a congenital aneurysm of the sinus of valsalva and two had a mycotic aneurysm of the ascending aorta.

The most common organisms were *Viridans Streptococci* in 30 patients, *Staphylococcus aureus* in 24, *Enterococcus* in 12 and *Staphylococcus epidermidis* in 12. Only one patient had a fungal infection (*Torulopsis glabrata*). No patients were known to be addicted to drugs.

Endocarditis occurred on the native aortic valve in 66 patients and on a previously placed replacement device in 42 patients (allograft 27, mechanical 13 and bioprosthesis in two). Autopsy was undertaken in 19 of the hospital deaths and in 18 of the 30 late deaths.

The type of valve inserted at the operation for active endocarditis was an aortic allograft in 78, a stented allograft in one, a mechanical prosthesis in 16 and a bioprosthesis in 13.

During the period a freehand allograft was the preferred replacement device. The reasons for not using an allograft were not stated in 12 patients and in two a suitable allograft valve was not available. In three operations a prosthetic valve was placed as the surgeon was also replacing the mitral valve with a prosthetic valve. In 12 instances selection was in favour of a prosthetic valve as the patient required a Bentall operation because the aortic root was too large for an allograft.

No patient was lost to follow-up. The follow-up ranged up to 242 months and averaged 79 months.

Prince Charles Hospital group

The Brisbane group (6) looked at the performance of various valve types in active endocarditis but their patient group is diluted by the inclusion of patients who had healed and in most cases had remote endocarditis.

This study had two groups. One with an acute life-threatening illness ($n = 128$) with active or possibly active infection and one with a more standard elective valve replacement procedure ($n = 81$).

Table 3 describes the patient characteristics in this study.

The most frequently occurring organisms were *Staphylococcus aureus* and *Viridans Streptococci*. The types of valve used are shown below.

The valves chosen were according to surgeon preference and an allograft aortic valve was a more a common choice in the latter part of the experience. Concomitant procedures were performed in 42 patients and these included mitral valve replacements (13 patients), mitral valve repair (12 patients), coronary artery bypass operation (five patients), aortic root replacement (three patients) and miscellaneous procedures (nine patients).

Median follow-up was 91.6 months (range 1.7 to 258.3 months). This group had very careful follow-up as they only lost one patient to follow-up (this patient was known to be alive 5 months after operation). In addition a mode of death was able to be assigned for each patient dying after operation. All patients dying with

Table 3. Patient characteristics of those in the Prince Charles Hospital series (Brisbane)

	Infection status Active/possible active	Infection status Healed
Characteristic	$n = 128$	$n = 81$
NVE	100	63
PVE	28	18
NYHA 3 and 4	55	36
NYHA 5	16	2
Indication for operation		
Heart failure	81	58
Sepsis	48	1
Emboli	19	2
Vegetations	32	4
Increasing aortic incompetence	101	70
Other organ dysfunction		
Hepatic	6	1
Renal	27	10
Respiratory	6	1
DIC	2	0
Aortic annular infection	61	15
DIC = Disseminated intravascular coagulopathy		

Table 4. The types of replacement valve used in the Prince Charles Hospital (Brisbane) series

Valve type	Number inserted
Xenograft	74
Mechanical	67
Allograft	53
Discontinued biologic	15

Xenograft valve (Hancock, Carpentier-Edwards, or Intact)
Mechanical valve (Lillehei-Kaster, Bjork-Shiley, or St Jude Medical)
Allograft aortic valve in 53 patients (4 °C stored in 18 and cryopreserved in 35)
Discontinued (in 1972) biologic valves (calf or pig heterografts, fascia lata valves, and a frame-mounted allograft).

infection had an autopsy, and this meant that the presence of PVE was accurately determined.

Combination and comparison of the two studies

It is interesting to compare the data from the two studies. Although they have clearly different patient groups the outcome for each group of patients is similar in many ways. The Green Lane group only contains those with active endocarditis whereas the Brisbane group contains those with active and also healed endocarditis (a lower risk group overall).

Survival

The survival figures from each institution are seen in Table 5.

It is clear from these data that endocarditis is a lethal condition both on the short- and long- term. Early mortality is high in both study groups whereas the later drop off is much less severe. Dominating as a risk factor for early death was the level of NYHA class and whether the operation was a redo procedure. In the Brisbane group the use of an allograft was a factor that reduced the likelihood of early death whereas it was not so for the Green Lane group. In the Green Lane series the allograft was the valve of choice and used for a much bigger percentage of patients (73.1%) than that in the Brisbane series (25.4%). When used liberally like this it would appear that the allograft may not be truly protective against early death but there may be an underestimation of the advantages of the allograft as in the Green Lane group those with the most destruction tended to receive an allograft valve. The Brisbane group have also noted that the presence of an allograft as negative coefficient risk factor for early death in their series may be due to subtle patient selection.

Freedom from recurrent endocarditis

The overall freedom from recurrent endocarditis is remarkably similar between institutions and this is depicted in Table 6. Despite the fact that in the Brisbane series 25.4% were allografts whereas in the Green Lane series the figure was 73.1% the freedom from endocarditis is virtually identical.

Table 5. Survival figures for the two series of patients

Survival	Green Lane active endocarditis	Brisbane any endocarditis
1 month	82%	92%
1 year	73%	86%
5 years	64%	76%
10 years	52%	60%
15 years	36%	43%

Table 6. Freedom from endocarditis in the two patient groups

Freedom from recurrent endocarditis	Green Lane	Brisbane
1 year	94%	96%
5 years	88%	92%
10 years	80%	80%
15 years	65%	66%

If allografts are truly protective against recurrent infection then one would have expected the freedom from recurrent endocarditis to be highest at Green Lane Hospital as this group used allografts three times as frequently as the group in Brisbane. This is where the difference between the two patient populations becomes important. In the Green Lane series 100% of the patients had active endocarditis as opposed to only 61% in the Brisbane group. Over 95% of the patients in the Green Lane series had organisms cultured during their surgical admission whereas only 55% were positive in the Brisbane series (assuming that the 81 patients having healed remote endocarditis were culture negative during their surgical admission). This would suggest that the allografts were in general placed in a more provocative setting in the Green Lane series as compared to the Brisbane series and this would blunt any

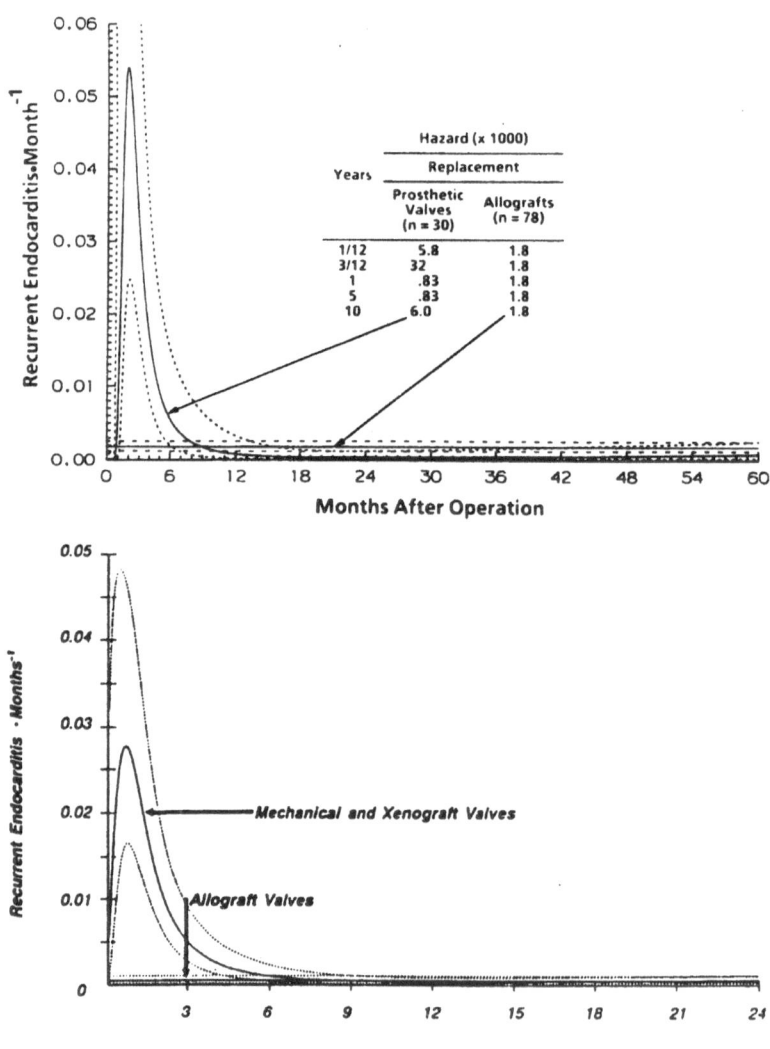

Fig. 1. The hazard function curves (solid lines) and the 70% confidence limits (dotted lines) for Green Lane Hospital patients on the top and Brisbane patients on the bottom. (Reproduction by permission).

obvious advantage of allografts when comparing the ultimate freedom from recurrent infection between the two groups. The fact there is no difference between the two groups despite the more provocative environment in the Green Lane group would therefore be supportive for the concept that the use of an allograft is beneficial in preventing recurrent endocarditis.

Another way to dissect the data further is to compare the hazard function curves from both series that documents the risk of recurrent infection for the different valve types. This information is depicted in Fig. 1 and is virtually identical from each institution. This data, because of its consistency between two independent institutions, is very persuasive with the obvious conclusion being that allograft valves resist infection well in the early phase (6–12 months) reaching the constant hazard phase from the time of implantation. The mechanical and xenograft valves however have a much greater likelihood of recurrent infection in the first 3 to 6 months.

Summary

How does this help the surgeon facing a patient with endocarditis requiring surgery? Although none of the above patients were randomized to an allograft versus another valve there would appear to be a few points that can be made from this data.

1) Because of the high early surgical mortality in endocarditis the first challenge is to allow patient survival and this has to take precedence over other factors that may determine the surgeon's choice of valve type for replacement. It is most likely that the use of an allograft does not alter the surgical survival and it is very unlikely that use of an allograft is disadvantageous.
2) Choosing an allograft valve replacement is associated with good results and offers a number of technical advantages. In the situation where there are cavities to cover over from paravalvular abscesses, false aneurysms and fistulas then allograft tissue is available for this purpose rather than having to use synthetic material in addition to a prosthetic valve.
3) In the first 6–12 months after valve replacement in the aortic position there would appear to be an increased freedom from recurrent endocarditis. The advantages in the later period are less certain. From this would be inferred that the worse the infection in and around the valve then the greater would be the advantage conferred by the use of an allograft. The extreme situation is where there has been complete destruction of the aortic root in the presence of a prosthetic valve. Often these patients have already had multiple procedures in an attempt to eradicate the infection. This would appear to be the situation par excellence where the surgeon and patient can be rescued from further disaster by total allograft/autograft root replacement.
4) There is conflicting evidence on what benefits are conferred on the allograft patient after the first postoperative year when compared to those patients receiving another type of valve. The number of cases with long-term follow-up in the above series are too small to make any definite conclusions about the freedom from reoperation figures in comparison to other valve types. The lack of durability of the allograft has to be weighed against its extremely low thromboembolic rate and lack of need for anticoagulant.

References

1. David T, Bos J, Christakis G, Brofman P, Wong D, Feindel C (1990) Heart valve operations in patients with active infective endocarditis. Ann Thor Surg 49: 701–5
2. Haydock D, Barrett-Boyes B, Macedo T, Kirklin J, Blackstone E (1992) Aortic valve replacement for active infectious endocarditis. J Thorac Cardiovascular surgery 103: 130–9
3. Kirklin J, Barratt-Boyes B (1993) Aortic valve disease. In: Kirklin J, Barratt-Boyes B (eds) Cardiac Surgery. Churchill Livingstone Inc. New York, 491–572
4. Lau J, Robles A, Cherian M, Ross D (1984) Surgical treatment of prosthetic endocarditis. Aortic root replacement using a homograft. J Thorac Cardiovasc Surg 87: 712–716
5. Lupinetti F, Lemmer J (1991) Comparison of allografts and prosthetic valves when used for emergency aortic valve replacement for active infective endocarditis. Am J Cardiol 68: 637–641
6. McGiffen D, Galbraith A, McLachlan G, Stower R, Wong M, Stafford G, Gardner M, Pohlner P, O'Brien M (1992) Aortic valve infection. Risk factors for death and recurrent endocarditis after aortic valve replacement. J Thorac Cardiovasc Surg 104, 2: 511–520.
7. Oswalt J, Dewan S (1993) Aortic infective endocarditis managed by the Ross procedure. J Heart Valve Disease 2, 4: 380–384
8. Saldanha R, Raman J, Feneley M, Farnsworth A (1989) Homograft aortic root replacement to correct infective endocarditis requiring seven open cardiac procedures. Ann Thorac Surg 47: 300–1
9. Sweeney M, Reul G, Cooley D, Ott D, Duncan M, Frazier O, Livesay J (1985) Comparison of bioprosthetic and mechanical valve replacement for active endocarditis. J Thorac Cardiovasc Surgery 90: 676–680
10. Tuna I, Orszulak T, Schaff H, Danielson G (1990) Results of homograft aortic valve replacement for active endocarditis. Ann Thor Surg 49: 619–24
11. Wallace AG, Young WG, Osterhout S (1965) Treatment of acute bacterial endocarditis by valve excision and replacement. Circulation 31: 450
12. Yankah C (1994) Surgical management of infective endocarditis: Pulmonary autograft or allograft. J Heart Valve Disease 3, 4: 380–383
13. Zwischenberger J, Shalaby T, Conti V (1989) Viable cryopreserved aortic homograft for aortic valve endocarditis and annular abscesses. Ann Thor Surg 48: 365–70.

Author's address:
D.-A. Haydock, MD
Cardiothoracic & Vascular Surgeon
Cardiothoracic Surgical Unit
Green Lane Hospital
Green Lane West
Auckland 3
New Zealand

Allograft aortic root surgery. The infected aortic root

A. C. Yankah, Y. Weng, J. Hofmeister, H. Siniawski, R. Hetzer

German Heart Institute Berlin, Berlin, Germany

Introduction

The major early anatomical complication of native aortic valve endocarditis is valve regurgitation (or jet lesion) and the onset of ventricular failure followed by aortic ring and burrowing root abscesses during treatment at which the indication for operative intervention becomes very necessary and urgent. Prosthetic valve endocarditis is more insidious in the onset and with an organism of high virulence like *Staphylococcus epidermidis*, the clinical course is likely to be complicated by suture dehiscence resulting in paravalvular leakage and burrowing root abscesses, myocarditis and onset of ventricular failure. In a prospective study in 1991, the incidence of post-operative infection of prosthetic valve substitutes in a sterile aortic root was found to be 0.9% (12/1393 cases) as compared to 14.4% (16/111 cases) in infected roots (15). Surgical management simply designed to replace the infected native valve or prosthesis including local debridement is likely to fail due to the persistence of residual infected tissue retained within the blood circulation (3, 8, 15). Since 1988, we have adopted the technique of surgical exclusion of infected aortic root tissue from the blood circulation by homograft aortic valve and root replacement instead of using synthetic material (2).

Patients and methods

Between March 1988 and March 1996, 94 patients underwent homograft aortic valve and root replacement for active infective aortic valve endocarditis at the German Heart Institute Berlin. There were 17 females and 77 males at the ages of 9 to 75 years (mean 48 years). Of these, 47 had ring abscesses, 17 with previous prosthetic valve replacements. Additional procedures were performed in 12 patients; mitral replacement in four, mitral reconstruction in three, tricuspid reconstruction in one and replacement of the ascending aorta in four patients.

Procurement of homografts

Homograft conduits were obtained from our Institution-based bank or from the Bio-Implant Service of the Eurotransplant in Rotterdam, Netherlands. The homograft valves were harvested under sterile conditions from cardiac transplant recipients and multiorgan donors processed and cryopreserved as described elsewhere (5, 10, 13).

Operation techniques

The primary aim of homograft root and valve replacement is to exclude all infected root tissue from the blood circulation and to allow free drainage of abscess cavity and infected tissue after debridement into the pericardial mediastinum (3, 8). The secondary aim is to replace the valve with antibiotic-impregnated homograft tissue, resistant to infection, which exudes antibiotic into the surrounding tissue during the immediate postoperative period. The third aim is to restore the anatomic units of the aortic root without geometric distorsion, particularly when the aortic root is destroyed by abscess formations. The third aim can only be achieved by root replacement technique. After excising the infected aortic valve and completely removing all the periannular infected and necrotic tissues the abscess cavity is well opened and disinfected. The lower end of the homograft root is anastomosed to the host viable aortic annulus by multiple interrupted 4/0 prolene single or pledgeted mattress sutures. The mattress sutures can be placed as interlocking to achieve perfect hemostasis. The mobilized coronary ostia with 2–3 mm of aortic wall cuff are anastomosed to the site of the coronary ostia of the homograft using continuous 5/0 prolene sutures. The distal end of the homograft is anastomosed to the ascending aorta. Root infection without abscess formation was managed with subcoronary freehand valve implantation using the Ross technique, i.e., scalloped homograft with preserved non-coronary sinus (4, 7, 13, 16). Details of implantation techniques are described in the appendix on "Different techniques of homograft aortic valve implantation". Forty-seven patients each received aortic root and subcoronary freehand aortic valve replacements. Seven patients with abscess formation of the aortic mitral septum received subcoronary freehand implant with reconstruction of the destroyed aortic mitral septum with the anterior mitral leaflet of the homograft. The described operation techniques preserve the anatomical and functional units (valve, annulus, commissures and sinuses) of the homograft aortic root (10, 12), the left ventricular outflow and the sino-tubular ridge.

Early and late clinical results

The hospital death rate in patients without root abscesses was 8.7% and with root abscess was 12.7%. New York Heart Association functional class IV and sepsis were

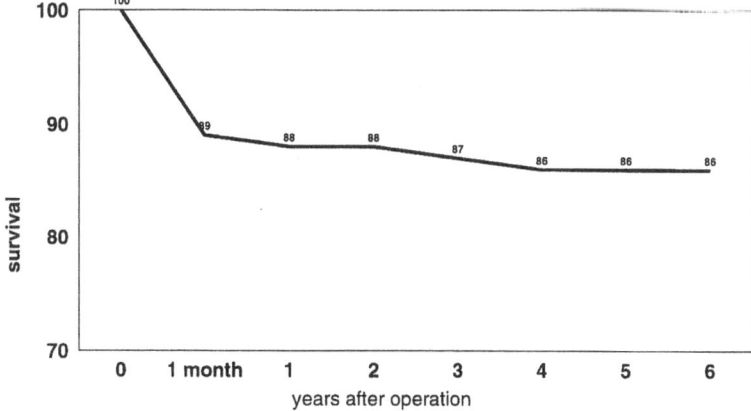

Fig. 1. Actuarial survival including 30-day mortality after homograft subcoronary freehand aortic valve (AVR) and root replacement (ARR) in infected aortic roots.

risk factors for early death. Among the patients receiving cryopreserved homograft valves for subcoronary freehand aortic valve and root replacement techniques the actuarial 1 and 5 years survival was 88% and 86%, respectively (Fig. 1). During a period of follow-up ranging from 1 to 96 months the actuarial survival at 8 years for patients without root abscesses was 91% and 73% for root abscesses.

Structural and non-structural deterioration

During the period of follow-up ranging from 1 to 96 months, one patient with root replacement developed early tissue degeneration within 44 months after operation due to undersized conduit. Two other patients with intact subcoronary valve replacement developed pseudoaneurysm from the right and left coronary subannular abscess cavities 4 and 18 months after surgery, respectively. None of the seven patients

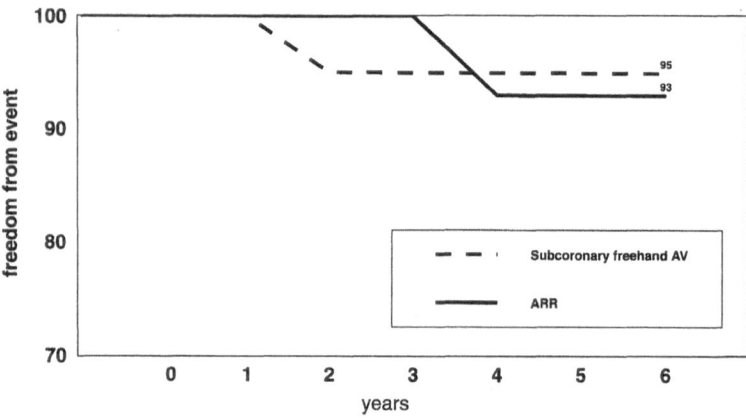

Fig. 2. Actuarial freedom from reoperation for reinfection or psudoaneurysm formation after homograft subcoronary freehand aortic valve (AVR) and root replacement (ARR) in infected aortic roots.

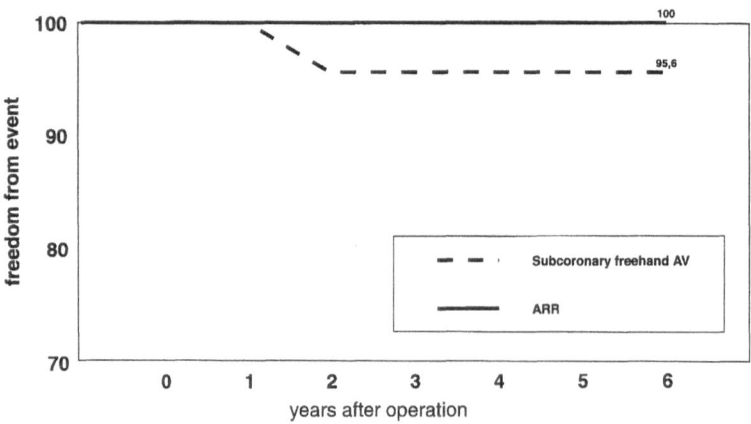

Fig. 3. Actuarial freedom from pseudoaneurysm formation after homograft subcoronary freehand aortic valve (AVR) and root replacement (ARR) in infected aortic roots (ref. 17).

with subcoronary freehand valve implant for the management of the root infection with abscess formation of the aortic mitral septum developed either reinfection or pseudoaneurysm. Freedom from non-structural deterioration (pseudoaneurysm) for the subcoronary implantation technique was 95% and for the root replacement technique was 100%, whereas freedom from reinfection for root replacement technique was 93% at 8 years respectively (Fig. 3).

Reoperation

Five patients underwent reoperation at intervals varying from 4 to 50 months after the first operation. Actuarial freedom from reoperation for subcoronary freehand implantation technique was 95.6% and 93% for root replacement technique at 8 years (Fig. 2).

Appendix

Different implantation techniques of aortic root replacement in an infectious aortic root

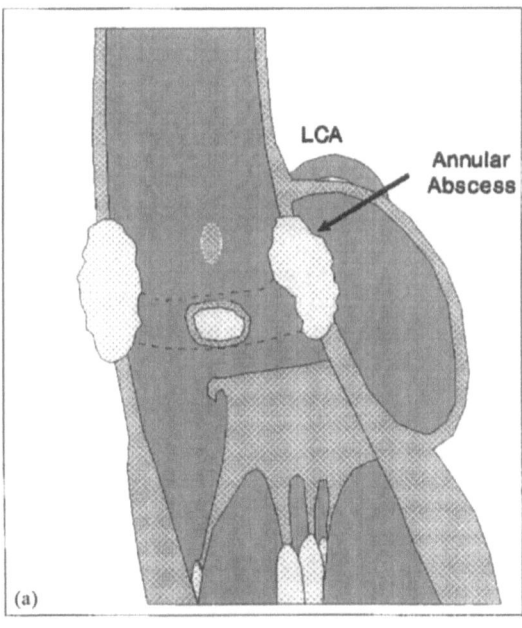

Fig. A1a and b. Demonstration of aortic root infection and complications. a) Native aortic valve endocarditis with extensive aortic root abscess formation which has developed ventricular–aortic dehiscence or discontinuity, b) prosthetic aortic valve endocarditis and pseudoaneurysm formation (LCA = left coronary artery).

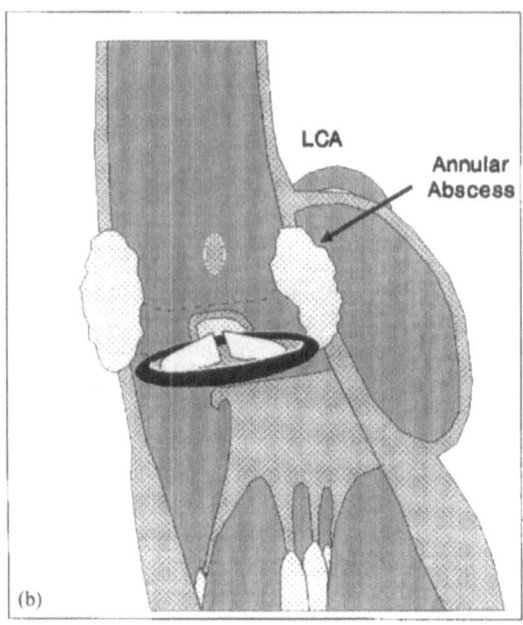

Fig. A1b.

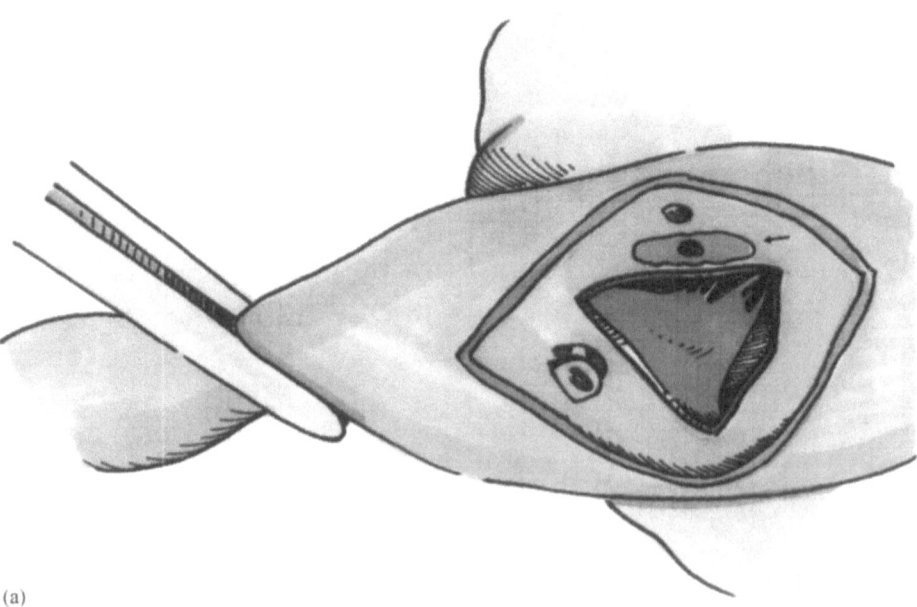

(a)

Fig. A2a and b. Septic aortic root. a) infected aortic root with formation of a ventricular septal defect in a necrotic muscular septum (two arrows), b) closure of supraannular, subcoronary VSD (arrow) before the proximal anastomosis and dissected coronary artery buttons (arrow).

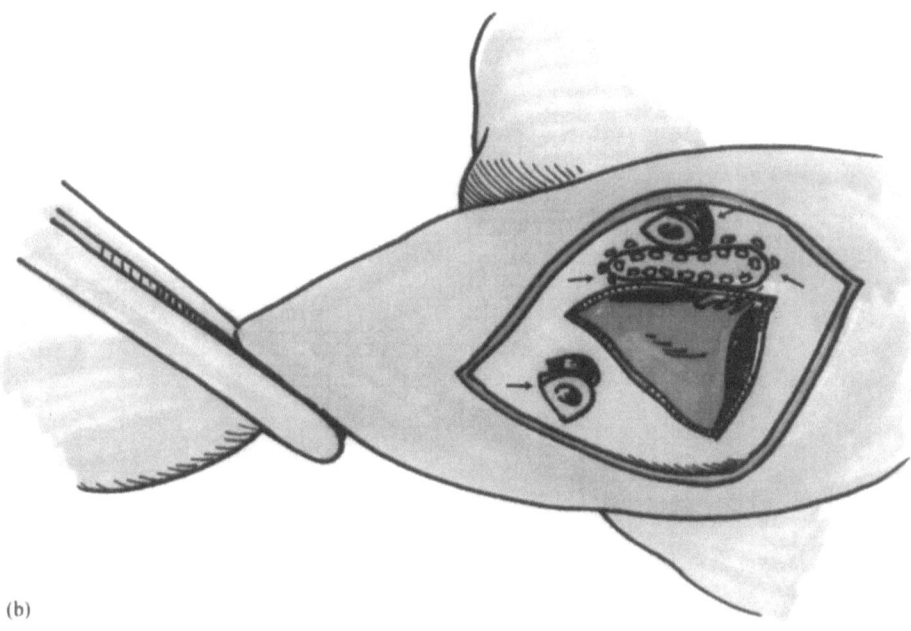

(b)

Fig. A2b.

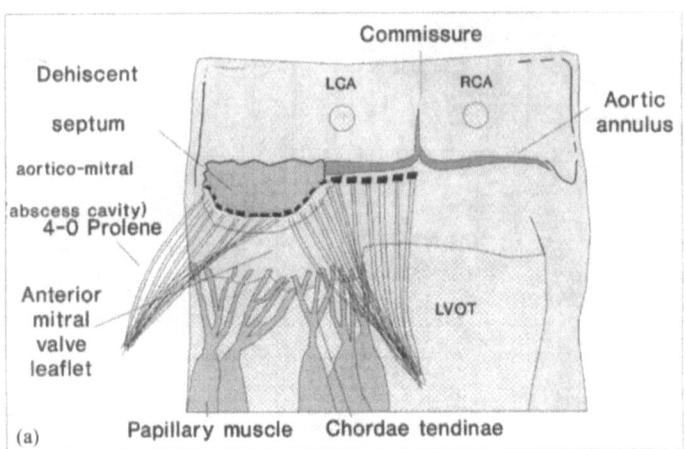

(a)

Fig. A3a and b. Technique of proximal anastomosis in a septic destroyed aortic root. a) Demonstration of an abscess cavity of the aortic-mitral septum. Suturing technique to exteriorize the abscess cavity by placing horizontal multiple single 4/0 prolene mattress sutures with pericardium pledgets at the host anterior mitral annulus along the lower abscess cavity wall up to the aortic annulus from the ventricular to aortic aspect, b) the sutures are passed through the allograft anterior mitral valve leaflet.

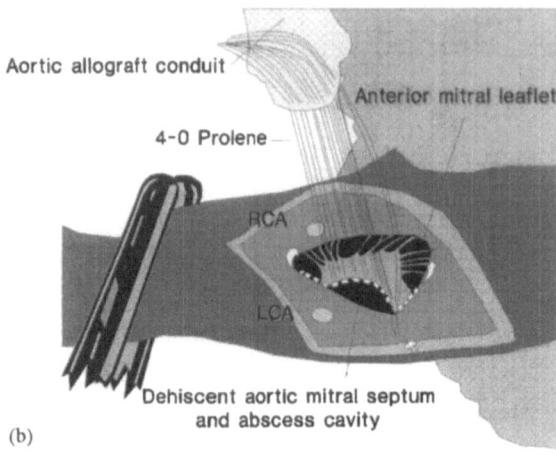

(b)

Fig. A3b.

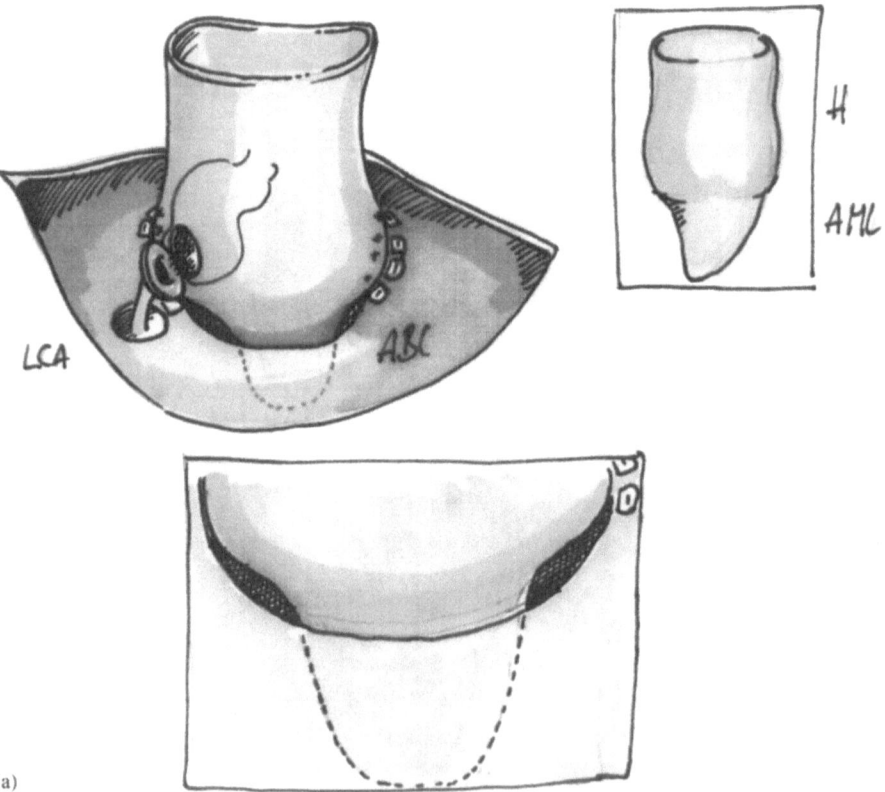

(a)

Fig. A4a–c. a) The allograft is lowered down and the allograft anterior mitral valve leaflet is fixed onto the host anterior mitral annulus and the abscess cavity is exteriorized. The allograft annulus is therefore positioned anatomically for completion of the proximal anastomosis, b) the proximal anastomosis is completed followed by reimplantation of the coronary button. The dissected left and right coronary buttons are sutured side-to-side with 5/0 prolene. The distal allograft conduit is being anastomosed with the host ascending aorta after tailoring to match the allograft size (LCA = left coronary artery), c) completed freestanding allograft aortic root with reimplantation of the coronary arteries (LCA = left coronary artery).

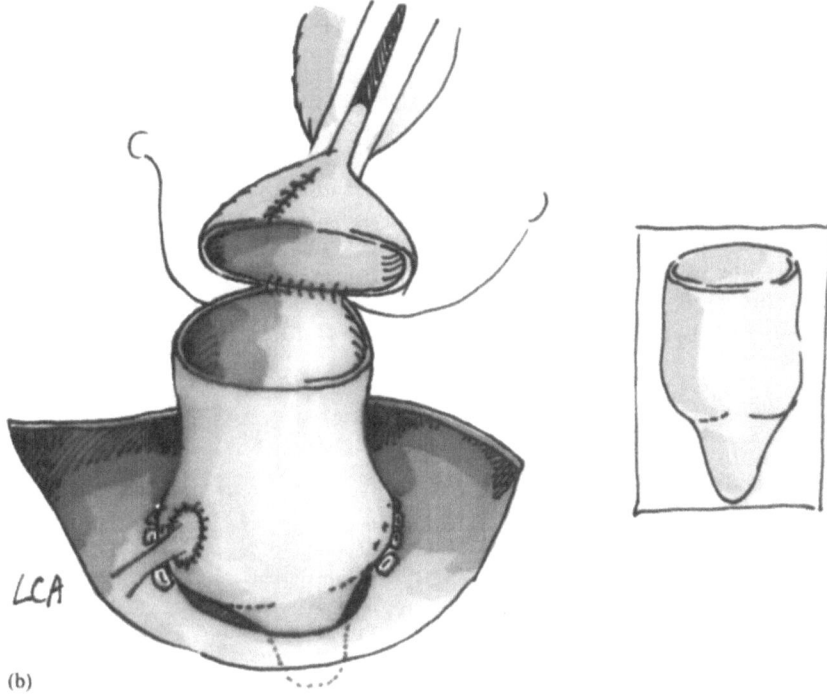

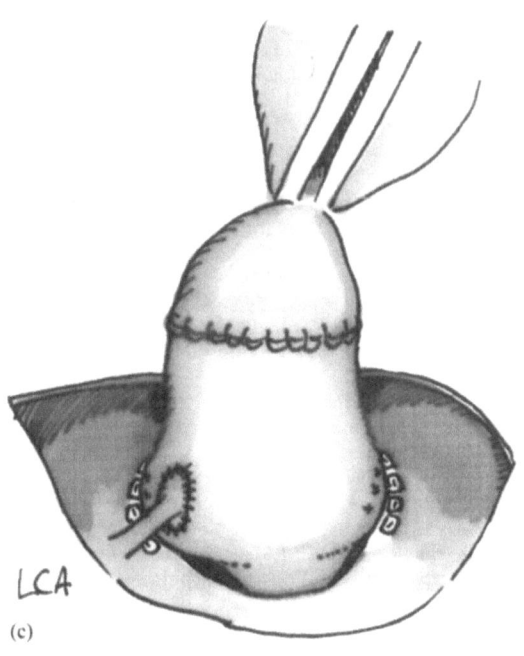

Fig. A4b and A4c.

Discussion

In our previous studies the rate of reinfection of prosthetic valves in infected aortic root was six times higher than that of homograft valves (15). This experience has shown that homograft aortic root replacement or subcoronary valve replacement to exclude infected root or periannular tissue from the blood circulation is an effective surgical method of treating patients with acute infective aortic valve endocarditis. Aortic root replacement is designed for the management of cmplicated aortic root infections with abscess formation which are always associated with geometric distortion of the root (1, 3, 4–11, 15, 16). The results have confirmed our concept and encouraged us to extend the indication to all forms of aortic infection.

References

1. Albertucci M, Wong K, Petrou M, Mitchell A, Somerville J, Theodoropoulos S, Yacoub M (1994) The use of unstented homograft valves for aortic valve reoperations. Review of a twenty-three-year experience. J Thorac Cardiovasc Surg 107: 152–161
2. Bentall HH, DeBono A (1968) A technique for complete replacement of the ascending aorta. Thorax 23: 338–339
3. Donaldson RM, Ross DN (1984) Homograft aortic root replacement for complicated prosthetic valve endocarditis. Circulation 70 (Suppl 1): I179–I182
4. Matsuki O, Robles A, Gibbs S, Bodnar E, Ross DN (1988) Long-term performance of 555 aortic homografts in the aortic position. Ann Thorac Surg 46: 187–191
5. O'Brien MF, Finney RS, Stafford EG, Gardner MAH, Pohlner PG, Tesar PJ, Cochrane AD, Gall KL, Smith SE (1995) Root replacement for all allograft aortic valves: preferred technique or too radical? Ann Thorac Surg 60: S87–S91
6. Okita Y, Franciosi G, Matsuki O, Robbles A, Ross DN (1988) Early and late results of aortic root replacement with antibiotic-sterilized aortic homograft. J Thorac Cardiovasc Surg 95: 696–704
7. Petrou M, Wong K, Albertucci M, Brecker SJ, Yacoub MH (1994) Evaluation of unstented aortic homografts for the treatment of prosthetic aortic valve endocarditis. Circulation 90 (Suppl 2): II198–II204
8. Ross DN (1988) Aortic root replacement with a cardiac allograft. The infected root. In: Cardiac valve allografts 1962–1987. (AC Yankah, R Hetzer, DC Miller, DN Ross, J Somerville, MH Yacoub, eds.). Steinkopff Verlag, Darmstadt, Springer Verlag, New York, pp 167–171
9. Somerville J, Ross DN (1982) Homograft replacement of aortic root with reimplantation of coronary arteries. Br Heart J 47: 473–482
10. Yacoub MH (1988) Allograft aortic root replacement. In: Cardiac valve allografts 1962–1987. (AC Yankah, R Hetzer, DC Miller, DN Ross, J Somerville, MH Yacoub, eds.). Steinkopff Verlag, Darmstadt, Springer Verlag, New York, pp 149–55
11. Yacoub M, Rasmi NRH, Sundt TM, Lund O, Boyland E, Radley-Smith R, Khaghani A, Mitchell A (1995) Fourteen-year experience with homovital homografts for aortic valve replacement. J Thorac Cardiovasc Surg 110: 186–194
12. Yankah AC, Sievers HH, Bürsch JH, Radtke W, Lange P, Heintzen PH, Bernhard A (1984) Orthotopic transplantation of aortic valve allografts. Early hemodynamic results, Thorac Cardiovasc Surgeon 32: 92–95
13. Yankah AC, Wottge HU, Müller-Hermelink HK, Feller AC, Lange P, Wessel U, Dreyer H, Bernhard A, Müller-Ruchholtz W (1987) Transplantation of aortic and pulmonary allografts, enhanced viability of endothelial cells by cryopreservation, importance of histocompatibility. J Cardiac Surg 2 (Suppl): 209–220
14. Yankah AC, Hetzer R (1989) Valve selection and choice in surgery of endocarditis. J Cardiac Surg 4: 324–330

15. Yankah AC, Weng Y, Schiessler A, Warnecke H, Fleck E, Hetzer R (1991) Comparison of mechanical vs. bioprosthetic vs. allograft valve substitute for infective aortic root. Proceedings 5th annual meeting European Assoc. for Cardiothoracic Surgery, Abstr. Nr. 65, p 166
16. Yankah AC, Siniawski H, Lange PE, Fleck E, Hetzer R (1995) Connaissances de Base. Allogreffes et autogreffes valvulaires cardiaques. Conservation et chirurgie (D. Metras ed.) Masson, Paris, Milan, Barcelone, pp 49–78
17. Yankah AC, Weng Y, Hofmeister J, Alexi-Meskhishvili V, Siniawski H, Lange PE, Hetzer R (1996) Freehand subcoronary aortic valve and aortic root replacement with cryo-preserved homografts: Intermediate term results. J. Heart Valve Dis. 5: 498–504

Author's address:
A. Charles Yankah, MD, PhD
Consultant, Assistant Professor
Deutsches Herzzentrum Berlin and Humboldt University
Dept. Cardiothoracic and Vascular Surgery
Augustenburger Platz 1
D-13353 Berlin
Germany

Cryopreserved aortic homografts for mycotic aneurysms and infected arterial grafts

P. R. Vogt, M. I. Turina

Clinic for Cardiovascular Surgery, University Hospital, Zurich, Switzerland

Introduction

The treatment of mycotic aneurysms and infected arterial grafts is a special challenge to the vascular surgeon. As late as 1967, Benett considered infected aneurysms of the abdominal aorta to be invariably fatal (4). Today, almost 30 years later, the management of mycotic aneurysms and infected arterial grafts remains a difficult problem. Complete removal of all infected prosthetic material and reconstruction with extra-anatomic bypass is widely recommended as the only possible solution, although prosthetic *in situ* replacement of mycotic aneurysms and infected grafts, with local and systemic antibiotics, has also been tried. A large variety of treatment modalities has been developed and overall results improved in recent years. Nevertheless, mortality rates of up to 50% and amputation rates of up to 60% are reported (5, 33, 34, 36, 48, 57). Above all, the surgery for mycotic aortic aneurysms and aortic graft infections remains the most demanding technical challenge, due to operative difficulties encountered in heavily scarred, infected regions.

Having substantial experience with extra-anatomic bypass grafting in vascular infections (45), we have been encountering late problems with such reconstruction's, consisting mainly of late thrombotic closure and of a sometimes difficult reversal of the procedure, i.e., anatomic reconstruction of the previously resected aorta. Favourable experience with homograft valves in the treatment of infective aortic valve endocarditis and the excellent long-term survival of implanted cryopreserved human cardiac valves (3, 28, 40, 41, 43, 58) led us to attempt the use of cryopreserved arterial homografts for a single-stage, *in situ* repair of thoracic and abdominal aortic mycotic aneurysms and infected arterial grafts.

The use of arterial homografts in vascular surgery is not new and has been reported by Gross (21), Dubost (13) and Oudet (44). Due to inevitable late aneurysm formation of homografts, Szilagyi (52) confirmed their "unsuitability to serve as vascular substitutes". Subsequently, the use of homografts was abandoned and replacement with vascular prosthesis became the method of choice in aneurysmal and obstructive aortic disease. We believe that their use might be warranted in special occasions, i.e., in presence of a vascular infection, and this report summarises our present clinical experience with the use of cryopreserved arterial homografts.

Material and methods

Patients

Between January 1991 and October 1995, cryopreserved arterial homografts were implanted in 20 consecutive patients with major vascular infection. The mean age was 59 ± 17 years (range, 28 to 85). Mycotic aneurysm and prosthetic graft infection was found in 10 patients each. Emergency surgery was performed in nine patients (45%). Blood cultures were positive in twelve patients (60%) in whom preoperative sepsis was diagnosed. In 18 patients (90%) the antibiotic treatment had been started before the operation. Twelve patients (60%) had undergone between 1 to 10 previous vascular operations. In 13 patients (65%) massive infection or pus accumulation was found intraoperatively. Arterial vessel wall, perigraft tissue or graft cultures were positive in all except two patients (90%). For patients with infected arterial grafts, the mean interval between the first procedure and the insertion of a homograft was 62 months (range, 1 month to 24 years).

Thoracic aorta

The thoracic aorta was affected in 7 patients (35%) (Table 1); four had a mycotic aneurysm and three had prosthetic aortic graft infection: two patients with mycotic aneurysm of the descending thoracic aorta presented with acute massive hemoptysis from aorto-bronchial fistula (Fig. 1). In one of them preoperative transoesophageal echocardiography demonstrated a large false aneurysm of the descending thoracic aorta. In one patient, infectious spondylodiscitis of the 6th thoracic vertebral body was diagnosed 2 months before operation (Fig. 2). Another patient with chronic type A dissection had a history of acute cholecystitis and developed a mycotic aneurysm of the ascending aorta (Fig. 3). One patient presented with an infected vascular prosthesis and bacterial aortitis of the transverse aortic arch after graft replacement of the proximal descending thoracic aorta for acute type B dissection.

Abdominal aorta

The abdominal aorta and distal vessels were affected in 13 patients (65%) (Table 2); five had a mycotic aneurysm of the infrarenal aorta and one of the left common iliac artery; seven had prosthetic aorto bifemoral graft infection. In five patients (38%) persistent bleeding or sinus tracts draining through the groin were found, originating

Table 1. Mycotic aneurysms and infected arterial grafts: Thoracic aorta

- Mycotic aneurysm of the ascending aorta after chronic type A dissection
- Mycotic aneurysm of the descending aorta after spondylodiscitis
- Mycotic aneurysm of the descending aorta with aorto-bronchial fistula
- Mycotic aneurysm + large false aneurysm of the descending aorta with aorto-bronchial fistula after repair for coarctation of the aorta
- Infected supracoronary aortic graft after repair for acute type A dissection
- Infected composite graft after repair for anulo-aortic ectasia
- Infected descending aortic graft and infectious aortitis of the transverse arch after repair for chronic type B dissection

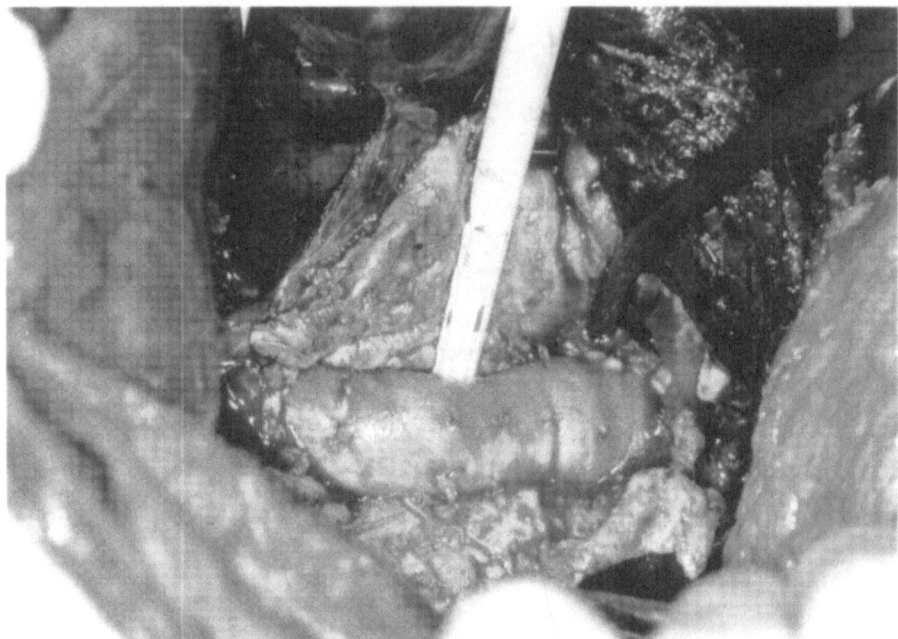

Fig. 1. Sixty-nine-year-old patient: intraoperative view of an aneurysm of the descending thoracic aorta with aorto-bronchial fistula. Infectious agent: *Mycobacterium tuberculosis. In situ* repair with a cryopreserved aorta descendens homograft.

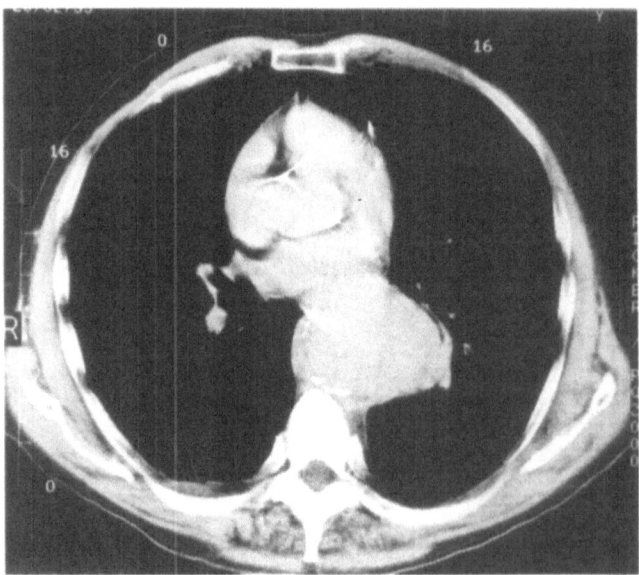

Fig. 2. Sixty-one-year-old patient with a mycotic aneurysm of the descending thoracic aorta, 2 months after spondylodiscitis with *Streptococcus penumoniae.*

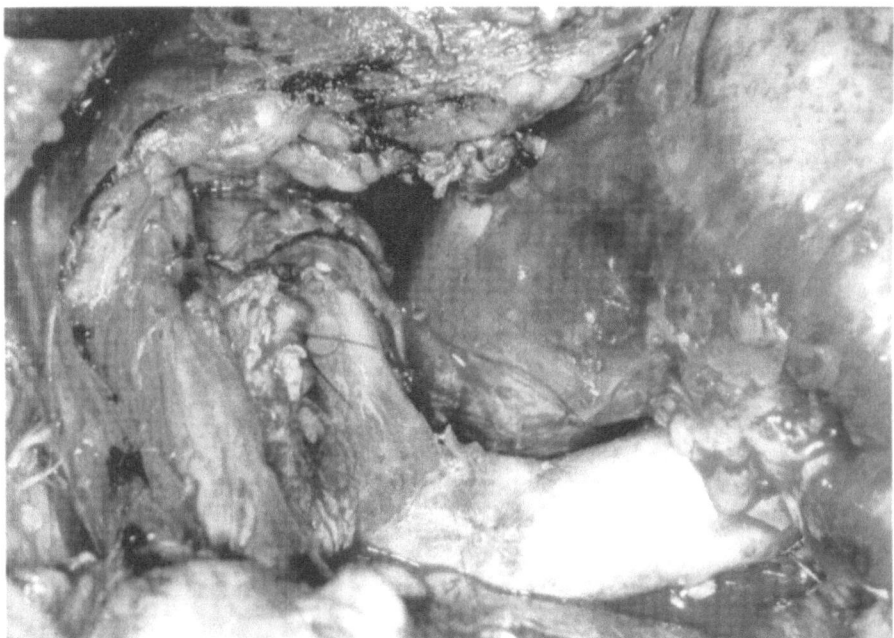

Fig. 3. Seventy-three-year-old patient with a mycotic aneurysm of the ascending aorta after chronic type A-dissection, 1 month after acute cholecystitis. Infectious agent unidentified. *In situ* repair of the ascending aorta with a cryopreserved aorta descendens homograft.

Table 2. Mycotic aneurysms and infected arterial grafts: Abdominal aorta

- Mycotic aneurysm of the infrarenal aorta
- Mycotic aneurysm of the left common iliac artery
- Mycotic aneurysm of the infrarenal aorta and the right common iliac artery combined with perforated diverticulitis
- Mycotic, inflammatory aneurysm of the juxtarenal aorta
- Mycotic aneurysm of the infrarenal aorta, combined with an infected false aneurysm and an infected prosthetic graft of the left iliac artery
- Mycotic, symptomatic aneurysm of the infrarenal aorta, combined with sepsis from bacterial knee joint arthritis and urosepsis
- Bacterial aortitis of the infrarenal aortic stump, combined with infected right axillofemoral and femorofemoral grafts
- Infected aorto-bifemoral (superficial femoral artery) graft
- Infected aorto-bifemoral graft with uretero-cutaneous fistula
- Infected aorto-biiliac graft
- Infected aorto-bifemoral graft: two patients
- Infected retroperitoneal space after inadvertent intestinal lesion after aorto-biiliac graft replacement for chronic aortic occlusion

from the prosthetic material. One patient had uretero-cutaneous fistula draining along the right leg of the aorto-bifemoral prosthesis. One patient with a 14-day history of abdominal pain had combined symptomatic infrarenal aortic aneurysm and perforated diverticulitis of the sigmoid colon. Another patient presented with an inflammatory juxtarenal aortic aneurysm which became infected. A 55-year old patient had aorto-bifemoral Dacron prosthesis 7 years ago. Due to prosthetic graft infection, he had 10 subsequent reoperations and finally presented with acute bleeding through the left groin. He had six different prosthetic grafts reaching from the infrarenal aorta to the distal part of the superficial femoral artery on the right as well on the left side (Fig. 4). Two patients were on dialysis due to diabetic end-stage nephropathy. One was hospitalised continuously during the 6 months prior to homograft insertion (renal transplantation, removal of a necrotic renal graft, aorto-iliac reconstruction and extra-anatomic bypass with secondary infection). The other was repeatedly hospitalised during the 2 years prior to the implantation of the homograft. He had a mycotic aneurysm of the infrarenal aorta, an infected aorto-iliac Dacron prosthesis and a huge infected spurious aneurysm, extending into the left retroperitoneal space, containing *Pseudomonas aeruginosa* (Figs. 5 and 6).

Preoperative antibiotic treatment

Preoperative antibiotic treatment was already instituted in 12 (60%) patients and was either empirical, or based on microbiological results. Seven patients (35%) had a history of prolonged preoperative antibiotic treatment up to 2 years prior to homograft implantation using multiple combinations of different antibiotics.

Homograft selection and preparation

Large arteries are procured under sterile conditions from brain-dead multi-organ donors or cadavers, aged from 18 to 40 years. All donors who fulfil heart valve

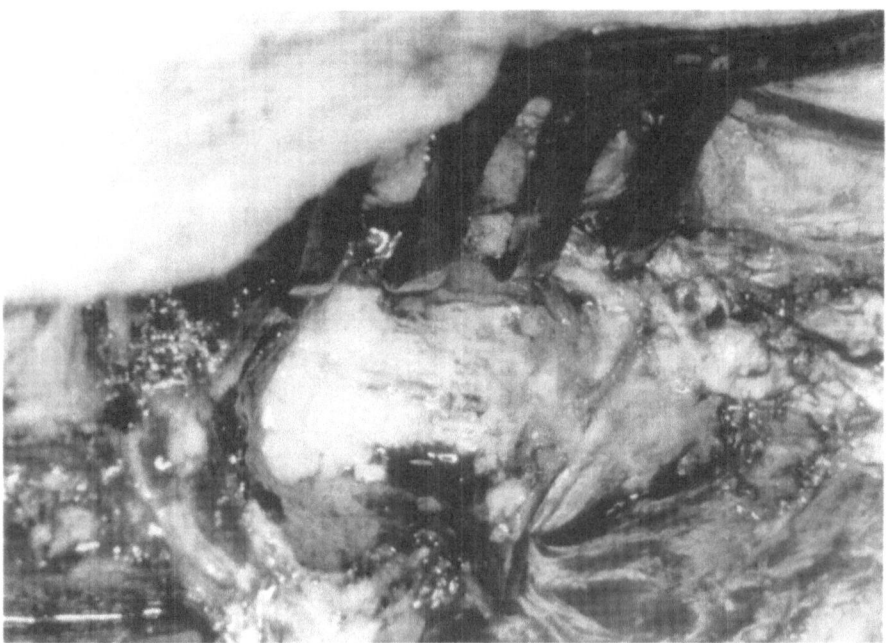

Fig. 4. Fifty-eight-year-old patient with an infected arterial bifurcation graft, extending from the infrarenal aorta to the distal superficial femoral artery on the right as well on the left side: Right groin, infected with *Staphylococcus aureus* and *Candida parapsilosis*.

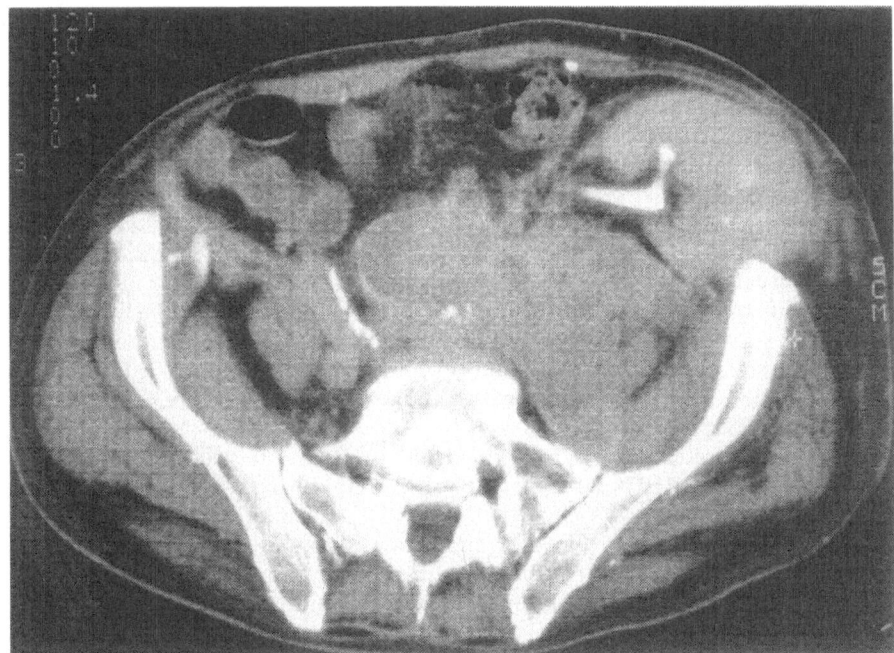

Fig. 5. Preoperative CT scan: 59-year-old man with a mycotic aneurysm of the infrarenal aorta, combined with an infected arterial graft of the left iliac artery and a large false aneurysm extending into the left retroperitoneal space. Infectious agent: *Pseudomonas aeruginosa.*

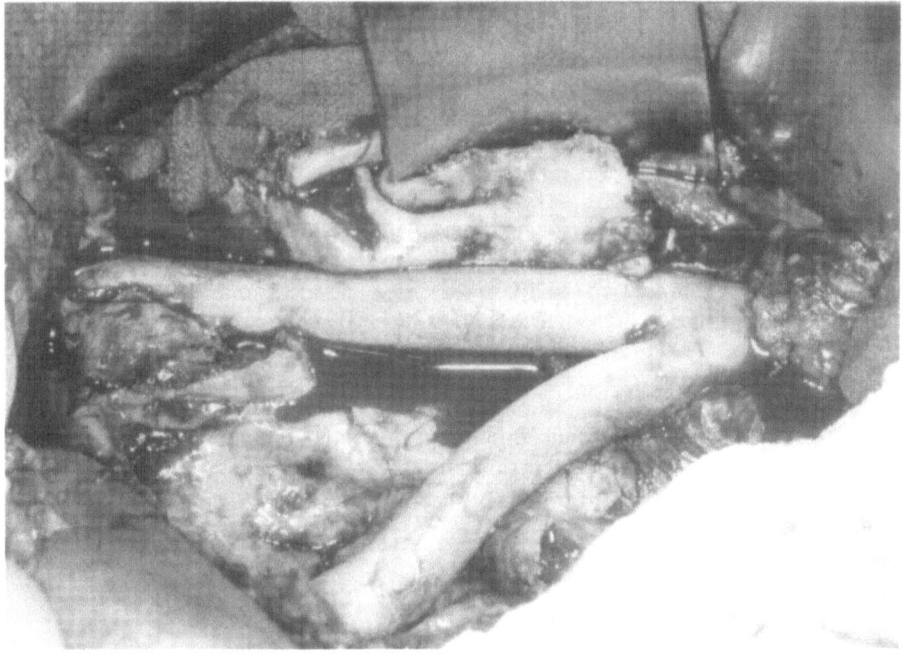

Fig. 6. Cryopreserved aorto-biiliac bifurcation homograft in the patient, described in Fig. 5. Note the severely altered retroperitoneal tissue after four previous operation.

selection criterias according to the European standards for cryopreserved heart valve homografts (16) are candidates for donation of the ascending aorta with or without transverse aortic arch, of the descending aorta, aortic bifurcation, iliac and femoral vessels including the superficial femoral artery and the proximal part of the profunda femoris. All vessels are procured in an aseptic fashion. They are packed in ice-cold sterile transport solution and sent to the European Homograft Bank, Brussels, where they are prepared inside a first grade laminar flow room.

There, further dissection of the vessels is performed. Internal diameters of the distal and proximal end of the vessels are measured with a calibrated Hegar dilatator. The exact length of each vessel will be recorded. Intraluminal alterations are looked for by angioscopy. Finally, specimens for histological examination are taken. All vessels are recorded on a standardised form comprising schematic drawings and accompany the homograft at distribution. Decontamination is achieved by means of a low concentrated antibiotic cocktail at 4 °C during 24 h and for 48 h when the donor was kept on artificial ventilation for more than 2 days.

Thereafter, cryopreservation is performed: all vessels are transferred to an ice-cold cryoprotective solution (10% DMSO) and sealed in double pouches. The pouches are frozen in liquid nitrogen vapour to −100 °C, according to an electronically monitored program and stored in the vapour phase of liquid nitrogen at −180 °C. Cryopreservation media, time and temperature of incubation as well as freezing rates and control-rate freezing endpoints that produce a clinically suitable homograft are noted. The pouches are transported with a cryogenic dry shipper maintaining a temperature of the frozen tissue below −130 °C for the entire time. The grafts are thawed and washed immediately before implantation according to a well defined protocol.

Operative technique

Thoracic aorta

The ascending aorta and the transverse arch are approached through a median sternotomy. Cardiopulmonary bypass is instituted through a right femoral artery and a right atrial venous cannula. Cardiac arrest is achieved by retrograde application of cold blood cardioplegia. For deep hypothermic circulatory arrest, retrograde cerebral perfusion is used. The mycotic aneurysm or the infected graft of the ascending aorta or the transverse arch are excised. Minimal periaortic debridement is performed and the homograft is inserted end-to-end to the normal aorta, using a single non-absorbable running polypropylene suture (Fig. 3). In the case of aortic arch replacement, the arch vessels are anastomosed each separately end-to-end to the homograft.

The descending aorta is approached through a left-sided posterolateral thoracotomy. The left groin vessels are cannulated, partial cardiopulmonary bypass with a heparin-coated oxygenator and moderate hypothermia (30 °C) is used. After clamping, the aneurysm is opened longitudinally and resected. The posterior aortic wall is tailored to preserve the most important intercostal arteries. A tube homograft is inserted end-to-end to the normal aorta with a single non-absorbable running polypropylene suture (Fig. 1). Important intercostal arteries are implanted into the homograft.

Abdominal aorta

For mycotic aneurysms of the infrarenal aorta/iliac arteries, a standard midline incision is performed. The infected aneurysmatic tissue is resected. The posterior wall of the aneurysm is left *in situ*. A cryopreserved tube or bifurcation homograft is inserted, anastomoses are performed in an end-to-end fashion to the normal aorta above and distal arteries below the mycotic aneurysm, utilising a non-absorbable running polypropylene suture (Fig. 6). In the case of the infected juxtarenal, inflammatory aneurysm, the proximal anastomosis is sutured directly at the ostia of the renal arteries. The thick inflamed aortic wall containing parts of the retroperitoneal duodenum is only minimal derided. A sigma resection according to Hartmann's technique was performed in the patient with the 14-day old perforated diverticulitis. As there were dense adhesions, only those parts of the huge, aorto-iliac aneurysm were resected which were easily accessible. An aorto-biiliac bifurcation homograft was inserted.

For infected prosthetic grafts, a retroperitoneal approach is used to replace infected infrarenal prostheses. A tube or bifurcation homograft is inserted as described. In the case of an infected extra-anatomic right axillo-femoral and femoro-femoral prosthetic bypass, the infrarenal aorta was reconstructed first and then the extra-anatomic bypass was removed. The large defects of the axillary and femoral arteries were reconstructed with homograft patches. For one patient, homografts from four donors were used to reconstruct both aorto-ilio-femoral axes in one step.

Microbiology and postoperative antibiotic treatment

Appropriate intraoperative collection of aspirates of pus, perigraft exudates, biopsies and tissue specimens is arranged with the infectious disease consultant. Rapid gram staining and reading for aerobes and anaerobes is performed. Appropriate culture medias and conditions, especially for anaerobes, fungi and mycobacterias, are secured in advance. The responsible infectious agents were identified in 90% of cases and are listed in Table 3.

Postoperative intravenous antibiotic treatment was chosen according to the microbiological results including antimicrobial susceptibility testing. The duration of antibiotic treatment was decided individually for each patient and was influenced by the type of the infectious agent and by the extension of the infection as determined intraoperatively. None of the patients received long-term or indefinite antibiotic treatment.

Table 3. Intraoperatively identified microorganisms

Staphylococcus coagulase-negative
Staphylococcus aureus
Streptococcus pneumoniae
Pseudomonas aeruginosa
Aspergillus fumigatus
Mycobacterium tuberculosis
Candida albicans
Candida parapsilosis
Propionibacterium acnes
Escherichia coli
In 90% of patients, the responsible infectious agent has been identified. Three patients had vascular infection with more than one microorganism: one with *Mycobacterium, Staphylococcus aureus* and *Aspergillus fumigatus*; one with *Staphylococcus aureus* and *Candida parapsilosis* and one with *Staphylococcus aureus* and *Candida albicans*

Follow-up

Early and medium-term follow-up information were obtained from the referring hospital or from the primary care physician. Computed tomography (CT), magnetic resonance imaging (MRI), transoesophageal echocardiography (TEE) and/or intravenous digital subtraction angiography were performed routinely at the end of this follow-up. The average follow-up was 18.6 ± 17.4 months (range, 2 to 58).

Results

There was one early postoperative death, for a hospital mortality of 5%: a 75-year-old patient had a perforation of the sigmoid colon with faecal peritonitis 6 days after implantation of an aorto-bifemoral bifurcation Dacron-prosthesis. The prosthesis was replaced by an aorto-bifemoral homograft; he had subsequent laparotomies for abscesses and died 3 weeks later from multi-organ failure.

The mean hospital stay was 23 ± 18 days (6 to 48). Hospital stays above 21 days were entirely due to prolonged intravenous antibiotic treatment. Neurologic complications were not observed. Reoperations were necessary in four patients: a femoropopliteal vein graft for associated peripheral vascular disease; an iliaco-femoral vein graft for ongoing infection of an external iliac artery segment; splenectomy for delayed spleen rupture on the 2nd postoperative day; stabilisation for accidental hip fracture. Delayed wound healing was observed in 4/19 survivors (21%). No delayed operative wound closure was necessary.

The mean duration of the postoperative antibiotic treatment was 34 ± 14.6 days (range, 4 to 72). Antibiotic treatment for more than 6 weeks was carried out only in the

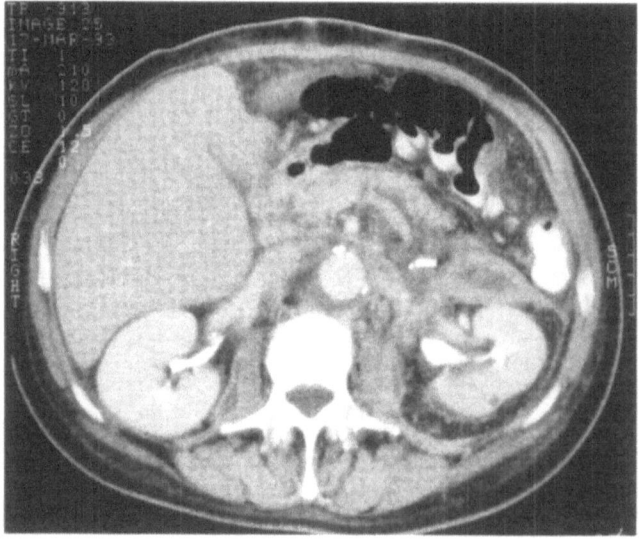

Fig. 7. Postoperative CT-scan: 59-year-old patient 1 month after replacement of a mycotic aneurysm of the infrarenal aorta with a cryopreserved aortic tube homograft.

case of fungal infection. Postoperatively, neither septic nor homograft-related complications were observed. There were three late deaths (16%), of which only one (5.6%) was homograft related: an 85-year-old patient with an aorto-bifemoral homograft died 7 months later due to acute upper gastrointestinal bleeding. On autopsy, there was an inferior mesenterico (homograft)-duodenal fistula. The second patient was a 41-year-old patient who died 9 months later from severe diabetes-related complications; the reconstruction with homograft was intact and he was free from infection. The third patient died from coronary artery disease.

Postoperative MRI in eight patients, CT scan in nine, angiography in eight and TEE in four patients were normal. There were no false aneurysm nor homograft leakage. Neither peri-homograft exudation, unusual scar formation or intraluminal mural thrombi of the homografts could be detected by MR-angiography or CT-scan (Fig. 7). All patients had normal peripheral circulation and were free of infection with normal hematologic findings.

Discussion

Present treatment of vascular infections

Cryopreserved arterial homografts are an effective treatment for mycotic aneurysms and prosthetic graft infection of the thoracic aorta, the abdominal aorta and the iliaco-femoral arteries as well as for infected extra-anatomic bypass. In 1967, Benett predicted that all patients with mycotic aneurysms would finally succumb to their disease (4). In the same year, Fry and Lindenauer reported a 75% mortality and a 33% incidence of limb loss among survivors of aortic graft infection (20).

Since then, improvement in the treatment of vascular infection has occurred and has resulted in remarkably improved outcome. Nevertheless, 30 years later, the treatment of mycotic aneurysm and arterial graft infection remains a special challenge to the vascular surgeon and the microbiologist alike. Even in recent series mortality and amputation both range up to 58% with the highest mortality and morbidity resulting from thoracic and abdominal aortic infection (42, 49, 50).

Currently, *in situ* repair with vascular prostheses and extra-anatomic reconstruction, in particular the axillo-femoral bypass, are mainly used to treat these life-threatening conditions. Both techniques carry a substantial rate of mortality and morbidity and are associated with several potential complications (1, 23, 38). Extra-anatomic bypass techniques allow complete removal of all infected prosthetic material and has urgently been recommended in severe sepsis, in situations, where significant haemorrhage would be associated with the aortic anastomosis as well as in pangraft infections with virulent organisms like Pseudomonas or fungi (12). Nevertheless, this technique has several distinct disadvantages: first, depending on the site of infection, e.g. transverse aortic arch or paravisceral aorta, extra-anatomic reconstruction may be impossible; second, extra-anatomic grafts may become subsequently infected (1, 23, 38) and have lower overall patency rates than aorto-iliac or aorto-femoral reconstruction (9, 15, 32), necessitating multiple reoperations in the axilla, the groin and in the retroperitoneum; third, total graft excision has a high mortality (1, 23, 38) and amputation rate (53, 57) and fourth, aortic stump blow-out is associated with up to 43% of the early deaths and 71% of the late deaths (49).

In situ interposition of a vascular prostheses may prevent the complications of an extra-anatomic bypass and give satisfactory long-term results with early mortality rates as low as 14% to 17% (57). Nevertheless, suture line complications and secondary graft infections may occur (30). Prolonged antibiotic treatment is necessary and sometimes recommended as a life-long therapy (6, 11).

Previous experience with arterial homografts

The implantation of homografts for mycotic aneurysms and infected arterial grafts has occasionally been recommended (2, 29, 39). Kieffer reported the use of fresh allografts, stored at 4 °C for 48 h. The operative mortality rate was 13.8% (25, 26). After a mean follow-up of 19.6 ± 14.0 months (range, 1 to 53) 24% had pathologic changes in the allograft requiring reoperation in 9% (26). This might have been caused by inadequate homograft preservation methods which may result in shorter homograft survival (21, 46). This is supported by the excellent long-term survival of cryopreserved human cardiac valves (3) which have significantly superior long-term results than freshly implanted cardiac allografts valves (41).

Advantages of a one-stage repair

We believe that many complex techniques, like extended perigraft, mediastinal and chest wall debridement, mobilisation of viable tissue such as omentum or flaps of muscle as well as sacrifice of arteries and veins as autografts (7, 8), applied to treat mycotic aneurysms and graft infection (10, 18, 19, 22, 27, 31, 35, 37, 47, 51, 54, 56) can be replaced by the use of cryopreserved homografts.

This technique allows safe *in situ* repair and limits extended debridement at the site of infection. Local antibiotic treatment, producing resistant strains, is unnecessary. Cryopreserved homografts may achieve impressing results: this is demonstrated by the 55-year-old patient, whose 7-year-old aorto-bifemoral Dacron graft became infected and who had 10 subsequent reoperations during the following 2 years. Finally, he presented with massive purulent *Staphyloccocus aureus* and *Candida parapsilosis* infection of a graft which extended from the infrarenal aorta to the distal superficial femoral artery on the right as well on the left side. In this case, we think that the total graft replacement by homografts in one step, combined with limited antibiotic treatment, has been live-saving.

Reliable eradication of vascular infection was observed even in the presence of virulent or traditionally difficult to treat organisms like *Pseudomonas aeruginosa*, *Mycobacterium tuberculosis*, *Candida albicans* or *Aspergillus fumigatus*.

In this difficult patient population, the use of cryopreserved homografts has a mortality rate which compares favourably with the results for primary replacement of non-infected abdominal aortic aneurysms (14). In addition, there was no early or late amputation, a finding which is clearly confirmed by Kieffer (26).

Postoperatively, homografts do not produce the diagnostic problems seen in other vascular prostheses, such as prolonged postoperative pyrexia or unusual perivascular inflammatory responses like fluid accumulation and scar formation around the graft (55), avoiding troublesome investigations for presumed persistent or early recurrent infection.

Therefore, vascular reconstruction with cryopreserved arterial homografts is indicated in mycotic aneurysms and arterial infection of the thoracic and abdominal aorta, iliac and femoral vessels. Vascular prostheses infection at any site of the arterial tree, aorto-enteric fistula and contamination of retroperitoneal space by intestinal content represent ideal indications for the use of these grafts. Even aorto-bronchial fistula, a highly lethal condition (17), can be treated safely by homograft interposition.

Long-term concerns after implantation of an arterial homograft

However, several questions are yet unanswered: first, a main concern is the long-term behaviour of arterial homografts after implantation in the human body. Large arteries such as the descending aorta should maintain a good patency, even in the case of postoperative neo-intimal fibrous sheeting. Smaller-sized arterial homografts such as the distal part of the external iliac and the superficial femoral artery are more likely to become obliterated by neo-intimal proliferation and thrombosis. "Fresh" larger arteries (homografts preserved in antibiotics at 2–4 °C for up to 3 weeks) are completely devitalised and show superficial alteration, probably as a result of non-calcific medial degeneration (23). In contrary, cryopreserved homograft heart valves are reported to be viable up to 10 years after implantation (24). Although the exact role of graft viability is not clear, concerning the long-term results of cryopreserved valves, we are expecting satisfactory patency rates and long-term stability of our cryopreserved arterial homografts. Even if this should not be true, arterial homografts may help eradicate the infection and allow later implantation of a prosthetic graft without the fear for recurrent infection.

Homografts are resistant to infection

It has not yet been clearly elucidated why cryopreserved homografts appear more resistant to bacterial infection than other conduits. Viability early after implantation may be important, possibly allowing antibiotic drug diffusion into the homograft. Rejection phenomenons combined with allurement of immunocompetent cells, provoked by the implanted homograft, may support eradication of the infection. These are interesting hypotheses, but to date, are entirely speculative. Culture-specific antibiotic treatment, based on perioperative microbiologic investigations, is an important component in the treatment of vascular infections. In these patients, the antibiotic treatment is based on the experience gained with the use of cryopreserved cardiac valve homografts in the treatment of aortic valve endocarditis. Although the duration of antibiotic treatment has been consistently lowered during this study, it has not yet been exactly determined.

Summary

Although larger clinical series and longer follow-up will be necessary to estimate the true potential of cryopreserved arterial homografts in the surgery of mycotic aneurysms and infected vascular prostheses, our early results are very satisfactory. Homograft vascular replacements have a low early and late mortality, they allow safe *in situ* repair, shorten the hospitalisation, reduce postoperative antibiotic requirements and obviate the need for early or medium-term reoperations. The results of this study encourage the use of vascular homografts as the prostheses of choice in the surgery of mycotic aneurysm and infected prosthetic grafts.

References

1. Bacourt F, Koskas F (1992) Axillobifemoral bypass and aortic exclusion for vascular septic lesions: a multicenter retrospective study of 98 cases. French University Association for Research in Surgery. Ann Vasc Surg 6: 119–126
2. Bahnini A, Ruotolo C, Koskas F, et al. (1991) In situ fresh allograft replacement of an infected aortic prosthetic graft: eighteen-month follow-up. J Vasc Surg 14: 98–102
3. Belcher P, Ross D (1991) Aortic root replacement – 20 years' experience of the use of homografts. Thorac Cardiovasc Surg 39: 117–122
4. Benett D, Cherry J (1967) Bacterial infections of aortic aneurysms. Am J Surg 113: 321–326
5. Casali RE, Tucker WE, Thompson BW, et al. (1980) Infected prosthetic grafts. Arch Surg 115: 577–580
6. Chan FY, Crawford ES, Coselli JS, et al. (1989) In situ prosthetic graft replacement for mycotic aneurysm of the aorta. Ann Thorac Surg 47: 193–203
7. Clagett GP, Bowers BL, Lopez-Viego MA, et al. (1993) Creation of a neo-aortoiliac system from lower extremity deep and superficial veins. Ann Surg 218: 239–248
8. Clagett GP (1994) A new option for treatment of infected aortic prostheses: the NAIS operation. In: Calligaro KD, Veith FJ (eds) Management of Infected Arterial Grafts. Quality Medical Publishing, Inc. St. Louis, Missouri, pp 82–94
9. Colburn MD, Moorew WS (1994) Reoperative approach for failed aortofemoral, axillofemoral and femorofemoral bypass. In: Rutherford RB (ed.) Seminars in Vascular Surgery. W.B. Saunders Company, Philadelphia PA, pp 139–151
10. Colburn MD, Moore WS, Chvapil M, et al. (1992) Use of an antibiotic-bonded graft for in situ reconstruction after prosthetic graft infection. J Vasc Surg 16: 651–658
11. Crawford ES, Crawford JL (1984) Diseases of the aorta including an atlas of angiographic pathology and surgical technique. Williams & Wilkins, Baltimore London, pp 340–374
12. Curl GR, Ricotta JJ (1994) Total prosthetic graft excision and extra-anatomic bypass. In Calligaro KD, Veith FJ (eds) Management of Infected Arterial Grafts. Quality Medical Publishing, Inc. St. Louis, Missouri, pp 82–94
13. Dubost C, Allary M, Oeconomas N (1952) Resection of an aneurysm of the abdominal aorta. Re-establishment of the continuity by a preserved human arterial graft, with result after five months. Arch Surg 64: 405–408
14. Ernst CB (1993) Current concepts: abdominal aortic aneurysm. N Engl J Med 328: 1167–1172
15. Eugene J, Goldstone J, Moore WS (1997) Fifteen-year experience with subcutaneous bypass grafts for lower extremity ischemia. Ann Surg 186: 177–183
16. European standards for cryopreserved heart valve homografts. Annexe 1 in: Metras D. Allogreffes et autogreffes valvulaires cardiaques. Conservation et chirurgie. Masson, Paris Milan, Barcelona 1995; 107–112
17. Favre JP, Gournier JP, Adham M, et al. (1994) Aortobronchial fistula: report of three cases and review of the literature. Surgery 115: 264–270
18. Favre JP, Gournier JP, Barral X (1993) Trans-osseus ilio-femoral bypass. A new extra-anatomical bypass. J Cardiovasc Surg Torino 34: 455–459
19. Fokin AA, Zotov SP, Verbovetskii LP, et al. (1991) Replacement of infected vascular prosthesis by the femoral vein. Khirurgiia Mosk 6: 57–59
20. Fry WJ, Lindenauer SM (1967) Infection complicating the use of plastic arterial implants. Arch Surg 94: 600–609
21. Gross RE, Hurwitt ES, Bill AH Jr, et al. (1948) Preliminary observations on the use of human arterial grafts in the treatment of certain cardiovascular defects. N Engl J Med 239: 578–579
22. Haverich A, Hirt S, Karck M, et al. (1992) Prevention of graft infection by bonding of gentamycin to Dacron prostheses. J Vasc Surg 15: 187–193
23. Higgins RSD, Steed DL, Julian TB, et al. (1990) The management of aortoenteric and paraprosthetic fistulae. J Cardiovasc Surg 31: 81–86
24. Khanna SK, Ross JK, Monro JL (1981) Homograft aortic valve replacement: seven years' experience with antibiotic-treated valves. Thorax 36: 330–337

25. Kieffer E, Bahnini A, Koskas F, et al. (1993) In-situ allograft replacement of infected infrarenal aortic prosthetic grafts: results in forty-three patients. J Vasc Surg 17: 349–356
26. Kieffer E, Plissonnier D, Bahnini A, et al. (1994) Abdominal aortic graft excision and in situ allograft replacement. In: Calligaro KD, Veith FJ (eds) Management of Infected Arterial Grafts. Quality Medical Publishing, Inc. St. Louis, Missouri: 82–94
27. Kinney EV, Bandyk DF, Seabrook GA, et al. (1991) Antibiotic-bonded PTFE vascular grafts: the effect of silver antibiotic on bioactivity following implantation. J Surg Res 50: 430–435
28. Kirklin JK, Kirklin JW, Pacifico AD (1988) Aortic valve endocarditis with aortic root abscess cavity: surgical treatment with aortic valve homograft. Ann Thorac Surg 45: 674–677
29. Kniemeyer HW, Torsello G, Hennes N, et al. (1994) Frisches homologes Arterientransplantat als aorto-iliako-femoraler Gefässersatz bei Protheseninfektion. VASA 23: 268–273
30. Lai DT, Huber D, Hogg J (1993) Obturator foramen bypass in the management of infected prosthetic vascular grafts. Aust N Z J Surg 63: 811–814
31. Leather RP, Darling RC 3d, Chang BB, et al. (1992) Retroperitoneal in-line aortic bypass for treatment of infected infrarenal aortic grafts. Surg Gynecol Obstet 175: 491–494
32. LoGerfo FW, Johnson WC, Corson JD (1973) A comparison of the late patency rates of axillobilateral femoral and axillounilateral femoral grafts. Surgery 81: 33–40
33. Lorentzen JE, Nielsen OM, Arendrup H, et al. (1985) Vascular graft infection: an analysis of sixty-two graft infections in 2411 consecutively implanted synthetic vascular grafts. Surgery 98: 81–86
34. Martin-Paredero V, Busuttil RW, Dixon SM, et al. (1983) Fate of aortic graft removal. Am J Surg 146: 194–197
35. McCarthy WJ, McGee GS, Lin WW, et al. (1992) Axillary-popliteal artery bypass provides successful limb salvage after removal of infected aortofemoral grafts. Arch Surg 127: 974–978
36. McNamara MF, Roberts AB, Bakshi KR (1987) Gram-negative bacterial infection of aortic aneurysm. J Cardiovasc Surg 28: 453–455
37. Mehran RJ, Graham AM, Ricci MA, et al. (1992) Evaluation of muscle flaps in the treatment of infected aortic grafts. J Vasc Surg 15: 487–494
38. Monreal M, Callejas JM, Lisbona C, et al. (1993) Surgical wound infection in patients undergoing extraanatomical arterial surgery. A retrospective study. Angiologia 45: 199–202
39. Nevelsteen A, Goffin Y, Lacroix H, et al. (1995) Recurrent aortic infection: treatment by arterial homograft replacement. Cardiovasc Surg 3: 441–444
40. O'Brien M, Stafford G, Gardner M, et al. (1987) The viable cryopreserved allograft aortic valve. J Cardiac Surg 2(Suppl): 153–167
41. O'Brien MF, McGiffin DC (1990) Aortic and pulmonary allografts in contemporary cardiac surgery. In: Karpi RB, Kouckoukos NT, Laks H, Wechsler AS (eds) Advances in Cardiac Surgery. Chicago, Year Book Medical Publishers, Inc. 1: 1–24
42. O'Hara PJ, Hertzer NM, Beven EG, et al. (1986) Surgical management of infected abdominal aortic grafts: review of a 25-year experience. J Vasc Surg 3: 725–731
43. Okita Y, Franciosi G, Matsuki O, et al. (1988) Early and late results of aortic root replacement with antibiotic sterilised aortic homograft. J Thorac Cardiovasc Surg 95: 696–704
44. Oudot J (1951) La greffe vasculaire dans les thromboses du carrefour aortique. Press Med 59: 234
45. Pasic M, Carrel T, Tönz M, et al. (1993) Mycotic aneurysm of the abdominal aorta: extraanatomic *versus in situ* reconstruction. Cardiovasc Surg 1: 48–52
46. Penta A, Qureshi S, Radley-Smith R, et al. (1984) Patient status 10 or more years after "fresh" homograft replacement of the aortic valve. Circulation 70(Suppl I): 1182–1186
47. Perler BA, Kolk CA, Manson PM, et al. (1993) Rotational muscle flaps to treat localized prosthetic graft infection: long-term follow-up. J Vasc Surg 18: 358–564.
48. Reddy DJ, Shepard AD, Evans JR, et al. (1991) Management of aortoiliac aneurysms. Arch Surg 126: 873–879
49. Reilly L, Altman H, Lusby B, et al. (1984) Late results following surgical management of vascular graft infection. J Vasc Surg 1: 36–44
50. Ricotta JJ, Faggiolo GL, Stella A, et al. (1991) Total excision and extra-anatomic bypass for aortic graft infection. Am J Surg 162: 145–149
51. Soyka P, Favez C, Ganzoni N (1990) Treatment of an infected inguinal wound following vascular reconstruction with a sartorius muscle flap. Helv Chir Acta 57: 355–358
52. Szilagyi DE, Rodriguez FJ, Smith RF, et al. (1970) Late fate of arterial allografts. Observation 6 to 15 years after implantation. Arch Surg 101: 721–733
53. Taylor SM, Mills JL, Fujitani RM, Robison JG (1992) The influence of groin sepsis on extra-anatomic bypass patency in patients with prosthetic graft infection. Ann Vasc Surg 6: 80–684

54. Torsello G, Sandmann W, Gehrt A, et al. (1993) In situ replacement of infected vascular prostheses with rifampin-soaked vascular grafts: early results. J Vasc Surg 17: 768–773
55. Yamamoto K, Noisihiki Y, Mo M, et al. (1993) Unusual inflammatory responses around a collagen-impregnated vascular prosthesis. Artif Organs 17: 1010–1016
56. Yared SF, Masri ZH, Melo JC, et al. (1991) A unique inlet (the ascending aorta) for extraanatomic bypass of infected arterial prostheses. J Ky Med Assoc 89: 274–276
57. Yeager RA, Moneta GL, Taylor LM, et al. (1990) Improving survival and limb salvage in patients with aortic graft infection. Am J Surg 159: 466–469
58. Zwischenberger JB, Shalaby T, Conti ER (1989) Viable cryopreserved aortic homograft for the aortic valve endocarditis in annular abscess. Ann Thorac Surg 48: 365–369

Authors' address:
P.R. Vogt, MD
Clinic for Cardiovascular Surgery
University Hospital
Rämistr. 100
CH 8091-Zurich
Switzerland

The use of aortic allografts for surgical management of mycotic infections and aneurysms of the thoracic aorta

R. Hetzer, C. Knosalla, A. C. Yankah

German Heart Institute Berlin, Berlin, Germany

Introduction

The use of synthetic grafts for replacing abdominal and thoracic aorta became attractive to surgeons because of their ready availability and lack of developing aneurysmal dilatation and calcification. The latter complications were experienced in homografts used in the early and late 1950s after their introduction by Dubost in 1952 (1). However the high rate of prosthetic infections, despite long-term antibiotic therapy in the infected area became a great concern. Subsequently antibiotic-impregnated synthetic grafts were introduced with some improvements in the results (2, 3). Improved cryopreservation techniques and homograft banking have brought a renaissance of the old concept of arterial reconstruction with vascular homografts, especially in vascular surgical procedures involved with mycotic aneurysms and prosthetic infections (4–7). The low incidence of infections with homografts in our series of native and prosthetic valve endocarditis as well as other series (8–10) prompted us to use cryopreserved arterial allografts for replacing mycotic aneurysms and infected aortic grafts.

Patients and methods

Between March 1988 and July 1996 ten patients underwent surgical repair of mycotic aneurysms at the German Heart Institute, Berlin. There were six males and four females ranging in age from 47 to 80 years with a mean age of 62.5 years. Three patients underwent emergency operations.

Previous operations and predisposing conditions

Six patients had previously undergone cardiac surgery (Table 1): three were heart transplant recipients, one of them had developed mediastinitis 2 weeks after transplantation. Three other patients had prosthetic valve endocarditis (isolated aortic valve replacement in one patient and composite replacement of the ascending aorta in two patients) with extension of the infection to the composite ascending aortic graft. One of them had undergone aortic valve replacement for the third time due to recurrent prosthetic valve infection. At the last operation valve replacement was combined with in situ prosthetic graft replacement for a mycotic aneurysm of the ascending aorta. Of the four patients who had no previous surgery, one had renal failure, another was under cortisone and methotrexate for several years for chronic polyarthritis and the third patient had been under treatment for diabetes mellitus. The

Table 1. Characteristics of ten patients with mycotic aortic aneurysms who were treated with cryopreserved aortic allografts at the German Heart Institute, Berlin from March 1989 to July 1996

Patient no.	Age	Sex	Predisposing factor	Previous	Follow-up (months/days)
1	60	M	Immunosuppression, diabetes mellitus, mediastinitis	HTX	54 mon.*
2	59	M	PVE	AVR(3 times) + Ascending aortic replacement	29 mon.
3	66	M	PVE and graft infection	Ascending aortic composite graft	28 mon.
4	49	M	Alcoholism, mediastinitis, PVE	AVR	31 mon.
5	47	F	Immunosuppression	HTX	14 mon.
6	65	M	No	No	39 mon.
7	70	F	Chronic polyarthitis	No	5 days
8	80	F	Diabetes mellitus	No	2 mon.
9	32	M	Immunosuppression, mediastinitis	HTX	10 mon.
10	73	F	Renal failure	No	20 days

HTX, heart transplantation; PVE, prosthetic valve endocarditis; AVR, aortic valve replacement
* After first intervention

fourth patient exhibited no predisposing conditions (Table 1). Diabetes mellitus was found in two out of the entire patient population.

Localization

Mycotic aneurysms were found at the following sites. (1) The previous donor-recipient anastomotic and aortic cannulation sites in three patients, who received orthotopic heart transplants. (2) At the cannulation sites in three patients who underwent aortic valve replacements. (3) At the aortic arch in two patients without previous surgery. (4) At the descending aorta in two patients without previous surgery.

Bacteriology

The microorganisms responsible for mycotic infection and aneurysms in the ten patients are listed in Table 2. *Staphylococcus aureus* was the causative organism in four patients; Infection with *Staphylococcus aureus* and *Pseudomonas aeroginosa* was present in one, with *Salmonellae* in three other patients respectively. *Streptococcus faecalis* and pneumococci were each found in three patients respectively. *Mycobacterium avium* and *Candida albicans* were found in a heart transplant recipient.

Surgical technique

Surgical intervention was performed through median sternotomy in eight cases. A thoraco-abdominal approach was used in one case with mycotic aneurysm of the

Table 2. Microorganisms and causes of death (early and late deaths) of ten patients with mycotic aortic aneurysm operated at the German Heart Institute, Berlin from March 1989 to July 1996

Patient no.	Causative agent	Early death	Late death	Death related to infection
1	Staphylococcus aureus, Pseudomonas aeroginosa	−	−	−
2	Streptococcus faecalis	−	−	+
3	S. aureus	−	−	−
4	S. aureus	−	+	−
5	Mycobacterium avium, Candida albicans	−	+	+
6	Pneumococci	−	−	−
7	Salmonellae sp.	+	−	+
8	S. aureus	−	+	−
9	S. aureus, Salmonellae thyphimurium	−	+	−
10	Salmonellae sp.	+	−	−

descending aorta. If the aneurysm was located in the ascending or descending aorta, surgery was performed with cardiopulmonary bypass and moderate hypothermia. Patients with aneurysms in the aortic arch were operated in deep hypothermia at 15 °C with a reduced flow of 0.5 l/min. Cardiopulmonary bypass via femoral cannulation was applied in four patients. In the other cardiopulmonary bypass was instituted through cannulation of the ascending aorta and the right atrial drainage. Resection of the aneurysm and allograft patch reconstruction to maintain the continuity of the aorta was performed in four patients (Fig. 1, Table 3). Two patients with aortic valve endocarditis received allograft aortic root and ascending aortic replacements (Figs. 2, 3). In one case a combined allograft aortic root replacement and allograft patch reconstruction of the ascending aorta was performed (Fig. 5). Two patients with mycotic aneurysms of the aortic arch underwent allograft aortic arch replacement (Fig. 6). All patients were treated with appropriate parenteral antibiotics up to 6 weeks guided by C-reactive proteins and leucocyte counts. They were regularly followed-up until completion of the study on July 31, 1996. The mean follow-up was 27.8 months (range, 5 days to 4 years 8 months).

Results

There were two hospital deaths (30 days) and four late deaths. Underlying infection was successfully treated in seven patients. Recurrent aneurysmal formation developed in a heart transplant patient. At the third and final operation she received a complete replacement of the aortic root and ascending aorta with an aortic allograft conduit, unfortunately she developed candida sepsis during the intensive care period and died 8 days after surgery during the 29 months follow-up period. Two other patients died from *Salmonella* sp. sepsis. Autopsy findings of both patients indicated that the allograft aortic repair was intact without evidence of local active infection. Late deaths

Table 3. Localization, operations, and reoperations of mycotic aortic aneurysms in ten patients at the German Heart Institute, Berlin from March 1989 to July 1996

Patient no.	Localization	Type of operation	Reoperation
1	Ascending aorta	Allograft patch reconstruction	No
2	Ascending aorta	Allograft aortic root replacement + subtotal ascending allograft patch replacement	No
3	Ascending aorta	Allograft root and ascending aortic replacement, reconstruction of subaortic curtain with allograft mitral leaflet	No
4	Ascending aorta (cannulation site)	Allograft aortic root replacement	No
5	Ascending aorta	Patch reconstruction (2 times), ascending aortic replacement	Yes
6	Aortic arch	Allograft aortic arch replacement	No
7	Aortic arch	Allograft aortic arch replacement	No
8	Descending aorta	Allograft patch reconstruction	No
9	Ascending aorta	Patch reconstruction	
10	Descending aorta	Descending aortic replacement	No

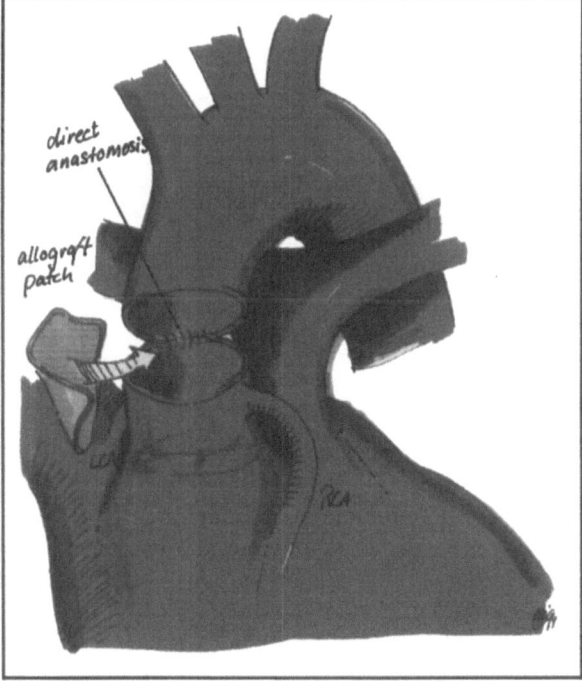

Fig. 1. Allograft aortic patch reconstruction of a mycotic aortic aneurysm at the distal ascending anastomotic site of a transplant recipient (patient no. 5). After resecting the aortic wall segment a direct end-to-end anastomosis of the posterior aspect was made. The remaining defect of the bilateral and the anterior aspect of the aorta was reconstructed with an allograft patch plasty. Reproduction by permission (ref. 16).

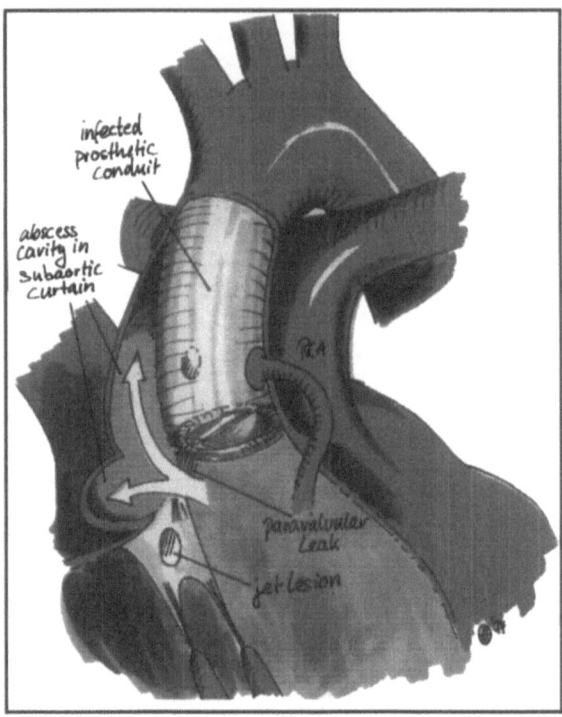

Fig. 2. Infected aortic valve and ascending aorta composite graft, paravalvular leaks, dehiscence of subaortic curtain and mitral valve jet lesion in patient no. 3. Reproduction by permission (ref. 16).

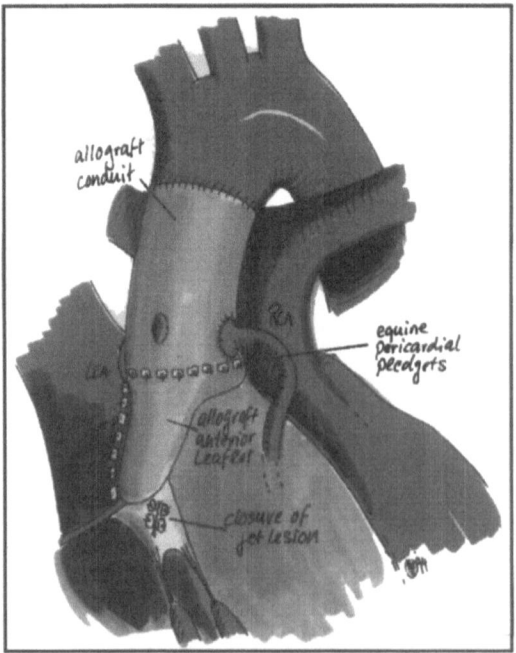

Fig. 3. Allograft aortic root and ascending aortic replacement, reconstruction of subaortic curtain with allograft mitral leaflet and closure of jet lesion in patient no. 3. Reproduction by permission (ref. 16).

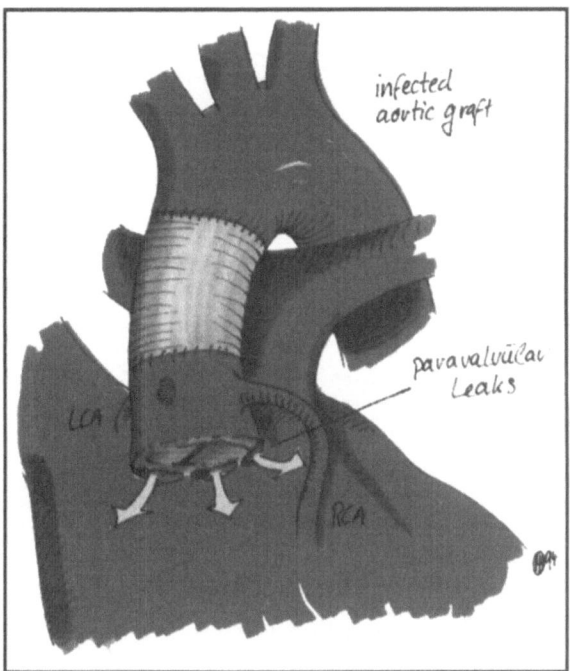

Fig. 4. Prosthetic valve endocarditis and infected prosthetic aortic graft in patient no. 2. Reproduction by permission (ref. 16).

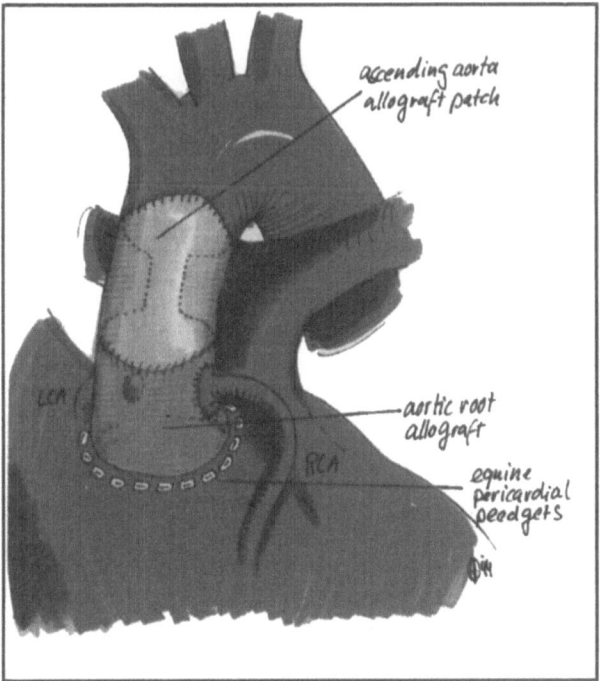

Fig. 5. Allograft aortic root replacement and subtotal ascending aortic allograft patch replacement in patient no. 2. Reproduction by permission (ref. 16).

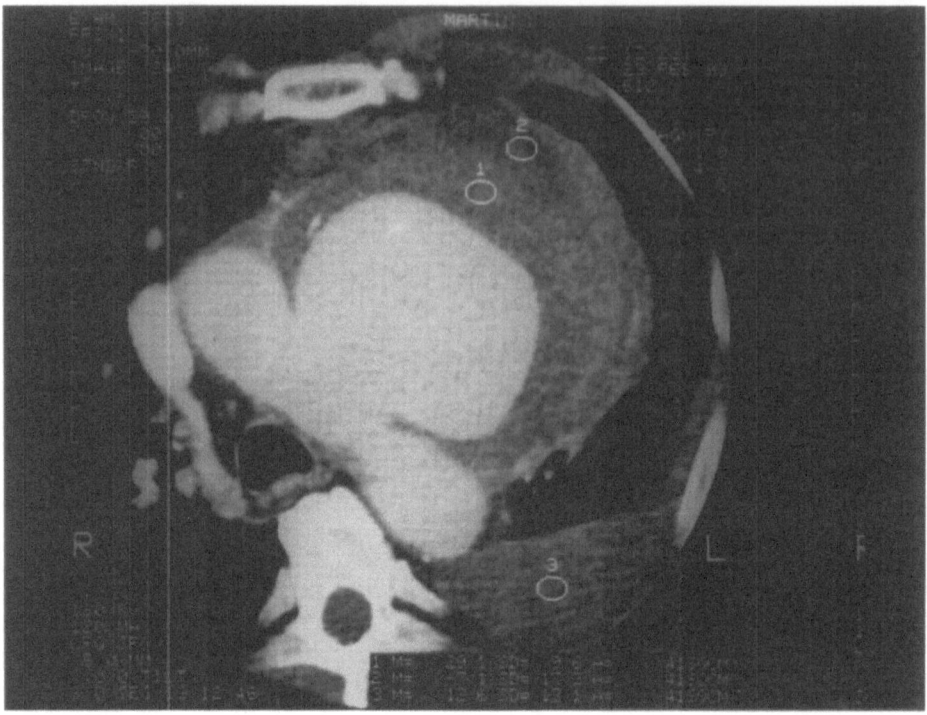

Fig. 6. Computer tomography (CT)-scan of a saccular mycotic aneurysm in the aortic arch in patient no. 6. Reproduction by permission (ref. 16).

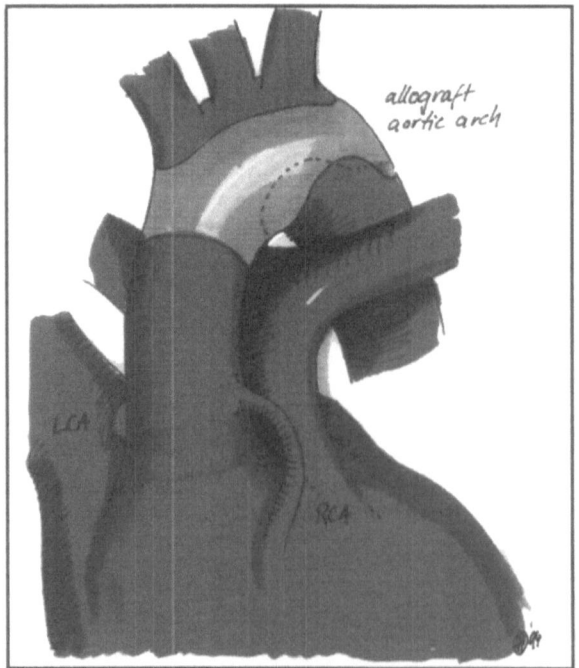

Fig. 7. Partial aortic arch replacement with allograft in patient no. 6 and 7. Reproduction by permission (ref. 16).

of causes unrelated to mycotic infections occurred in three of the four patients between two and 31 months after operation. At the time of death they exhibited no clinical signs of infection.

Discussion

Mycotic aortic aneurysms are rare, yet potentially life-threatening, lesions of the aortic wall. Kaufman reported in late 1970 mortality rates of 80% for such aneurysms (100% if the aneurysm was caused by *S. aureus* and *Escherichia coli*) (13). In other recent reports involving *S. aureus* infections, the mortality rate has improved significantly being 25% (4–6). As reported in other clinical series and by Vogt and associates in this book, the most common pathogens today are staphylococci, streptococci and *salmonella* sp., *Candida albicans, Aspergillus fumigatus* (4, 5, 11, 12). The microbiological findings of this study were similar to those in medical literature.

In recent years there have been reports of patients being successfully treated by in situ reconstruction of mycotic aneurysms of the aorta using prosthetic material in selected cases (2, 3), particularly in those of low virulent infections and negative blood or perigraft cultures (5, 6, 12, 13). Pasic and co-workers reported six in situ reconstructions of the thoracic aorta performed during 21 years (4). Repeat operations were performed in two patients, in one for acute rupture 1 cm distal to the previous repair of a mycotic aneurysm of the ascending aorta. Kieffer and associates (5) as well as Mestres and Pomar (6) have reported satisfactory results of their experiences with allograft replacement of infected infrarenal aortic prosthetic grafts with a recurrent rate of 2.3%. There were no early or late amputations in the entire series, an outcome that has not been reported before with any of the conventional methods.

Mycotic aortic aneurysms might result from septic embolization from endocarditis as has been experienced in three cases of our series. It might also develop at a previous aortic cannulation site or at the anastomotic region of the ascending aorta following a mediastinitis. As previously reported, infections of the aortic wall may occur at potentially weakened areas, such as suture lines or cannulation sites, where intimal and endothelial ischaemia or damage may have occurred (7).

Although antibiotic therapy may control the infection and septicaemia associated with mycotic aortic infections, it does not lead to complete healing of the lesion or prevent rupture (4, 5, 7). The required duration of antibiotic therapy remains a matter of opinion. Most authors advocate 4 to 6 weeks (4, 14) whereas we have been using C-reactive proteins and leucocyte counts as a guide to determine the termination of the antibiotic therapy. In high-risk patients in particular, such as transplant patients, mediastinitis might present a predisposing factor for mycotic infection and aneurysmal degradation of the anastomotic and cannulation sites of the aorta. Subsequently we recommend that patients with persistent chest pains and fever with or without positive blood cultures and presenting no ischaemic heart disease in the early or late postoperative period should undergo investigative chest computed tomographic scanning.

Allograft patch plasty can be performed on well-circumscribed mycotic aneurysms to repair the defect in the aortic wall. Complete debridement of all necrotic tissue and patch closure of the cavity to viable tissue without tension are essential features for preventing reinfection and recurrent aneurysmal formation (5, 13, 15). In cases involving greater inflammatory involvement of the aortic wall, we recommend replacement of the affected segment of the aorta with allograft material. Complete replacement of the aortic root and ascending aorta with allograft is recommended when composite prosthetic valve infections are present. Extensive infections of aortic cannulation and anastomotic sites should also be managed with replacement of the ascending aorta and proximal segment of the aortic arch. In conclusion, the use of aortic allograft to replace mycotic aortic infections and aneurysms is a promising and effective concept, capable of bringing thoracic aortic infections into complete remission.

References

1. Dubost C, Allary M, Oeconomos N (1952) Resection of an aneurysm of the abdominal aorta; re-establishment of the continuity by a preserved human arterial graft, with results after five months. Arch Surg 64: 405
2. Avramovic J, Fletcher JP (1992) Prevention of prosthetic vascular graft infection by rifampicin impregnation of a protein-sealed Dacron graft in combination with parenteral cephalo sporin. J Cardiovasc Surg 33: 70
3. Ney AL, Granja JA, Schuster PA, Tsukayama DT, Jacobs DM, Brubick MP (1994) The use of biodegradable amikacin microspheres to prevent vascular graft infection. J Surg Res 57: 698
4. Pasic M, Carrel T, Segesser von L, Turina M (1993) In situ repair of mycotic aneurysm of the ascending aorta. J Thorac Cardiovasc Surg 105: 321
5. Kieffer E, Bahnini A, Koskas F, Ruotolo C, LeBlevec D, Plissonnier D (1993) In situ allograft replacement of infected infrarenal aortic prostetic grafts: results in forty-three patients. J Vasc Surg 17: 349
6. Mestres CA, Mulet J, Pomar JL (1995) Large caliber cryopreserved arterial allografts in vascular reconstructive operations: early experience. Ann Thorac Surg 60: 105
7. Knosalla C, Weng Y, Warnecke H, Hummel M, Yankah AC, Hofmeister J, Hetzer R (1996) Mycotic aortic aneurysm after orthotopic heart transplantation—a three-case-report and review of the literature. J Heart Lung Transpl 15: 827
8. Knosalla C, Siniawski H, Weng Y, Yankah AC, Hetzer R (1995) Diagnosis and surgical treatment of active infective aortic valve endocarditis with associated priaanular abscesses. Cardiovasc Surg 3 (Suppl 1): 178
9. Donaldson RM, Ross DM (1984) Homograft aortic root replacement for complicated prosthetic valve endocarditis. Circulation 70 (Suppl 1): 178
10. Petrou M, Wang K, Albertucci M, Brecker SJ, Yacoub MH (1994) Evaluation of unstented aortic homografts for the treatment of prosthetic aortic valve endocarditis. Circulation 90 (Suppl 2): 198
11. Bennett D (1967) Primary mycotic aneurysms of the aorta – report of case and review of the literature. Arch Surg 94: 758
12. Jarrett F, Darling C, Mundth ED, Austen G (1975) Experience with infected aneurysm of the abdominal aorta. Arch Surg 110: 1281
13. Kaufman SL, White RI, Harrington DP, Barth KH, Siegelmann SS (1978) Protean manifestations of mycotic aneurysms. Am J Roentgenol 131: 1019
14. Mundth ED, Darling RC, Alvarado RH, Buckley MJ, Linton RR, Austen WG (1969) Surgical management of mycotic aneurysms and the complications of vascular reconstructive surgery. Am J Surg 117: 460
15. Fiore AC, Ivey TD, McKeown PP, Misbach GA, Allen MD, Dillard DH (1986) Patch closure of aortic annulus mycotic aneurysms. Ann Thorac Surg 42: 372
16. Knosalla C, Weng Y, Yankah AC, Hofmeister J, Hetzer R (1996) Using aortic allograft material to treat mycotic aneurysms of the thoracic aorta. Ann Thorac Surg 61: 1146–52

Authors' address:
Prof. Roland Hetzer, MD, PhD
German Heart Institute Berlin
Augustenburger Platz 1
13353 Berlin
Germany

Large-caliber arterial allografts

C. A. Mestres, J. L. Pomar

Cardiovascular Surgery, Hospital Clinico Provincial, University of Barcelona, Barcelona, Spain

Introduction

The early part of the 20th century saw the initiation of vascular surgery. The immense achievement of the Nobel Prize laureate Alexis Carrel must be considered as the foundation of vascular surgery as we know it today (5). His contributions and those of other pioneers in the surgery of blood vessels changed the surgical approach to cardiovascular disease (6, 14, 20). Almost a century later, just a few modifications have been introduced in the surgery for vascular replacement and reconstruction. The introduction in clinical practice of homotransplantation of arteries represented a mile-stone in the surgical treatment of vascular diseases. By the end of the 1940s and early in the 1950s, Gross (12) and Dubost (8) cleared the way with a number of significant clinical experiences when successfully attempting arterial homotransplantation as part of the treatment of coarctation of the aorta and abdominal aortic aneurysms. However, history also brought a number of major drawbacks that led to a progressive abandonment of arterial allografts as the substitute of choice in vascular surgery (13, 32).

It is also well known that secondary degradation of transplanted arterial segments, especially within the aortoiliac sector, in form of dilatation, calcification and thrombosis, added to the reluctance of surgeons in using this sort of biological material (7). The difficulties in ensuring consistent and continuous procurement, the lack of reliable methods of preservation and the inability of finding an adequate storage system beyond the time frame of a few weeks also contributed to the unavoidable disenchantment of surgeons regarding the use of biological material for vascular reconstruction. In addition, the advent of artificial vascular prostheses (35), with the advantages of being commercially available, easy to handle, available in all sizes and with no need for specific preoperative manipulation rapidly contributed to the progressive withdrawal of homologous vascular segments from the surgical armamentarium in spite of some long-term complications of vascular prostheses (19).

From the above-mentioned, one has to bear in mind that the use of biological material in the surgery of reconstruction and replacement within the vascular system is closely linked to the development of vascular surgery itself. These early attempts of using vascular allografts were later followed by the use of homologous valves to replace diseased cardiac valves as it has extensively been shown in the literature after the pioneering work of Lam (18), Duran and Gunning (9), Ross (29) and Barratt-Boyes (4). What has been common for vascular and cardiac valvular allografts is that in spite of theoretical advantages as cardiovascular substitutes, the difficulties in procurement, harvesting, processing and storage and in certain cases a number of technical problems precluded their widespread use.

It also became clear after a number of years that late primary tissue failure was the main influencing factor in allograft performance and patient morbidity and mortality.

The combination of late structural tissue degeneration and the lack of proper long-term storage systems was responsible for the low popularity of vascular allografts by the end of the 1950s. On the other hand, since the early experiences separately reported by Ross (29) and Barratt-Boyes (4) regarding aortic valve replacement using a human aortic valve, valvular allografts have progressively been incorporated by cardiovascular surgeons and the popularity of these replacement substitutes has already reach its peak, including use in all four valve positions.

A brief review of the history of allografts in cardiovascular surgery therefore confirms that valvular allografts became progressively more popular whereas vascular allografts were abandoned for a number of years (7). By the beginning of the present decade, the versatility and good results of valvular allografts in the treatment of valvular diseases of the aortic root, right ventricular outflow tract and at the atrioventricular level, has been shown. This is the result of the improvement in surgical technique, patient selection and a progressive modification of methodology in procurement, manipulation and storage of human tissues. The developments in cryobiology have been substantially influenced in this regard (25–27).

In other words, all of us actively involved in the use of valvular allografts have learned much about technique, indications, results and tissue manipulation. That has probably prompted us to use vascular allografts in certain vascular conditions. There is currently a renewed interest in using vascular allografts and we have to honestly recognize that without the previous experiences with fresh and cryopreserved valve allografts we would hesitate to use them otherwise. Consequently, we have reached a point at which vascular allografts must be considered as a reality in modern cardiovascular surgery. In any case, there is nothing conceptually new – we are simply returning to the early ideas of Carrel and others (5) – however, technology has helped us to reinitiate serious programs for using allograft tissue in vascular surgery.

Methodology

Procurement

As in many other institutions in Europe and the USA, vascular allograft procurement is performed by us following a protocol similar to that designed for allograft valves. In our country, all tissues are procured from brain-dead multiorgan donors through the Spanish National Organ Transplant Network (Organización Nacional de Transplantes – ONT). All vascular samples fulfill the legal requirements before processing with regard to predonation serologies such as Hepatitis B and C, Cytomegalovirus, Syphillis, Brucella and Human Immunedeficiency Virus. The allografts are immediately sent to our Cryopreservation Laboratory (Criobarna) at the Hospital Clinico, University of Barcelona. For allografts sent from outside the Hospital by plane and for those harvested at our Institution, warm ischemia seldom exceeds 30 min and cold ischemic time has rarely gone above 8 h.

We are currently harvesting the aortic bifurcation, iliac arteries and thoracic aortas on a routine basis. Adequate predonation coordination is mandatory as sometimes a conflict of interest among the transplant teams can be evident because of the need of specific cannulations for organ perfusion. More recently, carotid arteries and internal mammary arteries are being collected mainly for research purposes.

Manipulation

The allografts are dissected under a laminar flow hood in aseptic conditions. Excess tissue is eliminated and collateral branches are carefully doubly ligated with fine 5/0 silk sutures. That especially applies to the thoracic aortas as the intercostal branches must be carefully identified. The allografts are carefully inspected for atheroma, tear and dissection. This is an extremely important part of the whole process as we rigorously discard any artery with the suspicion of any abnormality.

Antibiotic decontamination

For arteries collected from a multiorgan donation performed under sterile conditions in the operating room, the antibiotic protocol is the same as that currently in use for allograft valve decontamination. In our Institution, penicillin 50 IU/l, streptomycin 50 IU/l and amphotericin B 10 mg/l for 24 h, is the protocol that has consistently been used for a number of years. Over the past 2 years, a new source of allografts has been patients dying in the emergency department upon arrival and who are maintained with organ perfusion instituted in the same area. Those "arrested hearts", as they are termed in our Hospital, are managed in a different way. Therefore, arterial allografts harvested from these donors receive the following protocol for 24 h: amphotericin B 10 mg/l (0.08 mg/l RPMI), vancomycin 50 mg/l (0.5 mg/l RPMI), amikacin 40 mg/l and metronidazole 20 mg/l (2 ml/l RPMI).

Cryopreservation

Large-caliber arteries are preserved using a cryoprotectant solution consists of RPMI, 10% DMSO (dimethylsulphoxide) and 10% bovine fetal calf serum (FCS). A computerized freezing chamber (Cryoson) is used and a freezing curve has been previously designed. Following this, a freezing rate of 1 °C per minute down to −40 °C and 3 °C every minute from −40 °C to −100 °C. The samples are then immersed in liquid nitrogen at −196 °C.

Small caliber arteries of the internal mammary are currently being used only for research purposes. Because of their different anatomy and pharmacological properties, they are more sensitive to external damage at the time of manipulation and preservation. They are technically more demanding because of the number of very small branches to be ligated in the laboratory. Cryoprotectant solution is slightly different and the methodology proposed by Müller-Schweinitzer is currently followed, using the Krebs-Henseleit cryoprotectant solution, incorporating 1.8 M DMSO, 0.1 M sucrose and no FCS.

Indications

A brief literature review shows that references regarding large series of patients undergoing arterial allograft implantation are still scanty. Many of them are true case reports from isolated experiences (1, 15, 17, 21, 31, 33). Others show a few data from limited series (3, 16, 23, 34). Therefore, there is no general agreement yet as to what the ideal indications for arterial allograft implantation are with the sole exception of vascular infection. According to our own clinical experience at the Hospital Clinico, University of Barcelona, the following is a list of possible indications to implant arterial allografts (22, 23). These might be a matter of controversy; because we are still in our learning curve and need for complete proper long-term follow-up, we certainly anticipate that some modifications will be accepted and some more indications will probably be incorporated in the future as more experience is gained. From the experience accumulated over the past 3 years, the following indications have been identified at our Institution: *Vascular infection* (primary, prosthetic); *Vascular trauma* (open/closed, Iatrogenic); *Complex vascular reoperations; Vascular reconstruction in patients with high risk of infection* because of underlying diseases or immunesuppression (transplant patients, end-stage renal disease, cancer, etc.).

In spite of all those factors, vascular infection, primary or prosthetic must probably be considered the ideal indication. There is some consensus regarding this matter in the literature (3, 16, 23, 34).

Clinical experience

Between October 1992 and October 1995, 28 patients underwent vascular replacement or reconstruction using a cryopreserved arterial allograft at the Hospital Clinico, University of Barcelona. Mean age was 54.4 years (25–72). Preoperative diagnosis is shown in Tables 1 and 2 with 50% of patients having aneurysmal disease. Several associated conditions were detected and are listed in Table 3. It can be seen

Table 1

Preoperative diagnosis (I)		
Aneurysmal disease		14
Aortoiliac	6	
Aortic	4	
Hepatic artery	2	
Iliac artery	1	
Superior mesenteric	1	

Table 2

Preoperative diagnosis (II)		
Vascular infections		5
False aneurysm	2	
Graft infection	2	
Aorta-caval fistula	1	
Arterial trauma		3
Arterial thrombosis		3
Hepatic	1	
Subclavian	1	
Renal	1	
Failed arterial reconstruction		3

Table 3

Associated conditions	
ESRF – Waiting list for renal transplant	7
Renopancreatic transplant	3
Liver transplant	2
Gastric cancer	2
Renal artery stenosis	1
Bladder tumor	1
Heparin-induced thrombocytopenia	1

ESRF = End-stage renal failure.

Table 4

Operations performed		
Composite allograft		3
Aortofemoral bifurcated	1	
Extranatomic ascending aorta-to-bifemoral	1	
Femoropopliteal	1	
Single allograft		24
Bypass allograft		12
Aortoiliac bifurcated	8	
Aortofemoral bifurcated	3	
Aortosubclavian	1	
Aortorenal	1	
Carotid-to-subclavian	1	
Interposition allograft		12
Iliac	4	
Abdominal aorta	3	
Hepatic	3	
Superficial femoral	1	
Superior mesenteric	1	

that eight (28.6%) of them had end-stage renal failure and were awaiting for renal transplantation. According to the preoperative diagnosis, different types of vascular reconstruction were performed (Table 4). Systemic heparinization with 5000 IU was achieved before clamping the involved artery. Standard vascular suturing technique was used (Fig. 1). Seven patients required eight associated procedures as shown in Table 5. Overall, 36 arterial allografts were used, namely 19 iliac arteries (average diameter 7.4 mm), 11 aortic bifurcations (average diameter 10.5 × 6.7 mm) and six thoracic aortas (average diameter 17.8 mm).

Results

Early

Two patients operated on for vascular infection died in the perioperative period from myocardial infarction (8 h) and disruption of aortotomy line (3 h), confirmed at

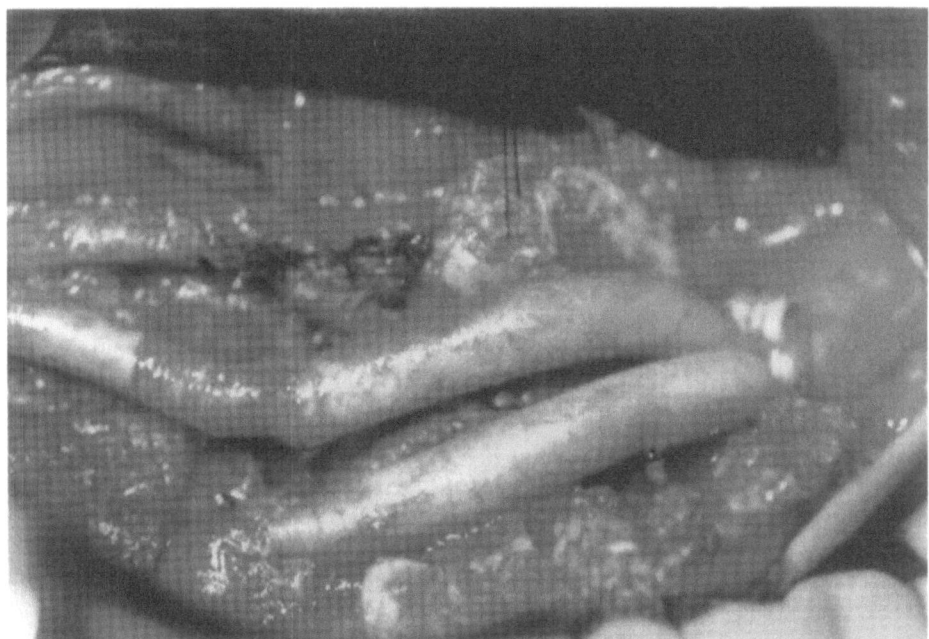

Fig. 1. Operative photograph showing a cryopreserved aortic bifurcation implanted in the aortoiliac position for aortoiliac aneurysm.

Table 5

Associated procedures	
Renal transplantation	2
Gastrectomy	2
Reimplantation of pancreatic allograft + appendectomy	1
Iliac endarterectomy	1
Cholecystectomy	1
CABG without CPB	1

CABG = Coronary Artery Bypass Graft; CPB = Cardiopulmonary Bypass.

postmortem study, for a 7.14% hospital mortality rate. Three patients had three early non-allograft-related postoperative complications (lower limb ischemia, rectus abdominis hematoma and upper gastrointestinal bleeding).

Late

One patient died 9 months after surgery because of acute myocardial infarction. Another patient died 22 months postoperatively from a ruptured anastomotic aneurysm in an interposition iliac allograft in spite of emergency reoperation. The 24 survivors are in good condition and follow-up is 100% complete. No relapsing vascular infections have been documented and no immunosuppression was given in non-transplanted patients.

Two patients had late complications in the form of prosthetic valve endocarditis at 10 months and colonic ischemia at 2 months. The first required allograft aortic root replacement according to Ross (30) and the second required colectomy. Aspirin is recommended on a routine basis. Angiography has been performed in 19 patients at an average of 10 weeks. Patency rate is 94.7% as one aortosubclavian allograft has not been visualized.

Allograft-related morbidity

From the above it can be seen that there were two cases (7.14% overall) of allograft-related mortality. One patient died 3 h after surgery from massive intrabdominal hemorrhage secondary to disruption of the aortotomy line. In this case a probably incomplete debridement of the infected aorta might be considered as the underlying cause of rupture. A second patient died 22 months after the operation from a ruptured anastomotic aneurysm on an iliac interposition allograft. This 31-year-old patient with a prior failed pancreatic transplantation had a severe calcification of the native vessels and chronic fatigue of the distal anastomosis; the poor quality of the recipient vessel was considered the cause of rupture. This is pure speculation as postmortem study was not allowed.

Comments

Vascular infection is an accepted indication for the use of arterial allografts. The experiences reported so far as isolated case reports (1, 15, 21, 31) and the only two large series from La Pitié in Paris, France (16) and the University Hospital in Zürich, Switzerland (34) seem to support this statement in spite of different methods of preservation used by these groups. The French group used fresh antibiotic-preserved allografts and the Swiss group used cryopreserved allografts. A number of advantages have been identified such as reduced morbidity and mortality, shortened hospitalization and reduced antibiotic requirements. With the obvious limitations of extrapolating these experiences based on the work done on infective endocarditis, there is a consensus on the advantages.

As stated earlier, we have been able to identify a few additional indications. To us, vascular trauma could be an interesting indication, especially in open cases. In our experience, one young patient underwent surgery because of a gunshot wound to the groin and two patients because of iatrogenic surgical trauma. We were able to implant an allograft as we have our own tissue bank with cryopreservation facilities. Immediate availability made the operations smooth. Therefore, true vascular emergencies in Institutions without a tissue bank might theoretically be difficult to be considered for allograft implantation.

Vascular reoperations were managed by us in three cases by implanting an arterial allograft. Whether these patients should be managed with a new prosthesis could also be a matter of controversy but the availability of human tissue made us consider an allograft. So far, the results in this small group of patients have been satisfactory in spite of a late cardiac death.

The group of patients with a theoretical higher risk of infection is particularly attractive. Three of them had different types of tumor, two gastric and one vesical managed concomitantly and sequentially together with the vascular condition. As gastric resection had to be performed, a combined operation was thought to be a better option to avoid a repeated laparotomy for aortic surgery. In the case of the patient undergoing endoscopic resection and due for 1-year sequential intravesical chemotherapy, it was thought that an allograft could be a better option than a prosthesis to diminish the risk of repeated vesical catheterization. Another subgroup of patients with a potential high risk for infection are those with a previous organ transplantation or those with end-stage renal disease and candidates for a future renal transplantation. The management of vascular complications in three patients with liver transplantation and three with renopancreatic transplantation has been satisfactory with an allograft. In addition, the eight patients waitlisted for renal transplantation and aortoiliac disease have greatly benefited from vascular repair before or during the transplantation procedure. Two of them had concomitant surgery and a renal allograft was implanted on an aortoiliac allograft (one cryopreserved, one homovital). Both previous arterial allograft repair and simultaneous aortoiliac transplantation can help to expand the indications in cases of complex renal transplantation as has been recently described by us (24).

From our experience and that from others we can say that clinical results with arterial allografts tend to be satisfactory, especially in cases of infection with some other indications awaiting more clinical work to confirm the early impressions. What else can be expected from cryopreserved allografts? First, cyropreservation itself makes the allograft different than with fresh antibiotic-preservation as viable fibroblasts and collagen production and extended viability have been confirmed (2, 11). In addition, experiences from Müller-Schweinitzer confirm preservation of biochemical properties in opposition to fresh allografts that lose their structural, physicochemical and mechanical properties (27). In our laboratory, recent experiences show the ability of a contractile response to norepinephrine in cryopreserved pig arteries. Another very important aspect of cryopreservation is that it allows for a prolonged storage of processed samples.

On the other hand, there is lack of information about the long-term behavior of arterial allografts. With the exception of the results reported by Bahnini et al. (3) with a maximum follow-up of 5 years and the average follow-up of 18 months reported by Vogt et al. (34) nothing more consistent is available today. The high 21% allograft-related morbidity shown by Bahnini et al. (3) might be related to the methodology of preservation which badly compares to the 9% allograft-related morbidity reported by the Zürich group (34) and our 4% overall late allograft-related morbidity with an average of a little less than 14 months of follow-up (23). This probably means that preservation methodology might play a fundamental role in long-term patient and allograft survival. The histological evidence supplied by Bahnini et al. (3) supports the impression that allograft failure could be related to a form of chronic rejection, as inflammatory infiltrates, phagocytes and intimal proliferation were found. Pharmacological intervention to diminish possible phenomena of chronic rejection have also been advocated through glutaraldehyde and sodium dodecylsulphate but this approach also needs further elucidation (10, 28).

There are a number of questions still open for discussion. If cryopreserved arterial allografts are viable, what does viability mean? To what extent will this affect our postoperative management? What is an acceptable level of antigenicity through an enhanced viability? Do the patients require routine immunosuppression? These and other questions will probably be answered as more experimental and clinical information is collected. In the meantime, the overall impression is that surgeons are in the process of favorably modifying their approach to certain cardiovascular conditions through the use of large-caliber cryopreserved arterial allografts. Time will enlighten us.

References

1. Abad C, Hurlé A, Feijoo J, Gómez-Marrero J, Abdallah A (1995) Total aortic arch replacement by a cryopreserved aortic homograft. Eur J Cardio-thorac Surg 9: 531–533
2. Allaire E, Guettier C, Bruneval P, Plissonnier D, Michel JB (1994) Cell-free arterial grafts: morphologic characteristics of aortic isografts, allografts and xenografts in rats. J Vasc Surg 19: 446–456
3. Bahnini A, Plissonnier D, Koskas F, Kieffer E (1994) Traitement des infections artérielles par allogreffe artérielle in situ. pp 209–219
4. Barratt-Boyes BG (1964) Homograft aortic valve replacement in aortic incompetence and stenosis. Thorax 19: 131–150
5. Carrel A (1910) Experimental surgery of the thoracic aorta by the method of Meltzer and Auer. JAMA 54: 28–29
6. Carrel A (1912) Ultimate result of aortic transplantation. J Exp Med 15: 389–398
7. Dennis C (1987) Brief history of developments of vascular grafts. In: Sawyer PN (ed) Modern Vascular Grafts. McGraw-Hill Book Company, New York, pp 1–25
8. Dubost C, Allary M, Oeconomos N (1952) Resection of an aneurysm of the abdominal aorta: re-establishment of the continuity by a preserved human arterial graft, with results after five months. 64: 405–408
9. Duran CMG, Gunning A (1962) A method of placing a total homologous aortic valve in the subcoronary position. Lancet 2: 487
10. Dumont CE, Plissonnier D, Guettier C, Michel JB (1993) Effects of glutaraldehyde on experimental arterial iso- and allografts in rats. J Surg Res 54: 61–69
11. Gournier JP, Adham M, Favre JP et al. (1993) Cryopreserved arterial homografts: preliminary study. Ann Vasc Surg 7: 503–511
12. Gross RE, Bill AH Jr, Pierce EC II (1949) Methods for preservation and transplantation of arterial grafts. Observation on arterial grafts in dogs: report of transplantation of preserved arterial grafts in nine human cases. Surg Gynecol Obstet 88: 689–694
13. Halpert B, DeBakey ME, Jordan GL et al. (1960) The fate of homografts and prostheses of the human aorta. Surg Gynecol Obstet 111: 659–674
14. Horsley JS (1915) Surgery of the blood vessels. The CV Mosby Company, St Louis, pp 31–45
15. Julia P, Jebara VA, Desgranges P et al. (1991) Management of infected vascular prostheses: the vascular homograft revisited. Texas Heart Inst J 18: 293–295
16. Kieffer E, Bahnini A, Koskas F et al. (1993) In situ allograft replacement of infected infrarenal aortic prosthetic grafts: results in forty-three patients. J Vasc Surg 17: 349–356
17. Kniemeyer HW, Torsello G, Hennes N, Grabitz K, Sandmann W (1994) Frisches homologes Arterientransplantat als aorto-iliako-femoraler Gefässersatz bei Protheseninfektion. Vasa 23: 268–273
18. Lam CR, Aram HH, Munnel ER (1952) An experimental study of aortic valve homografts. Surg Gynecol Obstet 94: 129–135
19. Lorentzen JE, Nielsen OM, Arendrup H et al. (1984) Vascular graft infection: an analysis of sixty-two graft infections in 2411 consecutively implanted synthetic vascular grafts. Surgery 98: 81–86
20. Makins GH (1919) Gunshot Injuries to the Blood Vessels. John Wright & Sons, Bristol, pp 1–5
21. Mestres CA, Miró JM, Pomar JL (1994) Cryopreserved homografts in the treatment of relapsing fungal cardiovascular infections. J Thorac Cardiovasc Surg 108: 990–991
22. Mestres CA, Pomar JL (1995) Indicaciones y resultados de los transplantes de segmentos vasculares homólogos criopreservados. In: Matesanz R, Miranda B (eds) Coordinación y Transplantes - El Modelo Español. ONT, Madrid, pp 251–255
23. Mestres CA, Mulet J, Pomar JL (1995) Large-caliber cryopreserved arterial allografts in vascular reconstructive operations: early experience. Ann Thorac Surg 60: S105–107
24. Mestres CA, Talbot-Wright R, Carretero P (1996) Simultaneous aortorenal homograft transplantation. Expanding the indications for renal and vascular replacement. Br J Surg (In press)

25. Müller-Schweinitzer E (1994) Applications for cryopreserved blood vessels in pharmacological research. Cryobiology 31: 57–62
26. Müller-Schweinitzer E (1994) Vascular tissue preservation techniques. In: Bevan RD, Bevan JA (eds) The Human Brain Circulation. Humana Press, pp 319–331
27. Müller-Schweinitzer E (1994) Arterial smooth muscle function after prolonged exposure to a medium containing dimethylsulfoxide (Me$_2$SO) and storage at $-196\,°C$. Cryobiology 31: 330–335
28. Petersen MJ, Abbott WM, H'Doubler PB et al. (1993) Hemodynamics and aneurysm development in vascular allografts. J Vasc Surg 18: 955–963
29. Ross DN (1962) Homograft replacement of the aortic valve. Lancet 2: 487
30. Ross DN (1987) Application of homografts in clinical surgery. J Cardiac Surg 2(Suppl): 175–181
31. Schuch D, Wolff L (1991) Repair of mycotic aneurysm of the innominate artery with homograft tissue. Ann Thorac Surg 52: 863–864
32. Szilagyi DE, Rodríguez FJ, Smith RF, Elliott JP (1970) Late fate of arterial allografts: observations 6 to 15 years after implantation. Arch Surg 101: 721–733
33. Vogt P, Pasic M, von Segesser LK, Carrel T, Turina M (1995) Cryopreserved aortic homograft for mycotic aneurysm. J Thorac Cardiovasc Surg 109: 589–591
34. Vogt P, von Segesser LK, Goffin Y, Pasic M, Turina M (1995) Cryopreserved arterial homografts for in situ reconstruction of mycotic aneurysms and prosthetic graft infection. Eur J Cardiothorac Surg 9: 502–506
35. Voorhees AB Jr, Jaretzki AL III, Blakemore AH (1952) The use of tubes constructed from Vynion "N" cloth in bridging arterial defects. Arch Surg 135: 332–336

Author's address:
Carlos-A. Mestres, MD, PhD
Cardiovascular Surgery
Hospital Clinico Provincial
University of Barcelona
Villarroel 170
08036 Barcelona (Spain)

Allograft reconstruction of the right ventricular outflow tract: Techniques and results

D. R. Clarke, D. A. Bishop

The Children's Hospital and University of Colorado Health Sciences Center, Denver, Colorado, USA

Introduction

A variety of valved and non-valved conduits have been used to establish right ventricle to pulmonary artery continuity in pediatric patients with complex congenital anomalies of the right ventricular outflow tract. Ross and Somerville originally described right ventricular outflow tract reconstruction with an extra-cardiac valved aortic allograft in 1966 (15). As early as 1968, aortic allograft calcification and degeneration were reported and attributed to then current methods of allograft collection, processing and storage (6). The disappointing results with the use of aortic allografts led to a search for more promising options for right ventricular outflow tract reconstruction. Mechanical valve prostheses were implanted in older children who were at a stage of physical development that would allow implantation of the relatively large valves. However, the inherent risk factors associated with thromboembolism and anticoagulation led most cardiac surgeons to avoid the use of a mechanical valve in the right ventricular outflow tract of pediatric patients. Favorable results with porcine valved bioprostheses implanted in adults led to their use in children in the early 1970's. Unfortunately, it was not long before multiple problems presented themselves. Early valvar calcification and degeneration, conduit rigidity, and formation of intimal peel quickly curtailed enthusiasm for the use of porcine bioprostheses in the pediatric population (1, 10). As the popularity of porcine bioprostheses for pediatric use declined, interest in aortic valve allografts resurfaced. New methods of preservation and storage including antibiotic sterilization and cryopreservation resulted in increased cell viability and implied increased allograft durability (2, 4). In spite of less toxic preservation and storage methods, aortic valve allograft calcification continued to plague certain subsets of patients; younger children and patients with pulmonary hypertension (14, 16). The calcification problem along with the limited availability of aortic allografts prompted the use of pulmonary allografts for right ventricular outflow tract reconstruction in the mid 1980s. Pulmonary valve allografts with comparable viability demonstrated several potential advantages over aortic allografts (13). Pulmonary allograft anatomy and physiology accurately simulate the native right ventricular outflow tract, branch pulmonary arteries are available for distal reconstruction, and pulmonary allograft conduit calcium content is less than that of aortic conduits. Results with pulmonary allografts have been consistently superior to aortic allografts for reconstituting the right ventricle to pulmonary artery connection (3). However, recent follow-up of infants who received pulmonary allografts for right ventricular outflow tract reconstruction reveals that there is still room for improvement. Allograft calcification and degeneration that require reoperation are persistent problems for 16% of the infant population within ten years after implantation (9).

Materials and methods

From April 1985 through July 1995, at The Children's Hospital and the University of Colorado Health Sciences Center in Denver, 225 cryopreserved valve allografts have been implanted in pediatric patients to reconstruct the right ventricular outflow tract. One-hundred-and-ninety-five pulmonary and 30 aortic allografts were used. Allograft recipients consisted of 119 males (53%) and 106 females (47%) who ranged in age from 6 days to 18 years at the time of operation.

One-hundred-and-sixty-nine allograft recipients were 13 months to 18.4 years of age at the time of surgery (mean age: 5.0 years). Fifty-six children were infants, 12 months old or younger, at the time of allograft implantation (mean age: 4.4 months). Preoperative diagnoses by age group are listed in Table 1. Only eight of the older patients (5%) versus 43 of the infants (77%), had undergone no previous cardiac operations (Table 2).

Implantation of aortic allografts in the right ventricular outflow tract occurred early in the experience with the use of allograft tissue. Aortic valve conduits currently

Table 1. Preoperative diagnosis

Diagnosis	Patient age group	
	>1 Year	≤1 Year
Complex tetralogy of Fallot	45	7
Tetralogy of Fallot	27	5
Pulmonary atresia and ventricular septal defect	32	7
Conduit replacement	34	1
Truncus arteriosus	–	29
Complex transposition of the great arteries	16	4
Double outlet ventricle	15	1
Ebstein's anomaly, atrial and ventricular septal defects, pulmonary stenosis	–	1
Aortic atresia, hypoplastic aortic arch, ventricular septal defect	–	1
Total	169	56

Table 2. Previous cardiac surgical procedures

Operation	Patient age group	
	>1 Year	≤1 Year
Unilateral systemic → pulmonary artery shunt	93	8
Bilateral systemic → pulmonary artery shunt	16	–
Ventricle → pulmonary artery conduit	40	1
Tetralogy of Fallot repair	32	–
Valvotomy or right ventricular outflow tract patch	8	–
Repair coarctation of the aorta	5	1
Arterial switch	2	1
Miscellaneous	7	1
No previous surgery	8 (5%)	43 (77%)

are used only when additional length is required or if an appropriate pulmonary valve conduit is unavailable. Prior to surgery, a cryopreserved valve conduit of appropriate size as determined by patient weight, is selected (7). Ranges and mean values for patient weight at operation and implanted allograft internal diameter are presented in Table 3.

Allograft thawing procedures as defined by CryoLife Cardiovascular, Inc. (Heart Valve Allograft (Homograft) Thawing and Dilution Instructions) are used. The triple pouch that contains the allograft is immersed in a 37° to 42 °C waterbath. The valve conduit is thawed until ice crystals are completely dissolved which normally takes 15 to 22 min. The outer pouch is dried, cut open with scissors, and the second peel-back pouch is extracted. The peel pouch is opened and the innermost, third pouch is passed aseptically onto the sterile surgical field. The top of the third pouch is cut open with sterile scissors and the allograft is removed and placed into a large sterile basin containing 1 l of room temperature, 5% dextrose and lactated Ringers. After the tissue is allowed to passively dilute for at least 5 min, the allograft is ready for implantation.

As the allograft thaws, the patient's chest is opened through a median sternotomy incision and cardiopulmonary bypass is established using bicaval and ascending aortic cannulation. If additional intracardiac repairs such as atrial or ventricular septal defect closure or infundibular muscle resection are required, or if distal pulmonary artery reconstruction is anticipated, the aorta is crossclamped and cold blood cardioplegia is infused into the aortic root with reinfusion every 20 to 30 min throughout that portion of the procedure. The entire surgery can be accomplished without clamping the aorta and with mild hypothermia to thus retain normal cardiac rhythm if the distal pulmonary arteries are normal and if outflow tract reconstruction is done as an isolated procedure as in conduit change or pulmonary valve replacement for regurgitation.

A vertical right ventriculotomy provides access for intracardiac repairs. If an outflow tract is present, the ventriculotomy is extended through the pulmonary annulus and into the main pulmonary artery. Distal allograft anastomosis is accomplished first using one of three surgical options. If the distal pulmonary arteries are normal, a circular allograft to main pulmonary artery anastomosis is performed (Fig. 1a). When unilateral distal obstruction is present, an allograft conduit flap extension enlarges the affected artery (Fig. 1b). A bifurcated pulmonary allograft is anastomosed to right and left pulmonary arteries in the presence of discontinuous or severely distorted branch pulmonary arteries (Fig. 1c). Almost two-thirds of the reconstructions have been accomplished with a main pulmonary artery connection (Table 4). The proximal anastomosis is initiated by suturing the allograft into the right ventricular outflow tract or onto the right ventricular surface (Fig. 2a).

Table 3. Patient weight at operation and internal diameter of implanted allograft

Patient age group	Patient weight at operation (kg)	Allograft internal diameter (mm)
>1 Year	Range: 5.0–71.7 Mean: 16.5	Range: 12–26 Mean: 21
≤1 Year	Range: 1.7–8.2 Mean: 4.8	Range: 9–21 Mean: 15

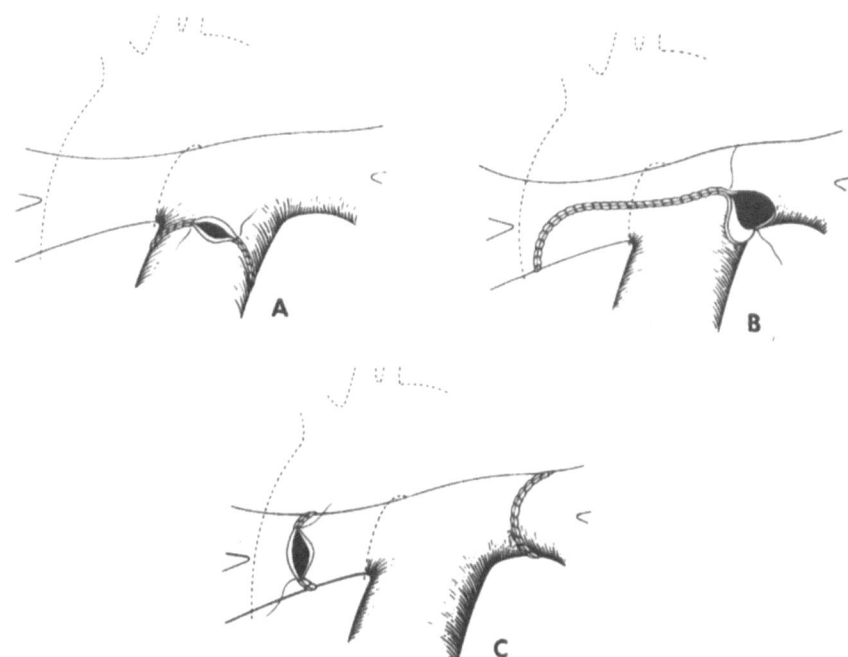

Fig. 1. A) A standard circular anastomosis is performed between the distal pulmonary allograft conduit and the main pulmonary artery. B) A pulmonary allograft conduit flap is extended onto the distal pulmonary artery to relieve obstruction. C) A pulmonary allograft with bifurcated conduit is anastomosed to the right and left pulmonary arteries. (From: Clarke DR, Campbell DN, Pappas G (1989) Pulmonary allograft conduit repair of tetralogy of Fallot. An alternative to transannular patch repair. J Thorac Cardiovasc Surg 98: 730–737.)

Table 4. Operative variations for pulmonary valve allograft reconstruction of the right ventricular outflow tract

Type of distal anastomosis	Patient age group		
	>1 Year	≤1 Year	Total
Allograft to main pulmonary artery	109	35	144
Allograft to distal pulmonary artery:			
– bifurcated allograft	29	19	48
– flap extension	31	2	33
Total	169	56	225

A shield-shaped patch forms a hood that connects the anterior extent of the allograft to the ventriculotomy (Fig. 2b).

Rewarming is begun as the proximal connection is performed. If the aorta was clamped, a warm dose of blood cardioplegia is administered and the clamp is removed. When the patient is completely rewarmed, bypass is weaned and the procedure is concluded in routine fashion.

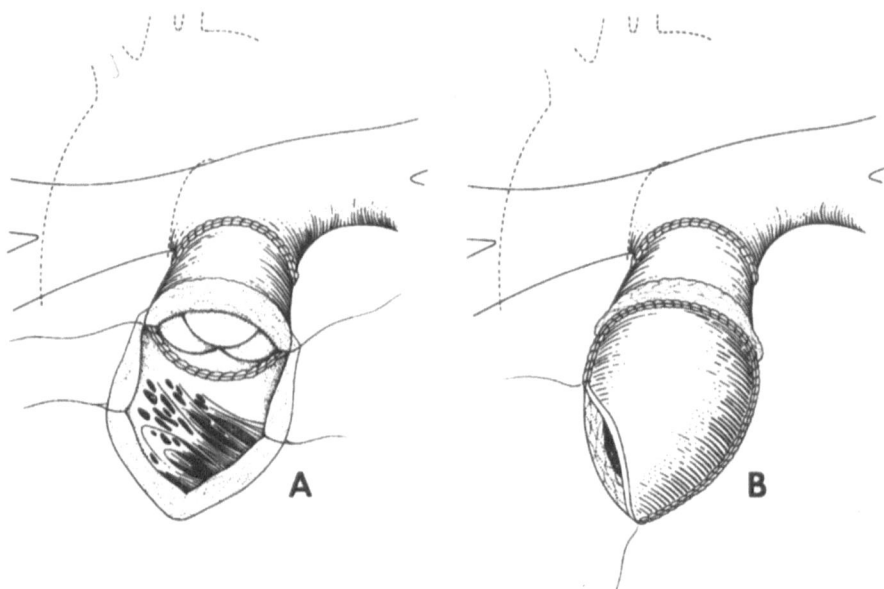

Fig. 2. A) The proximal pulmonary valve allograft is sutured into the right ventricular outflow tract. B) A shield-shaped patch completes the anterior ventricular connection (From: Clarke DR, Campbell DN, Pappas G (1989) Pulmonary allograft conduit repair of tetralogy of Fallot. An alternative to transannular patch repair. J Thorac Cardiovasc Surg 98: 730–737.)

Results

There were 16 hospital deaths (9%) among the children who were older than 1 year of age at surgery. Cause of death is defined in Table 5. Although 36% of operative survivors experienced a completely benign recovery, numerous early postoperative complications were encountered and are listed in Table 6. Of interest is one patient who underwent cardiac transplantation on the second postoperative day. Her original diagnosis was tetralogy of Fallot and she had a transannular patch repair at 3 years of age followed by pulmonary allograft reconstruction 2 years later. Severe pulmonary insufficiency developed and she underwent reoperative pulmonary allograft placement in addition to a bidirectional Glenn shunt and tricuspid annuloplasty for tricuspid regurgitation. She could not be weaned from cardiopulmonary bypass and was placed on extracorporeal membrane oxygenation until a donor heart became available for transplantation 2 days after implantation of the second allograft. One complication was technique related and occurred in a 2.5 year old male with pulmonary atresia, ventricular septal defect and multiple pulmonary collaterals. The child required balloon dilation of his distal pulmonary artery beyond the anastomotic site 22 days after allograft implantation. A complicated postoperative course continued involving coil occlusion of pulmonary collaterals, renal failure, sepsis and unmanageable pulmonary hypertension that ultimately led to his death from a pulmonary hemorrhage 1.5 months postoperatively.

Table 5. Perioperative mortality

Cause of death	Patient age group	
	> 1 Year	≤1 Year
Right ventricular failure	4	5
Intraoperative cardiac failure	3	4
Sepsis	4	2
Myocardial failure	1	2
Aortic allograft dehiscence (left and right ventricular outflow tract reconstructions	1	
Acute myocardial infarction → right ventricular failure	1	–
Pulmonary vascular disease	–	1
Arrhythmia	–	1
Metabolic derangement → cardiopulmonary failure	2	–
Total	16 (9%)	15 (27%)

Table 6. Early postoperative complications

Complication	Patient age group	
	>1 Year	≤1 Year
Pulmonary	43	16
Sepsis, mediastinitis, endocarditis	18	13
Hemorrhage	16	9
Arrhythmia, heart block	16	5
Neurologic impairment	10	8
Postpericardiotomy syndrome	13	1
Renal insufficiency or failure	5	6
Unable to reapproximate sternum	3	6
Diaphragm paralysis	6	2
Right ventricular failure	5	2
Extracorporeal membrane oxygenator (ECMO)	1	1
Balloon angioplasty distal pulmonary arteries	1	1
Cardiac transplant	1	–
Revise right ventricular outflow tract repair	–	1
Miscellaneous	5	4
No complications	55/153 (36%)	7/41 (17%)

The 152 remaining children in the older patient group have been followed for a mean 4.9 years (follow up range: 1 month to 10.5 years). One child was lost to follow up at 11 months after surgery. Eight of the children (5%) have experienced late deaths. Two children developed seizures postoperatively with subsequent neurologic dysfunction and died 1.1 and 1.7 months after allograft implantation. Two other patients died of pulmonary hemorrhage 1.5 (described above) and 16 months after surgery. One child expired during surgery to replace her mitral valve, five months after receiving an allograft. Another patient died 15 months postoperatively after an arrhythmia induced by hypertrophic cardiomyopathy. One youngster succumbed to complications of human immunodeficiency virus 5 years after allograft surgery and an asymptomatic teenager died in an automobile accident 18 months postoperatively.

A 12-year-old boy with double outlet left ventricle and aortic valvar insufficiency underwent aortic allograft left and pulmonary allograft right ventricular outflow tract reconstructions. He underwent cardiac transplantation 3.7 years after double allograft placement due to myocardial dysfunction. At explantation, both valve allografts were fully functional.

Seven of the older children (5%) have required allograft valve replacement. A synopsis of each child's experience is presented in Table 7. Pathologic examination was performed on five of the explanted allografts and revealed calcification in every one and mild cellular infiltrates in two allografts. Reoperative results have been positive in patients with good ventricular function. Mild to moderate pulmonary allograft insufficiency is common but stable in echocardiographic follow up of the 144 remaining allograft recipients in the older age group.

In the group of 56 children who were 12 months of age or younger at the time of surgery, there were 15 perioperative deaths (27%) that are listed in Table 5. A majority of surviving patients in the younger age group experienced early complications (Table 6), the most prevalent being pulmonary problems and infection. Two children underwent allograft-related procedures in the early postoperative period. An 11-month-old female with tetralogy of Fallot underwent primary repair with a bifurcated pulmonary allograft to the distal right and left pulmonary arteries. She was reoperated on the second postoperative day to relieve anastomotic strictures to both distal pulmonary arteries. The remaining postoperative course was unremarkable. A male neonate with type I truncus arteriosus and severe truncal valve insufficiency developed mediastinitis when his sternum was left open following placement of aortic and pulmonary allografts for left and right ventricular outflow tract reconstructions respectively. The child required balloon dilation of small left and right pulmonary arteries 1 week postoperatively. He died of sepsis 3 months after double allograft valve placement.

Forty-one infant operative survivors have been followed for a mean of 3.4 years. Ten of the younger children (24%) have died; all within the first postoperative year. Three infants succumbed to chronic congestive heart failure. Four deaths were pulmonary related with two deaths secondary to pneumonia and one death each due to cytomegalovirus and pulmonary embolus. One infant experienced sudden death that was probably related to arrhythmia and one neonate died of sepsis and was described previously. A male infant with tetralogy of Fallot, absent pulmonary valve and atrial septal defect had a sudden cardiac arrest at home 3 months after allograft surgery. His death was attributed to right ventricular failure due to increased pulmonary vascular resistance aggravated by respiratory infection.

Eleven operative survivors in the younger age group (27%) have required allograft valve replacement. Reoperative details are chronicled in Table 8. Calcification was present in all explanted allografts and cellular infiltrates were noted in 6 of the 11 removed valve conduits. Thirty of the infant allograft recipients are without cardiovascular symptoms but as in the older patient group, mild to moderate allograft valvar insufficiency defined echocardiographically is common.

Discussion

Statistically significant differences in both operative and follow up results are noted when infant and older pediatric allograft recipients are compared. Table 9 summarizes

Table 7. Allograft replacement in patients older than one year of age

Patient	Diagnosis at first allograft repair	Age and allograft type-first repair	Complication	Reoperation	Months after first allograft repair	Outcome
AR	tetralogy of Fallot	1.8 years aortic	allograft valvar stenosis	pulmonary allograft RVOTR	77.0	well 4.1 yrs. postop
AJ	double outlet right ventricle, pentalogy of Cantrell	2.0 years pulmonary	allograft valvar stenosis and insuff.	redo pulmonary allograft RVOTR	118.0	well 7 mos. postop
TSM	tetralogy of Fallot	2.0 years pulmonary	allograft insuff. and left PA stenosis	redo pulmonary allograft RVOTR	38.0	well 4.2 yrs. postop
TT	tetralogy of Fallot	3.0 years pulmonary	allograft stenosis and insuff., distal anastomotic kink	redo pulmonary allograft RVOTR	36.0	well 4 mos. postop
TS	tetralogy of Fallot	3.2 years pulmonary	allograft valvar insuff. and distal PA stenoses	redo pulmonary allograft RVOTR	15.0	well 9 yrs. postop
HE	tetralogy of Fallot	5.0 years pulmonary	allograft insuff., TR, cardiomyopathy	redo pulmonary allograft RVOTR	74.0	cardiac transplant 2 days postop
TWM	pulmonary stenosis	5.0 years pulmonary	allograft insuff. and conduit obstruction	aortic allograft RVOTR	69.0	redo pulmonary allograft RVOTR → kinked conduit

RVOTR = right ventricular outflow tract reconstruction; insuff. = insufficiency; PA = pulmonary artery; TR = tricuspid regurgitation

Table 8. Allograft replacement in patients one year old and younger

Patient	Diagnosis at first allograft repair	Age and allograft type-first repair	Complication	Reoperation	Months after first allograft repair	Outcome
CW	truncus arteriosus type I	9 days pulmonary	mediastinitis →	aortic allograft RVOTR	2.5	died 4 mos.
SH	aortic atresia, hypoplastic aortic arch	9 days aortic	allograft infection allograft valvar stenosis	pulmonary allograft RVOTR	38.0	postop → RV failure well 2.2 yrs.
JS	truncus arteriosus type I	2.0 months pulmonary	allograft insufficiency	redo pulmonary allograft RVOTR	41.0	postop well 2.5 yrs.
TB	truncus arteriosus type II	2.0 months aortic	allograft insuff., distal PA stenosis	pulmonary allograft RVOTR	33.0	postop well 2.5 yrs.
DH	truncus arteriosus type I	2.5 months aortic	allograft calcification and stenosis left and right PA	pulmonary allograft RVOTR	45.0	postop well 6 mos.
TJ	truncus arteriosus type I	2.5 months pulmonary	stenosis	aortic allograft RVOTR	2.0	postop died intraop → biventricular failure
JE	truncus arteriosus type I	3.0 months pulmonary	allograft stenosis and insuff.	redo pulmonary allograft RVOTR	31.0	well 4.5 yrs. postop
AG	truncus arteriosus type I	7.0 months pulmonary	allograft stenosis and insuff.	redo pulmonary allograft RVOTR	21.0	well 4.8 yrs. postop
JK	tetralogy of Fallot	7.0 months aortic	allograft stenosis and insuff.	pulmonary allograft RVOTR	83.0	well 3.3 yrs. postop
MC	truncus arteriosus type I	7.0 months aortic	allograft stenosis and insuff.	pulmonary allograft RVOTR	95.0	well 2.7 yrs. postop
MM	pulmonary atresia, ventricular septal defect	9.0 months aortic	allograft conduit stenosis and left PA stenosis	pulmonary allograft RVOTR	48.0	well 4.8 yrs. postop

RVOTR = right ventricular outflow tract reconstruction; RV = right ventricular; insuff. = insufficiency; PA = pulmonary artery the age group comparison for operative mortality, early postoperative complications, late mortality and incidence of allograft replacement. Incidences of each adverse event are higher in the infant group in all categories. The differences are most significant when late mortality and allograft explant are compared. Children who are 1 year of age or younger at the time of aortic or pulmonary allograft right ventricular outflow tract reconstruction experienced an increased incidence of early allograft degeneration and failure. While the increased incidence of perioperative death and complication might be attributable to the relative severity of cardiac anomalies in the younger children who require early surgical intervention, the contrast in late results is more difficult to explain. Figure 3 is an actuarial event-free curve that illustrates freedom from hospital death, allograft related death or allograft replacement. At ten years of follow up, 76% of the older children are alive with the original allograft while only 35% of the younger children remain event-free.

The etiology of early allograft degeneration might be immunologic. The rationale is identical to that presented for early aortic allograft failure in left ventricular outflow tract reconstruction. It is discussed in the chapter on allograft aortic root replacement

Table 9. Comparison of older and younger patient groups in early and late postoperative follow up

Patient age group	Early mortality	Early postoperative complications	Late mortality	Allograft explant
>1 year	16/169 (9%)	98/153 (64%)	8/151 (5%)	7/151 (5%)
≤1 year	15/56 (27%)	34/41 (83%)	10/41 (24%)	11/41 (27%)
Combined	31/225 (14%)	132/194 (68%)	18/192 (9%)	18/192 (9%)
p value (>1 vs ≤1)	$p < 0.01^*$	$p < 0.05^*$	$p < 0.001^*$	$p < 0.001^*$

*chi square for independent samples

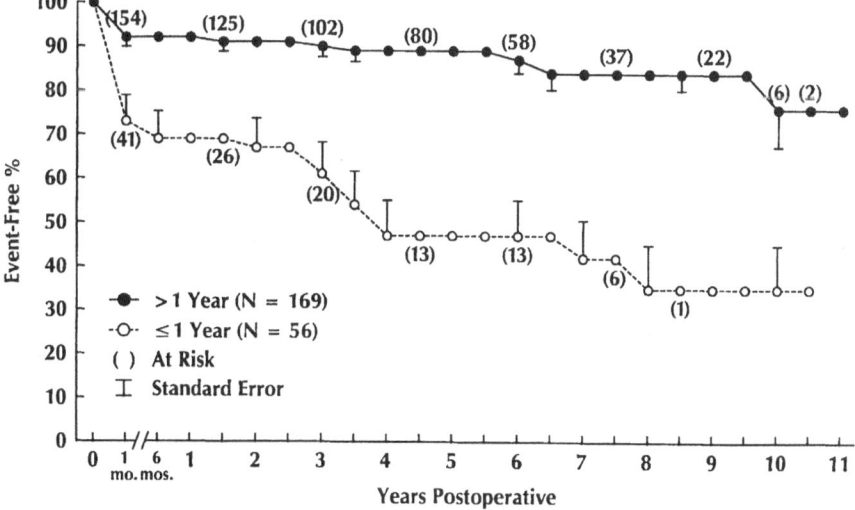

Fig. 3. Actuarial curves for older and younger patient groups illustrating freedom from hospital death, valve related death or valve explant.

Table 10. Use of pulmonary versus aortic allografts for reconstruction of the right ventricular outflow tract

Allograft type	Early mortality	Late mortality	Allograft explant
Pulmonary	24/195 (12%)	14/169 (8%)	11/169 (6%)
Aortic	7/30 (23%)	4/23 (17%)	7/23 (30%)
Combined	31/225 (14%)	18/192 (9%)	18/192 (9%)
p value (pulmonary vs aortic)	p > 0.10*	p > 0.10*	p < 0.001*

* chi square for independent samples

in children. In brief, an infant's immune system produces a generalized, all-or-none response to the antigenic stimulus of a viable allograft. A more mature immune system mounts a specific and dose-related response to allograft tissue.

Comparison of early and late results of aortic versus pulmonary valve allografts for right ventricular outflow tract reconstruction is of interest (Table 10). Duration of follow-up of the two allograft types is comparable with an aortic allograft mean follow up of 4.8 years and a pulmonary allograft mean follow up of 4.5 years. Incidences of early and late mortality between aortic and pulmonary allografts is not statistically different. A significantly higher percentage of aortic valve allografts has been ex-planted which corroborates previously published data and supports the use of pulmonary valve allografts to reconstruct the right ventricular outflow tract (2, 5, 11). An analogous but more exaggerated degenerative response has been documented with the use of aortic allografts for reconstruction of the left ventricular outflow tract in young children (8). Because aortic arterial walls are comprised of more elastin and calcium than are pulmonary arteries (12, 13), pulmonary allograft recipients might be partially protected from the response.

The ideal replacement conduit for right ventricular outflow tract reconstruction is not yet a reality. Although pulmonary allografts have both simplified the technique of right ventricular outflow tract reconstruction and made it an available option to children for whom there are no alternatives, they are not the perfect valved conduit replacements. The use of non-viable allografts or xenografts should be considered for infants who require right ventricular outflow tract reconstruction. If a viable pulmonary allograft must be implanted in a patient 12 months of age or younger, use of anti-inflammatory medication or a low dose immunosuppressant for 6 to 8 weeks postoperatively is suggested.

References

1. Agarwal KC, Edwards WD, Feldt RH, Danielson GK, Puga FJ, McGoon DC (1981) Clini-copathological correlates of obstructed right-sided porcine-valved extracardiac conduits. J Thorac Cardiovasc Surg 81: 591–601
2. Albert JD, Bishop DA, Fullerton DA, Campbell DN, Clarke DR (1993) Conduit reconstruction of the right ventricular outflow tract. Lessons learned in a twelve-year experience. J Thorac Cardiovasc Surg 106: 228–236
3. Al-Janabi N, Ross DN (1973) Enhanced viability of fresh aortic homografts stored in nutrient medium. Cardiovasc Res 7: 817–822
4. Angell JD, Christopher BS, Hawtrey O, Angell WM (1976) A fresh, viable human heart valve bank: sterilization, sterility testing, and cryogenic preservation. Transplant Proc 8(suppl I): 139–147

5. Bando K, Danielson GK, Schaff HV, Mair DD, Julsrud PR, Puga FJ (1995) Outcome of pulmonary and aortic homografts for right ventricular outflow tract reconstruction. J Thorac Cardiovasc Surg 109: 509–518
6. Brock L (1968) Long-term degenerative changes in aortic segment homografts, with particular reference to calcification. Thorax 23: 249–255
7. Clarke DR, Bishop DA (1995) Ten year experience with pulmonary allografts in children. J Heart Valve Dis (accepted for publication)
8. Clarke DR, Campbell DN, Bishop DA (1989) Homografts for congenital heart disease. In: Kron IL (ed) Cardiac Surgery: State of the Art Reviews. Hanley and Belfus Inc, Philadelphia, pp 1–17
9. Clarke DR, Campbell DN, Hayward AR, Bishop DA (1993) Aortic valve allograft degeneration in young recipients. J Thorac Cardiovasc Surg 105: 934–942
10. Jonas RA, Freed MD, Mayer JE Jr, Castaneda AR (1985) Long-term follow-up of patients with synthetic right heart conduits. Circulation 72(suppl): II77–83
11. Kay PH, Livi U, Parker R, Ross DN (1988) The pulmonary allograft for right ventricular outflow tract reconstruction. In: Yankah AC, Hetzer R, Miller DC, Ross DN, Sommerville J, Yacoub MH (eds) Cardiac Valve Allografts 1962–1987: Current Concepts on the Use of Aortic and Pulmonary Allografts for Heart Valve Substitutes. Springer-Verlag, New York, pp 189–193
12. Lansing AI (1959) Elastic tissue. In: Lansing AI (ed) The Arterial Wall. Williams and Wilkins, Baltimore, pp 136–160
13. Livi U, Abdulla AK, Parker R, Olsen EJ, Ross DN (1987) Viability and morphology of aortic and pulmonary homografts. A comparative study. J Thorac Cardiovasc Surg 93: 755–760
14. Moodie DS, Mair DD, Fulton RE, Wallace RB, Danielson GK, McGoon DC (1976) Aortic homograft obstruction. J Thorac Cardiovasc Surg 72: 553–561
15. Ross DN, Somerville J (1966) Correction of pulmonary atresia with a homograft aortic valve. Lancet 2: 1446–1447
16. Saravalli OA, Somerville J, Jefferson KE (1980) Calcification of aortic homografts used for reconstruction of the right ventricular outflow tract. J Thorac Cardiovasc Surg 80: 909–920

Author's address:
D. R. Clarke, MD
The Children's Hospital
Cardiothoracic Surgery, B200
1056 E. 19th Avenue
Denver, CO 80218
USA

Outcome of pulmonary and aortic allografts for reconstruction of the right ventricular outflow tract in congenital cardiac surgery

J. Weipert, J. C. Haehnel, H. Meisner

Department for Cardiovascular Surgery, German Heart Center Munich, Munich, Germany

Abstract

Between July 1982 and September 1995, a total of 280 patients (median age 6.4 years, range 1 month to 46 years, 68 patients younger than 1 year) underwent repair of the right ventricle to pulmonary artery connection by insertion of an allograft. The diagnoses were truncus arteriosus communis ($n = 84$, 30.0%), tetralogy of Fallot ($n = 62$, 22.1%), pulmonary atresia ($n = 76$, 27.1%), double outlet right ventricle ($n = 13$, 4.6%), complex transposition of the great arteries with pulmonary stenosis ($n = 31$, 11.1%), and others ($n = 14$, 5.1%). Either pulmonary ($n = 82$) or aortic ($n = 198$) cadaver allografts were implanted. *Results*: Follow-up was complete for 95.4% ($n = 267$, 1497 patient years). Thirty-day mortality was 13.2% ($n = 37$), late mortality 3.2% ($n = 9$). Kaplan-Meier analysis revealed that 64.0% patients with allograft valve diameter less than 15.0 mm underwent replacement of their conduit within 7 years, because these patients had outgrown their conduits. When the allograft was larger than 15.0 mm exchange was necessary in 17% at 10 years. Blood group compatibility and aortic or pulmonary origin of the allograft had no significant influence on allograft survival. *Conclusion*: 1) if it is possible to implant allografts with diameters greater than 15.0 mm, allografts of either pulmonary or aortic origin are the grafts of choice for restoration of the right ventricle to pulmonary artery continuation; and 2) 64.0% of the allografts with diameters less than 15.0 mm will require reoperation within 7 years. In these patients, xenograft implantation may also be indicated.

Introduction

Review of the literature regarding indications for and long-term follow-up of allograft implantation in neonates and infants reveals only few and contradictory reports. Yet, long-term evaluation is crucial for these patients to determine patient and allograft survival and quality of life. Albert and associates (1) and Livi and colleagues (7) discussed whether pulmonary allograft are less prone to calcification and subsequent exchange than are aortic allografts. Others have described an increased risk for aneurysm formation when pulmonary allografts were implanted in the right ventricular outflow tract (6). There is uncertainty with respect to the graft of choice for primary correction, especially in the newborn (9). To address the above questions, we analyzed our patients with allograft reconstruction of the right ventricular outflow tract during the time between 1982 to September 1995.

Methods and patients

Aortic and pulmonary valve allografts were harvested from healthy donors within 36 hours after death[1]. Preparation and antibiotic preservation of the allografts was standardized using the recommendations of the National Heart and Lung Institute, London, as described (8). One-hundred-ninety-six of the allografts were antibiotic preserved. Since January 1991, a new cryopreservation procedure was employed for standardized uniform cooling using heat sinks and defined package geometry in 84 allografts.

Figure 1a and b display the surgical inlay technique most suitable for patients with extensive dilatation of the pulmonary valve ring, e.g., tetralogy of Fallot with pulmonary insufficiency. The muscular rim at the base of the allograft is trimmed as short as possible, the distal portion is cut obliquely to ensure optimal adaptation to the pulmonary vessels (Fig. 1a). Usually, closure of the natural valve ring over the conduit cannot be attained and the sutures end on the upper end of the allograft. The allograft should be filled either by retrograde pulmonary flow or antegrade with a syringe, to demonstrate a competent valve in situ. To achieve optimal valve function proximal hood-like patch extension of the conduit is performed (Fig. 1b, see also ref. (8)).

Between July 1982 to September 1995, 280 patients (median age 6.4 years, range 1 month to 46.0 years, 68 patients below 1 year) had allografts implanted. The diagnoses were truncus arteriosus communis ($n = 84, 30.0\%$), tetralogy of Fallot ($n = 62, 22.1\%$), pulmonary atresia ($n = 76, 27.1\%$), double outlet right ventricle ($n = 13, 4.6\%$), complex transposition of the great arteries with pulmonary stenosis ($n = 31, 11.1\%$), and others ($n = 14, 5.1\%$). In 42 patients allograft exchange had to be performed once, in three patients twice. Follow-up was complete for 95.4% of the patients ($n = 267, 1497$ patient-years, median 6.4 years, range 1 month to 13.5 years). These patients were seen within the last year in the outpatient department[2], or patient data were gathered by their attending cardiologist.

Data are presented as median and range. Statistical analysis was performed with analysis of variance and chi-square test as indicated. Freedom from allograft failure analysis was done using the Kaplan-Meier method, with the calculations beginning at the end of extracorporeal circulation; differences were evaluated with the log-rank test. The preservation procedure was excluded from statistical evaluation because the median follow-up time for cryopreserved allografts was 2.5 years only.

---

[1] Institute of Forensic Medicine, University of Munich, Prof. Dr. Eisenmenger.
[2] Klinik für Herzerkrankungen im Kindesalter, Prof. Dr. K. Bühlmeyer.

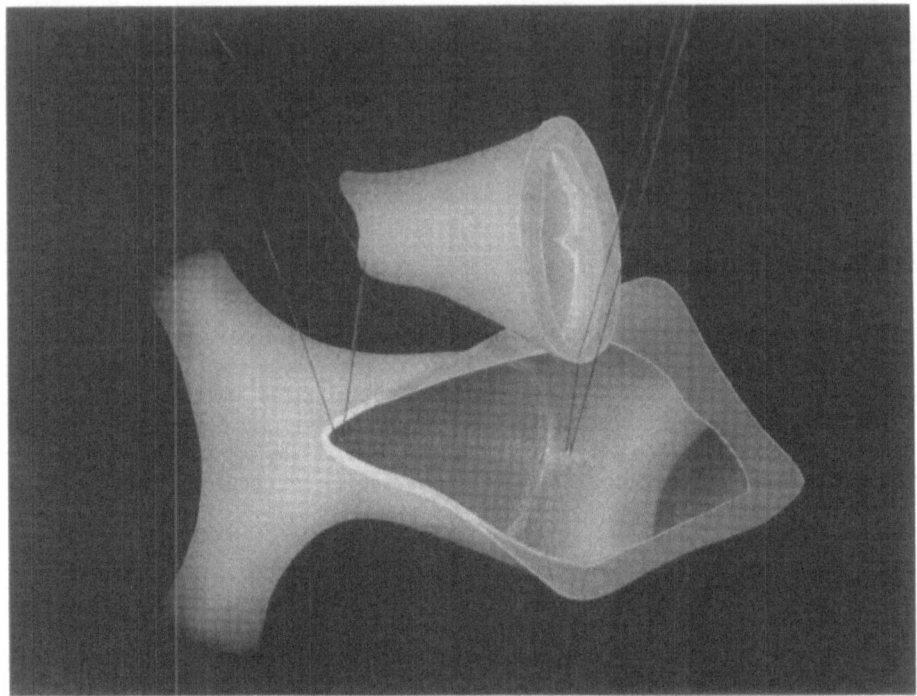

(a)

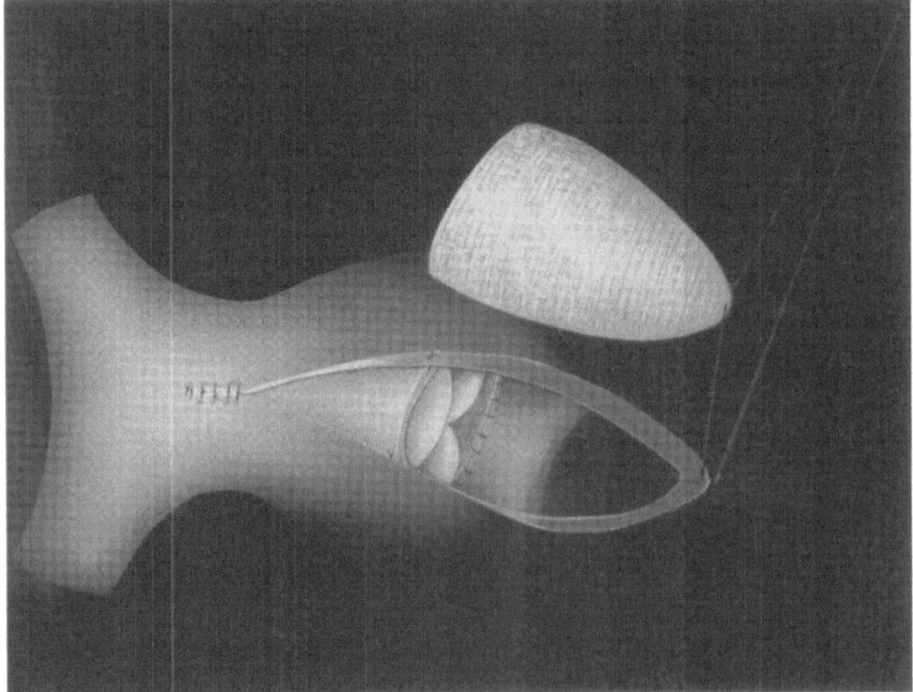

(b)

Fig. 1. (a) Demonstration of operative inlay technique for treatment of pulmonary incompetence. (b) After implantation of the allograft a patch is used for closing the gap to the right ventricle, thus avoiding traction on the valve.

Results

The median age of the allograft donors was 20 years (range 1 month to 42 years). Median storage time was 20 days for antibiotic-preserved allografts. Either aortic allografts ($n = 198$, 1188 patient-years) or pulmonary allografts ($n = 82$, 216 patient-years) were implanted. In 42 patients, a previously implanted xenograft had to be replaced after a median time of 5.1 years (range, 1 month to 12.2 years). Indication for replacement was seen with gradients above 60 mmHg over the allograft valve. Reoperation due to endocarditis or right ventricular aneurysm was necessary in 7 patients.

The estimated freedom from reoperation at 5 and 10 years after allograft implantation was $89.0 \pm 2.0\%$ and $73.0 \pm 4.0\%$ respectively. 13.5 years after allograft implantation 51% of the allografts are still in place (Fig. 2). 36% of allografts with diameters less than 15 mm are still in place 6.5 years after implantation, which is significantly ($p < 0.001$) shorter compared to allografts with diameters of 15 mm and more being 68% at 12.5 years (Fig. 3). Log-rank test with respect to blood group compatibility ($p = 0.76$) and origin of the allograft (aortic or pulmonary, $p = 0.51$) did not show any significant difference regarding allograft failure.

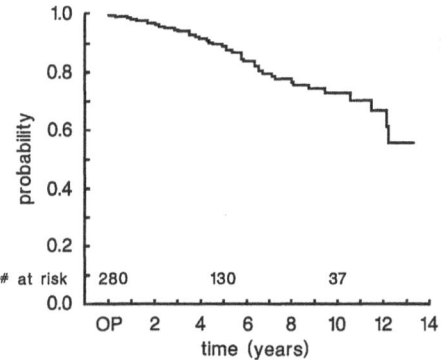

Fig. 2. Kaplan-Meier plot for overall freedom from allograft replacement in patients with right ventricular outflow tract reconstruction (7/1982–9/1995). # indicates number of patients at risk.

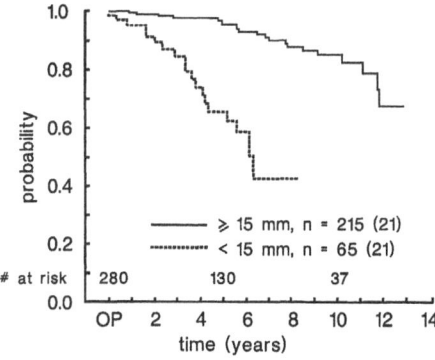

Fig. 3. Kaplan-Meier plot for freedom from allograft replacement according to allograft valve size. Numbers in parentheses indicate allograft replacements. # indicates number of patients at risk.

Discussion

Both antibiotic preserved (1982 to 1990) and cryo-preserved (since January 1991) allografts have been implanted. Livi and associates (7) and Bando and colleagues (2) suggested that pulmonary allografts in the right ventricular outflow tract position may be less prone to calcification. Among our patients who received pulmonary allografts, the reoperation rate due to valve failure was not significantly different from that in patients with aortic allografts.

Aneurysm formation after pulmonary allograft implantation – as described by others (6) – was found to be a minor problem in our patient population. The estimated freedom from reoperation at 5 and 10 years after allograft reconstruction of the RVOT was 89.0% and 73.0%, respectively (Fig. 2). These data are similar to the results from Albert and colleagues (1), but in contrast to data of Cleveland and co-workers (4) and Bull and associates (3). Although the demographic data of the patients are similar, only 55.0% ± 12.0% in the Cleveland group (4) were free of reoperation at 5 years. A possible explanation for the better results in our series might be the more recent time period, with general improvement of surgical technique and more standardized allograft procurement procedures.

We did not stratify our data according to patient age or diagnosis but to graft valve diameter at operation. At present, allograft survival seems to be determined mainly by the allograft diameter respectively the individual space for allograft implantation. Within 7 years, 64.0% of allografts with diameters less than 15.0 mm had to be replaced (Fig. 3). As we demonstrated earlier (10), these patients will require reoperation, because the diameter of their implanted allograft eventually became too small for their body surface area at the time of reoperation. These patients outgrew their conduit. Sano and co-workers (9) reported similar results with xenograft implantation in the right ventricular outflow tract. The authors suggested that initial xenograft implantation would facilitate subsequent graft reoperations by establishing a prosthetic sewing margin. Kaplan-Meier analysis revealed that 83.0% of patients with allograft diameters larger than 15.0 mm, were free from reoperation due to allograft failure at ten years (Fig. 3). Bull and associates (3) summarized the early experience of allograft and xenograft surgery at the Great Ormond Street Hospital and found no significant difference in function between the types. In their series, freedom from death or conduit obstruction at 5 and 10 years was 72.0% ± 6.5% and 25.0% ± 11.3%, respectively. In a recent retrospective study from our institution (5) freedom from reoperation significantly improved only for allografts with diameters greater than 20 mm as compared to xenografts. Yet no data from controlled, randomized, prospective studies are available.

We conclude that if it is possible to implant allografts larger than 15.0 mm, allografts of either pulmonary or aortic origin are currently the grafts of choice for right ventricular reconstruction. When the graft diameter is smaller than 15.0 mm, replacement will be necessary within 7 years in 63% of the patients. These patients outgrew their grafts. Xenografts may be equally effective in this situation.

References

1. Albert JD, Bishop DA, Fullerton DA, Cambell DN, Clarke DR (1993) Conduit reconstruction of the right ventricular outflow tract. J Thorac Cardiovasc Surg 106: 228–236
2. Bando K, Danielson GK, Schaff HV, Mair DD, Julsrud PR, Puga FJ (1995) Outcome of pulmonary and aortic homografts for right ventricular outflow tract reconstruction. J Thorac Cardiovasc Surg 109: 509–518

3. Bull C, Macartney FJ, Horvath P et al. (1987) Evaluation of long term results of homograft and heterograft valves in extracardiac conduits. J Thorac Cardiovasc Surg 94: 12–9
4. Cleveland DC, William WG, Razzouk AJ, Trusler GA, Rebeyka IM, Duffy L, Kan Z, Coles J, Freedom RM (1992) Failure of cryopreserved homograft valved conduits in the pulmonary circulation. Circulation 86 (suppl 2): II-150–II-153
5. Homann M, Haehnel JC, Wottke M, Meisner H, Mendler N, Sebening F (1995) Allograft vs. Xenograft-20 years experience with valved biologic conduits. Thorac Cardiovasc Surgeon 43: (suppl I), Abs 40, p. 60
6. Kadoba K, Armiger LC, Sawatari K, Jonas RA (1993) Mechanical durability of pulmonary allograft conduits at systemic pressure. J Thorac Cardiovasc Surg 105: 132–141
7. Livi U, Abdulla A-K, Parker R, Olsen EJ, Ross DN (1987) Viability and morphology of aortic and pulmonary homografts. J Thorac Cardiovasc Surg 93: 755–760
8. Meisner H, Hagl S, Sebening F (1987) Technique of inlay allografts into the RVOT to prevent pulmonary insufficiency. In: Yankah AC, Hetzer R, Miller DC, Ross DN, Somerville J, Yacoub MH, eds. Cardiac Valve Allografts 1962–1987. Berlin: Springer: 205–213
9. Sano S, Karl TR, Mee RBB (1991) Extracardiac valved conduits in the pulmonary circuit. Ann Thorac Surg 52: 285–290
10. Weipert J, Meisner H, Mendler N, Haehnel JC, Homann M, Paek S-U, Sebening F (1995) Allograft implantation in pediatric cardiac surgery: Surgical experience from 1982 to 1994. Ann Thorac Surg 60(2 suppl): S101–104

Author's address:
Dr. J. Weipert
Klinik für Herz- und Gefäßchirurgie
Deutsches Herzzentrum München
Lothstr. 11
80335 München, Germany

Long-term results of allograft conduits in the pulmonary circulation

J. L. Monro

Wessex Cardiothoracic Centre, Southampton General Hospital,
Southampton, UK

Introduction

Ross first reported the use of an aortic homograft for correction of pulmonary atresia with ventricular septal defect in 1966 (10) and this concept of a conduit to connect the right ventricle to the pulmonary artery has been expanded by others since. McGoon (4) reported correction of truncus arteriosus in 1968 and Rastelli correction of transposition with ventricular septal defect and pulmonary stenosis in 1969 (8). The early homografts were sterilised by a variety of methods but many failed and other surgeons started to use heterograft valves in Dacron tubes. Ebert obtained outstanding results using these valves although two-thirds of his valves needed replacing within 10 years (1). Others used heterografts but were not able to achieve the same early results. Perhaps because of the inevitable high reoperation rate within a fairly short space of time for replacement of the heterograft valve and their increased availability, there has been a return to preference for homograft valves in the right ventricular outflow tract and indeed the use of pulmonary valves has become more widespread. The author having witnessed the successful use of an aortic homograft by Barratt-Boyes in a young infant with truncus arteriosus in 1971 (2) has used almost exclusively the antibiotic sterilised aortic homograft for reconstruction of the right ventricular outflow tract during the last 21 years. The size and suturing qualities of the valve make it extremely suitable for right ventricular outflow tract construction in children of all ages. The experience gained with this valve is the subject of this chapter.

Material and methods

A homograft bank was first set up in Southampton in 1973 and was initially used to provide valves for aortic valve replacement (3). They have been sterilised in antibiotics (see Table 1) and stored at 4 °C. No valves have been cryopreserved. Since 1974 aortic homografts have been used in the right ventricular outflow tract and the author's personal experience is reported. Although a few pulmonary valves have been used in recent years, the experience has been very predominantly with aortic homografts and as these have functioned well their use has been continued and only aortic homografts are reported here.

Several different groups of patients have received a homograft in the right ventricular outflow tract and the groups are shown in Table 2.

Table 1. Composition of nutrient medium and antibiotic mixture

Nutrient medium Constituents		Quantity (ml)
Sterile distilled water		77.0
Medium 199 (bicarbonate free)		10.0
Preheated inactivated calf serum no. 1		8.0
Sodium bicarbonate (4.4%)		5.0
		100.0
Antibiotic mixture Constituents	Amount	Quantity (ml)
Nystatin	250 000 U	10.0
Methicillin	1000 mg	1.4
Erythromycin	600 mg	12.0
Gentamicin	400 mg	10.0
Streptomycin	20 000 U	0.1

Table 2. Total patients receiving aortic homografts in right ventricular outflow tract 1974–1994

Diagnosis	Total	Age range	Early deaths	%	Late deaths
Truncus Arteriosus	26	10 days–2 years	6	23	1
Pulmonary Atresia and VSD	21	10 months–23 years	1	4.8	4
Post Fallot Repair	10	3 years–29 years	0		0
Rastelli	6	1 year–18 years	0		3
Corrected TGA and PS	2	2 years–12 years	0		0
	65		7	10.8	8

Early deaths = within 30 days of operation; VSD = Ventricular septal defect; TGA = Transposition of the great arteries; PS = Pulmonary stenosis.

Truncus arteriosus

There were 26 patients with this condition and they have been operated on at a much younger age than the other groups. Only one patient was more than 1 year and 50% were less than 1 month of age. This has resulted in the use of smaller homografts, the mean diameter being 15.5 mm in diameter compared with 19.5 in the other groups. The diameter of the homograft was measured internally at the valve ring. Further-more, in those babies less than 1 month of age the mean size of homograft used was 14.1 mm in diameter, whereas in those between 1 month and 5 months it was 17.0 mm. In three small neonates the only homografts available were larger and these were tailored to a smaller diameter by excising one cusp and sewing the valve together longitudinally. This was first performed by the author in 1986 (7, 9) and has recently been reported by others (5, 11). This is a useful technique but it is also possible to get quite a large homograft in small infants. The largest used in the truncus arteriosus group was a size 22 mm valve in a 4-month-old child.

Pulmonary atresia and ventricular septal defect

There were 21 patients with this condition. The age range varied from 10 months to 23 years and in four patients who had absent or minute central pulmonary arteries Goretex tube grafts were used to connect the hilar pulmonary arteries to a homograft centrally.

Pulmonary regurgitation after previous correction of Fallot's Tetralogy with transannular patch

There were 10 patients in this group, five had previously been corrected by the author and five were referred from elsewhere.

Rastelli procedure for double outlet right ventricle or transposition of the great arteries with ventricular septal defect and pulmonary stenosis

There were six patients in this group. In one of these patients because of the distance from the right ventriculotomy to the pulmonary artery, a Dacron tube had to be used in addition to the homograft.

Corrected transposition with pulmonary stenosis

There were two patients in this group and in both because of the coronary anatomy a ventriculotomy had to be made fairly low down on the left ventricle and a Dacron tube used to connect to the homograft which was anastomosed to the pulmonary artery. These last three mentioned patients were the only ones in the group to have a Dacron tube although some patients needed an additional autologous pericardial patch. However, in most patients the anterior leaflet of the mitral valve was used to close the ventriculotomy.

Surgical technique

Truncus arteriosus

Having detached the pulmonary artery from the aorta and closed the resulting defect, a high transverse right ventriculotomy is made wherever possible and a semi circle of muscle cut out above it to give good exposure of the ventricular septal defect which is then closed (6). Dacron was used in the early part of the series for ventricular septal defect closure and more recently Goretex patch. It is important in closing the superior margin of this defect to avoid the truncal valve leaflets and the patch can be brought right up to the upper edge of the ventriculotomy. The distal pulmonary artery is then enlarged if necessary to match the distal end of the aortic homograft which is trimmed immediately above the homograft cusps posteriorly, although it may be angled so that the distance is a little longer anteriorly so that the valve tilts towards the ventriculotomy. 5/0 Prolene is usually used for the distal anastomosis or 6/0 in small infants. The proximal end is then sutured with 5/0 or 4/0 Prolene and the sutures start posteriorly going through the upper end of the ventricular septal defect patch, the right ventricular muscle and the posterior muscular part of the homograft. The homograft lies so that the anterior leaflet of the mitral valve comes down to cover the ventriculotomy. Usually the anterior leaflet neatly fills the ventriculotomy but particularly if the coronary anatomy has necessitated a longitudinal incision it may be necessary to insert a patch to complete it without distorting the outflow tract and autologous pericardium is suitable for this. Occasionally if the homograft is rather large the distal end can be narrowed to match the size of the pulmonary artery by taking a tuck in the homograft. As previously mentioned, if only a large homograft is available for a small infant the homograft can be tailored, narrowing the diameter by about a third.

Figure 1 shows a post operative right ventriculogram 4 years after insertion of a 16 mm homograft in a 3-month-old patient whose truncus arteriosus was corrected.

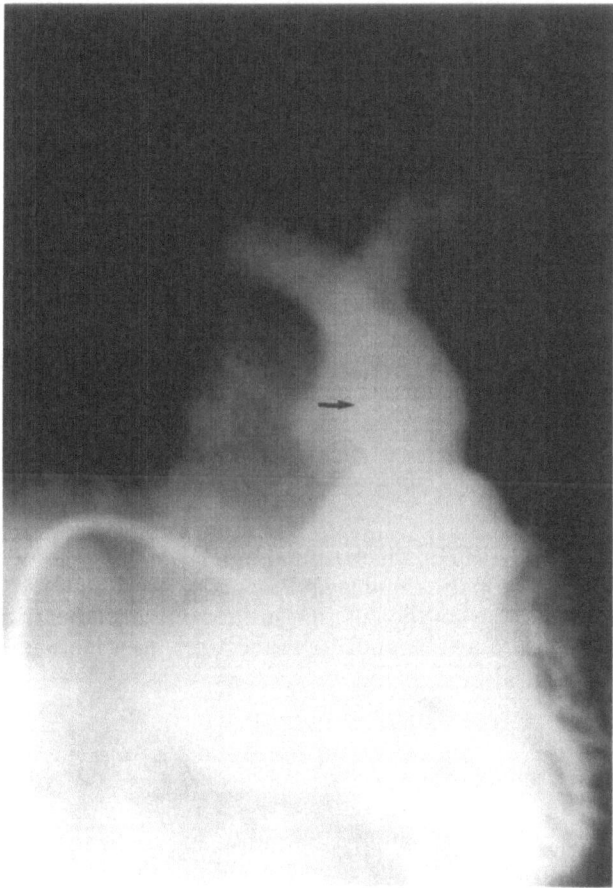

Fig. 1. A post operative right ventriculogram following repair of truncus arteriosus with a homograft (arrow).

Pulmonary atresia and ventricular septal defect

Again a transverse incision is very satisfactory with removal of a semi circle of muscle above it and this gives good exposure for closure of the ventricular septal defect. The upper margin of the ventricular septal defect patch is sutured to the infundibular septum, unlike in a truncus arteriosus. Again care must be taken not to catch the aortic leaflets. The pulmonary artery is opened to allow an orifice that matches the size of the homograft that is to be used and this is sutured as for the truncus arteriosus patient. However, the proximal end of the homograft is sutured to the right ventricular muscle, the ventricular septal defect patch being lower than this because of the infundibular septum. Again it may be necessary to use a patch to complete the ventriculotomy closure.

Conduit insertion for late pulmonary regurgitation following repair of Fallot's Tetralogy

Because of long standing pulmonary regurgitation the right ventricle is usually dilated and the pulmonary artery large and with good tissue. The distal main pulmonary artery should be transected and the distal end of the homograft sutured to it. The proximal end of the homograft should be attached to the outflow tract at the appropriate level. There is usually no need for much of the anterior leaflet of the mitral valve to be used.

Rastelli procedure

Because the right ventriculotomy may be a distance from the pulmonary artery it may occasionally be necessary to use a Dacron tube in addition to the homograft and a patch is usually necessary to widen the right ventricular outflow tract which would otherwise be narrow because of the ventricular septal defect patch.

Corrected transposition with pulmonary stenosis

In order to avoid damage to the bundle of His which runs anteriorly in this condition, it is not possible to transect the pulmonary annulus and therefore it is necessary to make a ventriculotomy fairly well down on the anterior surface of the left ventricle between the coronary arteries and use a tube graft to connect this to a homograft attached to the pulmonary artery.

Re-do procedure for removal of stenosed homograft

Since the homograft has been placed in the anatomical position and to the left of the mid-line and away from the sternum, although the usual precautions should be taken when opening the chest, the homograft itself is usually well out of the way to the left. The calcification can be felt and the homograft shelled out with dissection and a new homograft inserted exactly where the previous one was. It is, however, important to remember that the left coronary artery runs quite close behind the homograft and care must be taken not to damage this. If the pulmonary arteries are narrowed a patch can be used at the same time to widen them.

Results

Between 1974 and 1994, 65 consecutive patients have been operated on by the author for the insertion of an antibiotic sterilised aortic homograft into the right ventricular outflow tract. For completeness these patients are shown in Table 2. The high mortality in those patients undergoing correction of truncus arteriosus relates to the young age of patients, their pre-operative state, the presence of severe truncal regurgitation in four patients and post operative pulmonary vascular crises. In the patients with pulmonary atresia and ventricular septal defect, two of the late deaths resulted from long standing pulmonary hypertension relating to pre-operative palliation. In no patients was death related to the homograft.

In order to assess the long term function of these homografts (see Table 3) the progress of the 53 patients surviving more than 1 year after their initial operation is shown. One patient who is well lives abroad and the remainder have been followed regularly by cardiologists with frequent Doppler echo assessment. The longest follow up is 21 years in a patient who had repair of truncus arteriosus at 7 weeks of age and still has the same 17 mm homograft with a gradient of 22 mmHg across it. All homografts develop calcification in the wall of the aorta (see Fig. 2) and this has been seen as early as 3 months in younger patients. Heavy calcification of the homograft wall is shown in Fig. 3. This valve was explanted 4 years after insertion when the patient underwent truncal valve replacement because of severe regurgitation. The cusps were thin and pliable but acellular as shown in Fig. 4. The aortic wall was heavily calcified (see Fig. 5). Most homografts do ultimately develop calcification of the cusps and often shortening and all show at least mild or moderate regurgitation and a few show severe regurgitation. However, until now no valve in this series has been replaced because of regurgitation. With time increasing gradients develop partially because of the calcification of the homograft cusps but also because of growth of the patients. This is particularly so in the patients who had repair of truncus arteriosus (see Fig. 6). This obviously depends on the size of the homograft inserted initially and the length of follow up. In patients with pulmonary atresia and ventricular septal defect (see Fig. 7) the steady increase in the gradient with time is more clearly seen but these valves were larger.

It has been necessary to reoperate on 14 patients, as can be seen in Table 4. However, in only four of these patients was the reason for homograft replacement stenosis of the valve, although seven patients underwent homograft replacement. The four patients undergoing homograft replacement for stenosis were as follows.

1) A girl who had correction of truncus arteriosus at 3 months developed a gradient of 50 mmHg on echo across the homograft 12 years later and was becoming tired and the valve was therefore replaced. Figure 8 shows the gradient across her homograft during the last 19 years.
2) A girl with pulmonary atresia and ventricular septal defect who was 6 at original correction again became rather tired 12 years later. The gradient across the valve was 40 and this valve was replaced.

Table 3. Follow-up of patients surviving more than 1 year after homograft insertion

	Number of patients	Mean age at Op	Follow-up years	(Mean) years	Size of homograft (mm)	(Mean)	Homograft replacement operations	Current gradient (mmHg)	(Mean)
Truncus	19	67 days	1–21	(10.8)	12–22	(15.5)	3	0–50	(24.3)
Pulmonary Atresia and VSD	18	8.1 years	2–15	(9.0)	17–22	(19.4)	1	0–35	(16.7)
PVR (Post Fallot)	10	8.8 years	1–12	(6.5)	17–25	(20.5)	1	0–72	(19.2)
Rastelli	4	8.8 years	6–15	(10.5)	16–18	(17.5)	1	0–70	(29.0)
Corrected TGA	2	7.0 years	10–20	(15.0)	18–22	(20.0)	2	0	

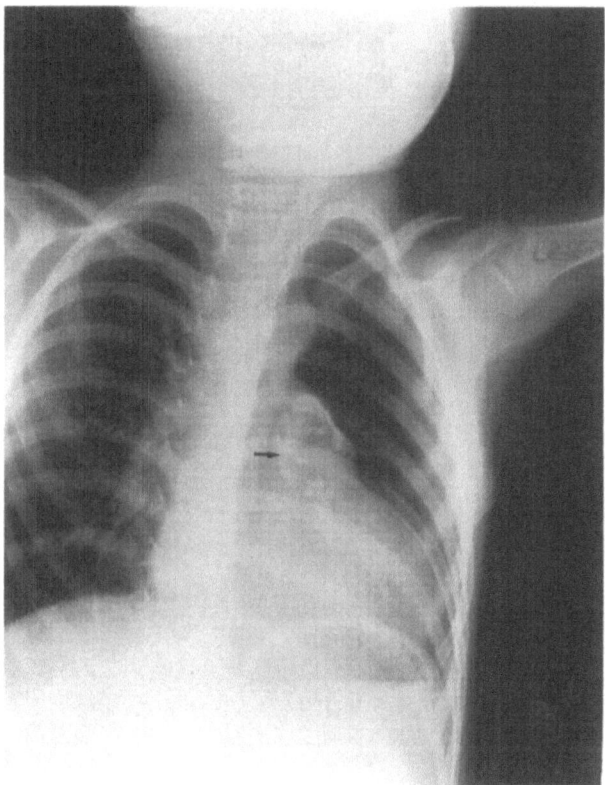

Fig. 2. Calcification is seen in the wall of the homograft (arrow) on plain chest x-ray. This homograft had been in position for 9 years.

3) A boy who had correction of Fallot's Tetralogy at the age of 3 with a transannular patch developed pulmonary regurgitation and a homograft was inserted at the age of 11. Eight years later it became stenotic with a gradient of 55 across it and was replaced with another homograft.

4) A girl who was 18 at the time of correction of double outlet right ventricle, developed ventricular tachycardias 13 years later. Although the gradient across the homograft was only 20 mmHg, she had important tricuspid regurgitation. The calcified homograft which was connected to the right ventricle by a Dacron tube graft was replaced and was stenosed to 1 cm.

All four valves showed stenosis of the cusps with calcification and central regurgitation. There is one further patient, 10 years post operatively who has a gradient across the valve of 70 mmHg and will probably need homograft replacement soon.

One patient who died 6 years after homograft insertion for double outlet right ventricle had a gradient of 70 across the homograft shortly before his death. He had developed both left and right ventricular failure. It is therefore possible that the narrowed homograft contributed to this death. The other late deaths were not related to homograft function.

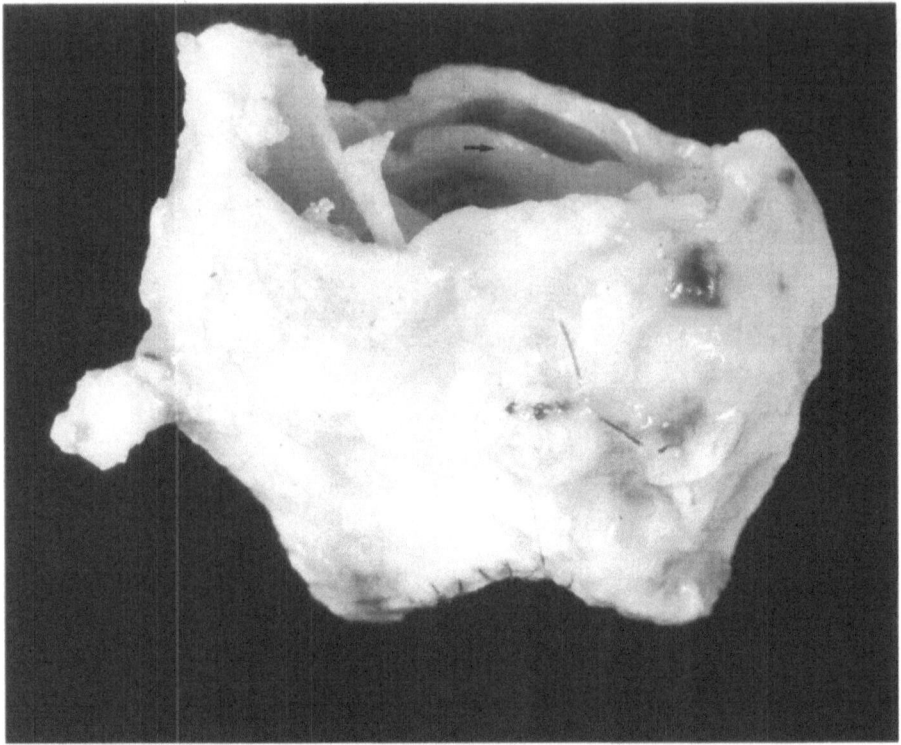

Fig. 3. A homograft removed 4 years after insertion for correction of truncus arteriosus, shows a completely rigid and calcified wall. However, the valve cusps (arrow) were thin.

Discussion

This is a small series but one of the longest reported. It is remarkable that the first patient in the series who was a girl of 7 weeks who received a size 17 mm homograft is extremely well at university, now $21\frac{1}{2}$ years later with the same homograft in position. Although one would anticipate replacement of these valves and indeed parents are always told to expect this, it is remarkable that a valve should have lasted so long and may well survive for many years to come. Calcification appears in the aortic wall of these conduits early on and progresses to complete calcification of the whole wall which is rock hard. It may well be that pulmonary valve homografts will not calcify to the same extent and indeed there may be other methods of preparation which reduce calcification. However, because this series was started with antibiotic sterilised aortic homografts kept at 4 °C this technique has been continued and this has been the method of choice throughout these 21 years. The aortic homograft also has the advantage of the anterior leaflet of the mitral valve forming a built in patch to close the ventriculotomy rather than a separate patch being needed in most cases. There has fortunately been an adequate supply of homografts and there has been no heterograft valve used during this time. Many surgeons have used heterograft valves either because homografts are not or were not available or for preference. However, they are

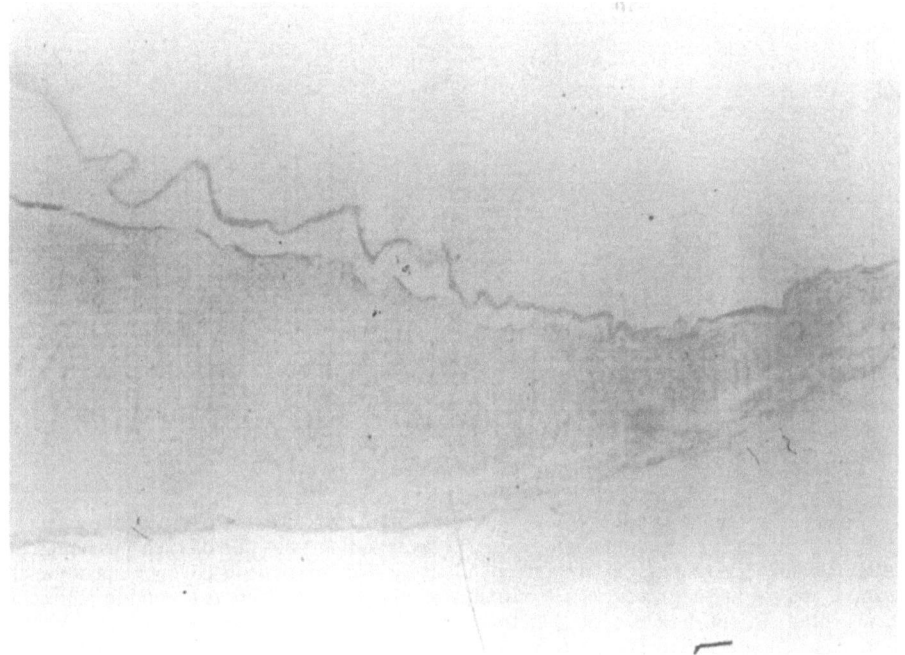

Fig. 4. The histology of the valve cusps from the valve shown in Fig. 3 shows complete acellularity.

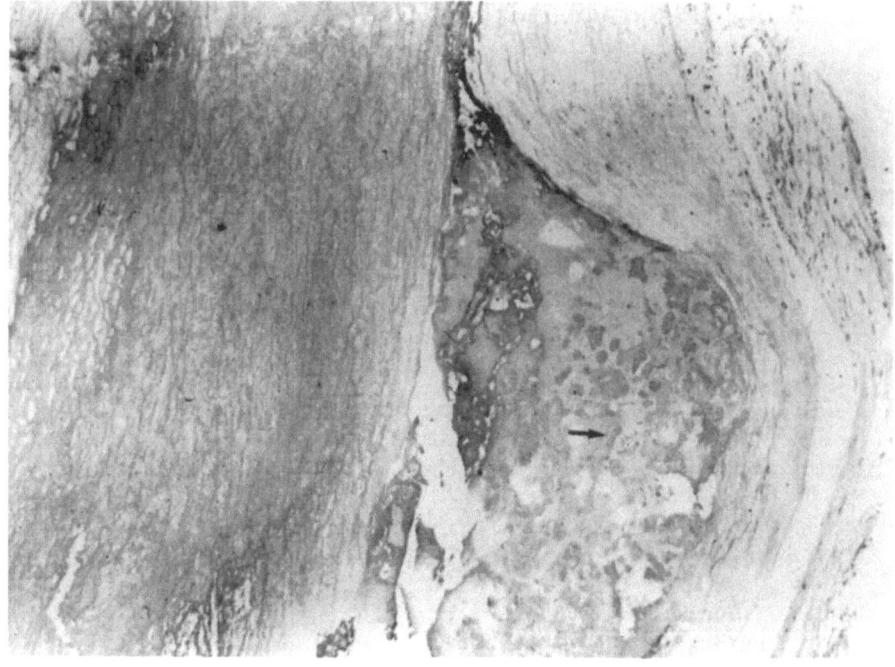

Fig. 5. Histology shows that the wall of the aorta of the valve shown in Fig. 3 contains calcification (arrow).

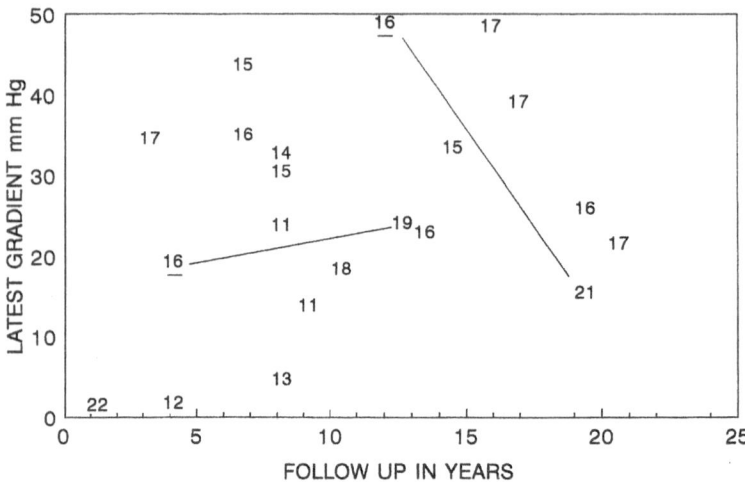

Fig. 6. Each patient surviving correction of truncus for more than 1 year is shown on the graph by a figure equal to the size of the homograft inserted at operation. The position on each axis represents the latest measured gradient and the duration of follow-up. The two patients having reoperation are underlined, and the line connects to their current size and gradient. There is a trend to increasing gradients with time, but there is a lot of scatter.

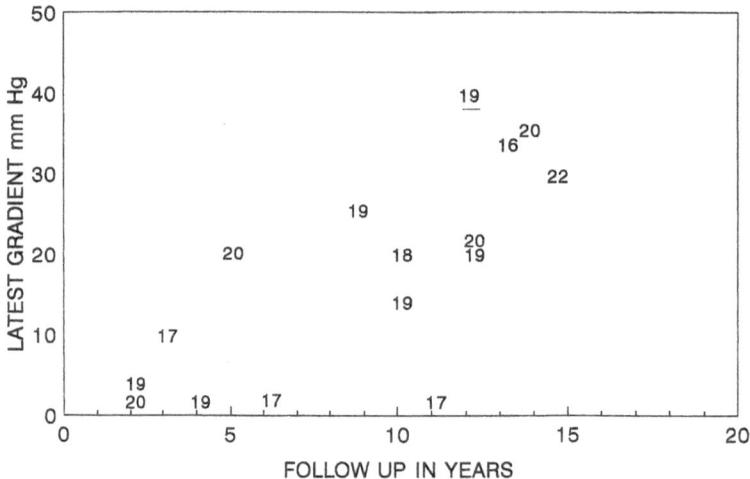

Fig. 7. This graph based on the same principles as Fig. 6 shows a steady increase in gradient across the homografts inserted for repair of pulmonary atresia and ventricular septal defect. One valve has recently been replaced.

more difficult to suture to, haemorrhage is more likely and they certainly do not last as long. Providing the conduit is placed in the anatomical position there is no problem replacing it when this is required.

Fortunately replacement of the homograft conduits has been rare in this series, only four valves being replaced for stenosis at a mean of 13.5 years after insertion.

Table 4. Reoperations

	Reason	Homograft replaced
Truncus arteriosus		
Time since operation	Reason	Homograft replaced
1.5 yers	Narrowed pulmonary artery	No
3 years	Truncal regurgitation	No
4 years	Truncal regurgitation	Yes
9 years	Truncal regurgitation	No
12 years	Narrowed homograft (Gradient 50 mmHg)	Yes
Pulmonary atresia and VSD		
Time since operation		
3 months	Narrowed pulmonary artery	No
1 years	Tricuspid valve replacement	No
3 years	TVR	No
9 years same patient	PVR and TVR	Yes
12 years	Narrowed homograft (Gradient 40 mmHg)	Yes
Fallot's Tetralogy		
Time since operation		
7 years	Narrowed homograft (Gradient 55 mmHg)	Yes
Corrected TGA		
Time since operation		
7 years	Narrowed Dacron tube	Yes
17 years	Narrowed Dacron tube	Yes
Rastelli		
Time since operation		
13 years	Narrowed homograft (Gradient 20 mmHg)	Yes

VSD = Ventricular septal defect; TGA = Transposition of the great arteries; TVR = Tricuspid valve replacement; PVR = Pulmonary valve replacement.

Homografts were replaced in other patients at the same time as another operation was being performed for either relief of stenosis of the pulmonary arteries or when the truncal valve was being replaced because of truncal regurgitation. Many patients have some regurgitation in these conduits but none has required replacement because of this alone.

Clearly truncus arteriosus is very different from the other groups as the patients are so much younger. The neonates required a valve that was about 3 mm in diameter smaller than older infants and the truncus group in turn required a mean size homograft 4 mm smaller than the other groups. Obviously as the patient grows even if the homografts do not narrow they will become relatively stenotic and if a small or tailored valve was used initially this will inevitably need replacement at some stage (Fig. 9). However, it is remarkable how large a homograft can be put into the right ventricular outflow tract in a baby with truncus arteriosus, and to narrow the distal end of the homograft to fit a rather small pulmonary artery a tuck can be taken in the homograft. Any patient over 6 months should certainly be able to receive a homograft from an adult donor.

Corrected transposition is a different situation where because of the inevitable increased distance between the ventriculotomy and the pulmonary artery a Dacron tube is necessary and this runs behind the sternum and may well get compressed, as

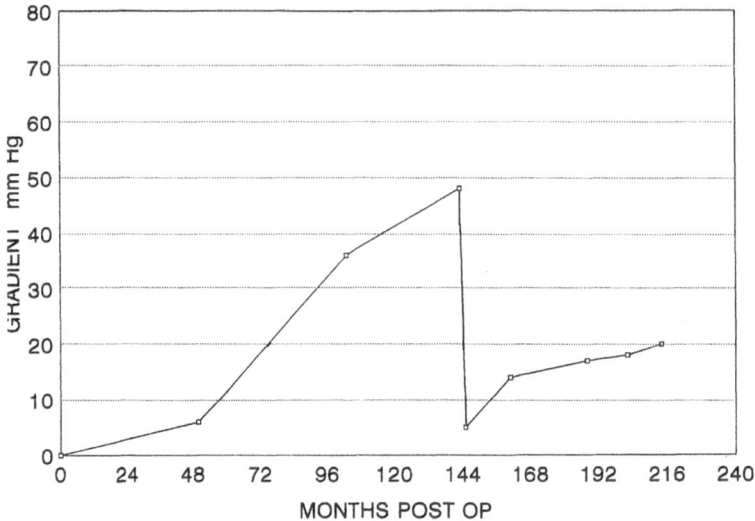

Fig. 8. The gradient across a 16 mm homograft in a patient who had correction of truncus arteriosus is shown to rise until replacement of the valve 12 years post operatively. There has been a steady but mild increase in gradient in the subsequent 7 years.

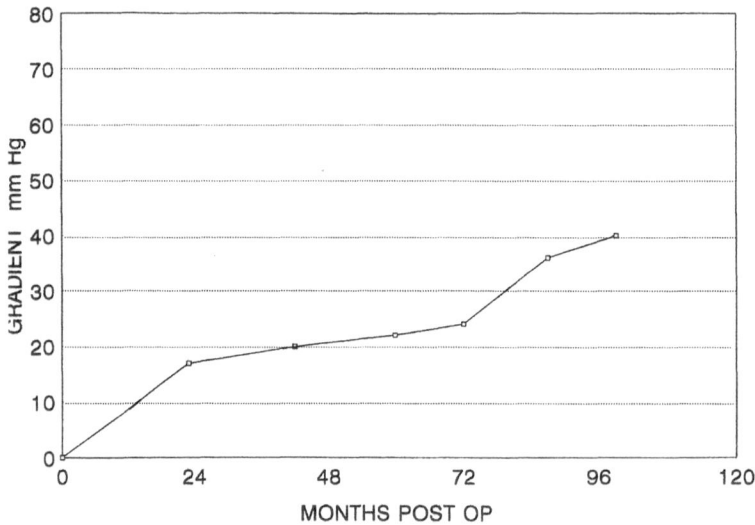

Fig. 9. This shows the steadily increasing gradient across a tailored homograft in a girl who had correction of truncus arteriosus as a neonate. There has been a steady increase in the gradient across the valve over the subsequent 9 years to 40 mmHg.

was the case in the two patients reported here. The homograft was therefore replaced in these two patients really because of the Dacron tube being narrowed rather than the homografts themselves. Only three patients required a Dacron tube extension, in all others direct continuity was established between the right ventricle and pulmonary artery with the homograft. The third patient with a Dacron tube extension had the homograft replaced 13 years later. This patient had double outlet right ventricle, and it was the narrowed homograft causing obstruction. The Dacron tube was perfect.

In summary it can be said that the antibiotic sterilised aortic homograft is an extremely satisfactory conduit for the creation of a right ventricle to pulmonary artery communication, although it will almost certainly leak and the wall of the homograft calcify. Despite this good function can be preserved for at least 20 years. Pulmonary homografts may calcify less and be an attractive alternative.

References

1. Ebert PA, Turley K, Stanger P, Hoffman JIE, Heyman MA, Rudolph AM (1984) Surgical treatment of Truncus Arteriosus in the first six months of life. Ann Surg 200: 451–456
2. Girinath MR (1973) Case presentation: Truncus arteriosus: Repair with homograft reconstruction in infancy with heart disease in infancy, Diagnosis and Surgical Treatment. eds. BG Barratt-Boyes, JM Neutze, EA Harris. Churchill Livingstone, Edingburgh. p 234
3. Khanna SK, Ross JK, Monro JL (1981) Homograft aortic valve replacement; seven years' experience with antibiotic-treated valves. Thorax 36: 330–337
4. McGoon DC, Rastelli GC, Ongley PA (1968) An operation for the correction of truncus arteriosus. J.A.M.A. 205: 59–63
5. Michler RE, Chen JM, Quaegebeur JM (1994) Novel technique for extending the use of allografts in cardiac operations. Ann Thorac Surg 57: 83–87
6. Monro JL, Shore G (1984) Correction of persistent truncus arteriosus in A Colour Atlas of Cardiac Surgery. Congenital Heart Disease. Wolfe Medical Publications, London. p 137–144
7. Monro JL, Tolan MJ, Slavik Z, Salmon AP, Keeton BR (1995) Downsizing of valve allografts for use as right heart conduits. Ann Thorac Surg 59: 789
8. Rastelli GC, Wallace RB, Ongley PA (1969) Complete repair of transposition of the great arteries with pulmonary stenosis. A review and report of a case corrected by using a new surgical technique. Circulation 39: 83–95
9. Raudkivi PJ, Sutherland GR, Edwards JC, Manners JM, Keeton BR, Monro JL (1990) Truncus arteriosus with Type B interrupted aortic arch: Correction in the Neonate. Pediatric Cardiology: 11: 117–119
10. Ross DM, Somerville J (1966) Correction of pulmonary atresia with a homograft aortic valve. Lancet 2. 1446
11. Santini F, Prioli A, Pessotto R, Mazzucco A (1995) Use of oversized homografts for right ventricular outflow tract reconstruction in infants. J Heart Valve Dis 4. 192–195

Author's address:
James L. Monro FRCS
Wessex Cardiothoracic Centre
Southampton General Hospital
Tremona Road
Southampton
Hampshire SO 16 4XY
UK

Techniques for repair of tetralogy of Fallot with pulmonary atresia using homografts – The Rotterdam Experience

T. P. Willems, A. J. J. C. Bogers, E. Bos

Department of Cardio-Pulmonary Surgery, University Hospital Sophia-Dijkzigt and Erasmus University, Rotterdam, The Netherlands

Introduction

Tetralogy of Fallot with pulmonary atresia (PA) comprises absence of functional continuity between the right ventricle and the pulmonary arterial tree, ventricular septal defect (VSD), and overriding of the aorta and right ventricular hypertrophy. In this setting the pulmonary blood flow may be supplied by the ductus arteriosus or by systemic-pulmonary collateral arteries (SPCA's) (3). In patients with a well developed pulmonary arterial system, treatment mostly consists of initial palliation with a modified Blalock-Taussig shunt and later complete repair (7). On the other hand, the presence of SPCA's is often associated with a diminutive central pulmonary arterial system (7). In this setting early and preferably complete unifocalization is necessary to attain an adequate pulmonary arterial system and to avoid imbalances of pulmonary vascular resistance. In both settings, the complete repair concerns closure of the VSD and establishment of the right ventricular-pulmonary arterial continuity with closure of previously constructed shunts. At present, the pulmonary homograft appears to be the conduit of choice for reconstruction of the right ventricular outflow tract (1, 2, 9).

This report describes our experience with homograft implantations in patients with pulmonary atresia and VSD. Because patients with SPCA's more often end up with an incomplete pulmonary arterial bed that may contain peripheral stenosis or areas with hypertensive vascular disease, we paid special attention to the results in PA, VSD and a normal pulmonary arterial bed versus PA, VSD and SPCA's.

Materials and methods

Patients

From 1987 to October 1995, 32 homografts (27 pulmonary and 5 aortic) were implanted in 29 patients for repair of PA with VSD at the University Hospital Sophia-Dijkzigt.

Fifteen patients (50%) had a well developed pulmonary arterial system (group A). Thirteen of these patients had undergone 19 previous palliative shunts and three patients had a previous repair of the right ventricular outflow tract. The actual pathology at the time of homograft implantation in these three cases was prosthetic non-valved conduit dysfunction ($n = 1$), homograft dysfunction ($n = 1$) and patch dysfunction ($n = 1$).

Fourteen patients (50%) with PA, VSD had a diminutive pulmonary arterial system with the pulmonary blood supply by SPCA's (group B). Nine of these patients had undergone reconstruction of the pulmonary arterial tree by bilateral unifocalization before total repair. Four patients had a failing previous repair of the right ventricular outflow tract at the time of homograft implantation (xenograft stenosis $n = 2$, homograft dysfunction $n = 2$).

The mean age of the 29 patients at the time of homograft implantation was 8.0 years (range 0.1–30.5 years), 50% of them being less than 5 years of age, 25% between 5 and 10 years, 10% between 10 and 20 years, and 15% 20 years of age or older. The mean weight of the patients was 21.8 kg (range 3.2–70.0 kg). The mean values of age and weight were similar in both patient groups (group A: 7.9 years, range 0.7–30.5 years, 21.0 kg, range 7.3–50.0 kg; group B: 8.0 years, range 0.1–26.7 years, 23.6 kg, range 3.2–70.0 kg).

Twenty-nine cryopreserved homograft valves were supplied by the Heart Valve Bank Rotterdam through Bio Implant Services. The technique for preparation and storage of these homografts has been described previously (8). Three fresh homografts were obtained from the National Heart Hospital London. The choice of conduit size was made on the basis of the patient's body surface area (5). In infants aged less than 1 year, an effort was made to insert a homograft somewhat larger than predicted from the tables of normal valve sizes. No attempt was made to achieve ABO blood type matching. The mean internal diameter of homografts in group A was 19.9 mm (range 16.0–26.0 mm) and in group B 21.3 mm (range 12–26). The mean donor age in group A was 26.1 years (range 6.4–54.7 years) and 22.0 years (range 2.2–50.4 years) in group B.

Operative technique

Surgical procedures were performed using standard cardiopulmonary bypass with moderate hypothermia, myocardial protection with crystalloid cardioplegia (St. Thomas Hospital solution). Topical cooling was used in adult patients only. The allograft was prepared according to protocol (8). Implantation of the homograft was done by interposition technique, using running polypropylene sutures for the distal and proximal anastomosis.

In the patients with a well developed pulmonary arterial system, nine procedures were performed with a standard circular anastomosis to the distal pulmonary artery and in seven procedures the donor pulmonary confluence was used to reconstruct the recipient confluent pulmonary artery. In the patients with a unifocalized pulmonary arterial system, the distal homograft anastomosis was made in an end-to-end fashion only in two procedures and in fourteen procedures the recipient confluent pulmonary artery was reconstructed by the opened bifurcation of the homograft as the distal anastomosis (Figs. 1 and 2).

A proximal extension of the conduit was considered and indicated in 19 operations. This was made using a homograft patch ($n = 9$), the anterior mitral valve leaflet in the case of aortic allografts ($n = 2$), a pericardial patch ($n = 6$) or a prosthetic patch ($n = 2$). In general, an attempt was made to position the allograft away from the sternum to prevent compression or distortion.

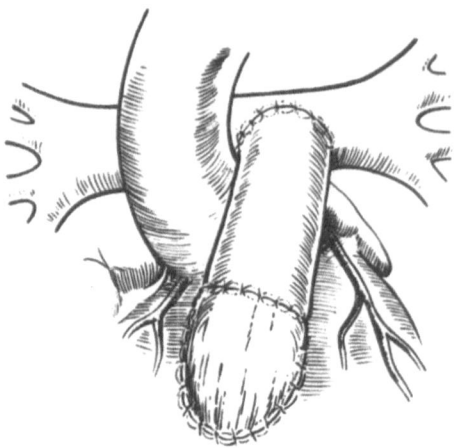

Fig. 1. Homograft implantation with a standard circular anastomosis to the distal pulmonary artery and with proximal extension of the conduit to the right ventricle.

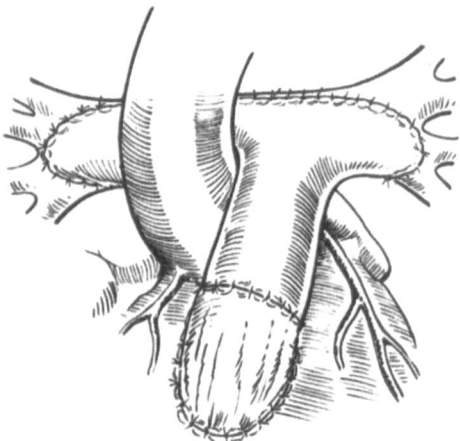

Fig. 2. Homograft implantation with reconstruction of the recipient confluent pulmonary artery by the opened bifurcation of the homograft and with proximal extension of the conduit to the right ventricle.

Follow-up

The mean follow-up for the homografts implanted in patients with a well developed pulmonary arterial system was 2.5 years (range 0.1–7.8 years) and 2.0 years (range 0.1–5.9 years) for the homografts implanted in patients with a unifocalized pulmonary arterial system. Postoperative homograft events were described according to guidelines of Edmunds (4). The nature of valve deterioration was determined at reoperation or autopsy. The decision to replace a homograft was based on symptoms attributed to pulmonary regurgitation or stenosis, confirmed by echocardiography or cardiac catheterization.

At last follow-up (mean 2.5 years; range 0.1–7.8 years) 23 echocardiograms of the patients with a homograft in-situ were available to evaluate the homograft competence. The severity of homograft regurgitation was graded semiquantitatively: "none" if there was no regurgitation, "mild" if a narrow regurgitation jet was visible, "moderate" if a broad regurgitation jet was visible extending into the right ventricular outflow tract, and "severe" if reverse flow was visible within the pulmonary branch arteries. The homograft was considered stenotic if the peak velocity was ≥ 2.5 m/s.

Statistical analysis

Survival and freedom from homograft failure were analyzed according to the method of Kaplan-Meier (6). Survival of a patient started at the time of homograft implantation and ended at death (event) or at last follow-up (censoring). Analysis of homograft survival started at implantation and ended at homograft failure (reoperation, valve related death) or at last follow-up. The differences between curves were evaluated using the log-rank test. The Mann-Whitney U-test was used to test for differences in homograft dysfunction on last echocardiogram. p-values less than 0.05 were considered significant.

Results

One out of 29 patients (3.4%) suffered early mortality. The primary cause of this death was respiratory insufficiency in a patient with a well developed pulmonary arterial system. There were two late deaths, one of them being valve related. This patient, with an originally diminutive pulmonary arterial system, died 3 months after homograft implantation due to sustained ventricular tachycardia. An echocardiogram performed 3 months before death showed dilatation of the right ventricle and severe allograft regurgitation. The other patient, with a unifocalized pulmonary arterial system, died suddenly, probably due to arrythmia. At 5 years the overall patient survival was 94% (95% CL 82–99%) for patients with a well developed pulmonary arterial system and 86% (95% CL 68–99%) for patients with a unifocalized pulmonary arterial system. This difference was not statistically significant ($p > 0.1$).

Three reoperations for homograft dysfunction were performed in three different patients. Two homograft failures were diagnosed as structural on the basis of operative findings, one as non-structural. One of the structural failures occurred in a patient with a normal pulmonary arterial system. The homograft showed stenosis at the proximal anastomosis and the pre-implant homograft diameter of 20 mm was reduced to 10 mm. The homograft leaflets were fibrotic. The other structural failure occurred in a patient with a unifocalized pulmonary arterial system. The homograft was replaced for regurgitation. In this regurgitant homograft a false aneurysm in one sinus was found at operation and confirmed microscopically. The non-structural failure occurred in a patient with a unifocalized pulmonary arterial system. In this case reoperation was necessary for stenosis of the distal anastomosis. All three homografts were explanted and replaced by another homograft. During follow-up one case of endocarditis was diagnosed, which was successfully treated with antibiotics.

Overall freedom from valve related events ($n = 5$, including one death, three reoperations, one endocarditis) was 71% (95% CL 44–97%) at 5 years. Freedom from reoperation for homograft failure in the patient group with a well developed pulmonary arterial system was 83% (95% CL 62–94%) at 5 years and was 86% (95% CL 60–99%) in the patient group with a diminutive pulmonary arterial system. This difference was not statistically significant ($p > 0.5$).

At the last echocardiographic follow-up three homografts (3/23) showed a moderate or severe regurgitation and seven other homografts (7/23) showed stenotis. There was no significant difference between homograft dysfunction in patients with a well developed (6/13) or a unifocalized pulmonary arterial system (4/10) ($p > 0.5$).

Discussion

The use of homografts for establishment of the continuity between the right ventricle and pulmonary arterial system in patients with PA and VSD is widespread. The pulmonary homograft is currently the conduit of choice (1, 2, 9). Especially because the donor bifurcation can be used for reconstruction of the confluent pulmonary arteries.

A limiting factor to successful complete repair of PA with VSD may be the degree of residual pathology of the pulmonary arterial tree. Because unifocalization procedures in a pulmonary artery system depending on SPCA's often result in a very acceptable but nonetheless an anatomically or functionally incomplete pulmonary arterial tree, an increased right ventricular pressure after repair cannot always be avoided (7). In this setting the homograft valve has to sustain elevated pulmonary arterial pressure, which may be a risk factor for homograft failure. However, in our series we did not find differences between homografts implanted in patients with a well developed pulmonary arterial system and homografts implanted in patients with a unifocalized pulmonary arterial system.

In our recent report (9), we have identified several risk factors for homograft failure. We could confirm known risk factors, such as young patient age at time of implantation, aortic allograft, small homograft diameter, but we also found a strong influence of younger donor age on homograft failure. We found a freedom from reoperation for homograft failure or valve related death 73% for aortic homografts and 93% for pulmonary homografts at 5 years.

In the present series of homografts used for correction of PA and VSD, the overall freedom from reoperation for homograft failure or valve related death was 83%. Because of the small number of patients and events the above-mentioned risk factors could not be confirmed.

Longer clinical follow-up could provide more definite information on the question of whether or not a unifocalized pulmonary arterial bed is an additional risk factor for homograft dysfunction in PA with VSD.

References

1. Albert JD, Bishop DA, Fullerton DA, Campbell DN, Clarke DR (1993) Conduit reconstruction of the right ventricular outflow tract: lessons learned in a twelve-year experience. J Thorac Cardiovasc Surg 106: 228–236

2. Bando K, Danielson GK, Schaff HV, Mair DD, Julsrud PR, Puga FJ (1995) Outcome of the pulmonary and aortic homografts for right ventricular outflow tract reconstruction. J Thorac Cardiovasc Surg 109: 509–518
3. DeRuiter MC, Gittenberger-de Groot AC, Bogers AJJC, Elzenga NJ (1994) The restricted surgical relevance of morphologic criteria to classify systemic-pulmonary collateral arteries in pulmonary atresia with ventricular septal defect. J Thorac Cardiovasc Surg 108: 692–699
4. Edmunds LH, Clark RE, Cohn LH, Miller DC, Weisel RD (1988) Guidelines for reporting morbidity and mortality after cardiac valvular operation. J Thorac Cardiovasc Surg 96: 351–355
5. Hopkins RA (1989) Cardiac Reconstructions with Allografts Valves. 1st edn. Springer-Verlag, New York, 189–190
6. Kaplan EL, Meier P (1958) Nonparametric estimation from incomplete observations. J Am Stat Assoc 53: 457–481
7. Kirklin JW, Barratt-Boyes BG (1993) Cardiac Surgery. 2nd edn. Churchill Livingstone, New York, 942–973
8. Thijssen HJM, Bos E, Konertz W, van Suylen RJ, de By TMMH (1992) Kryokonservierung humaner spenderherzklappen in der herzklappenbank in Rotterdam. Z Herz-, Thorax-, Gefäßchir 6 (suppl.1): 49–55
9. Willems TP, Bogers AJJC, Cromme-Dijkhuis AH, Steyerberg EW, Van Herwerden LA, Hokken RB, Hess J, Bos E (1996) Allograft reconstruction of the right ventricular outflow tract. Eur J Cardio-thorac Surg (in press)

Author's address:
T. P. Willems, MD
Department of Cardio-Pulmonary Surgery, Bd 156
University Hospital Sophia-Dijkzigt
Dr. Molewaterplein 40
3015 GD Rotterdam
The Netherlands

Use of allografts in the primary repair of Truncus arteriosus in early infancy and replacement of previous conduits revisited

K. Turley

California Pacific Medical Center, San Francisco, U.S.A.

The use of allografts in the treatment of complex congenital cardiac disease in early infancy, such as primary repair of truncus arteriosus and their use in replacement of previous conduits, has experienced remarkable expansion and change since our original symposium in 1987. At that time, our interest centered on aortic allografts and to paraphrase our introductory statement "there had been an enormous resurgence in their use" (14). This was due to reports of excellent long-term results of this technique, the advent of cryopreservation and the effects of increased donor availability at that time, secondary to infant transplantation. Since that original report a number of dramatic changes have occurred in the allograft experience and only a few of those initial impressions still hold true. In the current update of our experience, we continue to note excellent long-term results within specific categories. Cryopreservation has been demonstrated to markedly improve availability. However, a donor problem has persisted as increased use has impacted the donor pool. In the case of truncus arteriosus, neonatal repair has become the standard due to the availability of small-sized allografts for pulmonary artery reconstruction, tissue to tissue anastomoses, and the avoidance of pulmonary hypertensive crises by early repair. Experience has demonstrated the superiority of pulmonary allograft over aortic allografts, avoiding problems first noted in our original article with aortic allografts in the infant population. In the case of replacement conduits, again, pulmonary allografts have demonstrated excellent results in all subgroups. Finally, while the original allograft placements in early infancy have provided extended graft survival far beyond the Dacron conduits previously used, methods of patch repair for allograft stenosis, rather than allograft replacement, are possible in selective patients and may avoid subsequent allograft replacement. The entire field of allograft repair of complex congenital cardiac disease has seen significant changes in the past 8 years, none more dramatic than in primary repair of truncus arteriosus and the replacement of previous conduits.

Truncus arteriosus is a rare congenital lesion occurring in less than 1% of infants born with congenital heart disease. It is a condition in which the main pulmonary truncus is not related to the right ventricle but arises from a separate site on the aorta. The embryology of this lesion is important in understanding the approach to surgical repair and possible anatomic configurations which may influence and complicate such repair. The development of the main pulmonary trunk is related to the development of the proximal portion of the second through sixth aortic arches. These arches form the right and left pulmonary arteries and when they fuse, a transverse pulmonary artery and a ductus arteriosus are formed. As the truncus rotates in infancy, a spiral septum develops that separates the common trunk into the pulmonary and aortic components. If this does not occur the main pulmonary artery does not separate and no connection occurs between the transverse sixth arch and a separate main pulmonary artery. Thus, a transverse vessel connects directly to the trunk.

The natural history of truncus arteriosus, if unoperated, demonstrates that of 100 infants at birth, 75% die in the first year. Of the 25 remaining children, 35% are inoperable at age 4 due to pulmonary vascular disease. Of the 16 still operable at age 4 to 5, there is a 5% operative mortality. Of the 15 patients who survive, 20% progress to late pulmonary vascular disease. Thus, only 12 of the original 100 can be expected to live a relatively normal life.

Attempts at pulmonary artery banding have resulted in a natural history which is only slightly different. Of 100 patients banded, 50% die at the time of banding. Of those remaining, 10% die between 1 and 5 years of age and of the 45 still alive, 9% die following band removal and repair. Finally, of the remaining 40 patients, 25% develop late pulmonary vascular disease yielding only 30 relatively normal individuals. These findings, we think today, are quite optimistic. As many children with truncus die in the first few days to weeks of life, they do not fit within these natural history studies.

Thus, an aggressive approach to early repair in infancy was undertaken by our group in 1974. Initial medical management of patients of truncus was accomplished through the use of diuretics and digitalis and on many occasions through ventilatory support. Tracheostomy was avoided as it complicated the mediastinal surgical field and did not improve long-term survival, and since an operative repair was to be performed in early infancy, long-term respiratory support was not necessary, rather an approach of early referral and repair in early infancy was recommended.

The initial approach was repair in the first 6 months of life. This rapidly decreased to repair in the first 3 months, and by the time of our previous article, repair at approximately 6 weeks of age. Patients in this age group were the smallest in whom a Dacron conduit of 12 mm, the minimal sized conduit available, could be placed (Fig. 1). Our initial experience reported in 1984, with 100 consecutive patients resulted in 11% mortality (8). Sharma, Brawn, and Mee subsequently reported similar results, a 17% mortality in 23 patients in 1985 (12). In each of these series of Dacron heterograft repairs, close attention to post-operative care and in particular, techniques to prevent pulmonary hypertensive crises were stressed. Other centers did not experience such positive results. An example is Boston Children's Hospital, where from 1977 to 1981, mortality was 62%, while 91% of infants less than 3 months of age died. Results improved to 39% overall by 1986, however, 10 of 18 patients less than 3 months of age died during that period, reflecting the continued problems experienced in most centers (4).

With the advent of allograft reconstruction there has been a dramatic change in both the method, timing, and results of repair. Although our initial experience described in the 1987 article centered upon the use of larger sized aortic allografts in smaller infants (range 11–16 mm, mean 13.8 mm) in whom a 12 mm Dacron heterograft would have previously been used (1), it soon became clear that neonatal repair was possible using smaller allografts, appropriate for even the smallest neonate. This approach to correction could be performed while avoiding the risks of medical palliation and mortality in the first month of life, and tapping the special advantages of the allograft (i.e., hemostasis from tissue to tissue anastomosis, etc.) (Fig. 2). Improved results were observed. The Boston Children's experience demonstrated this; from 1987 to 1991, 57 patients underwent primary repair with 10 deaths, an 18% mortality, including 41 patients less than 3 months of age with 8 deaths, an 18% mortality, approaching our overall mortality of 15% reported in 217 patients as of 1988 (4).

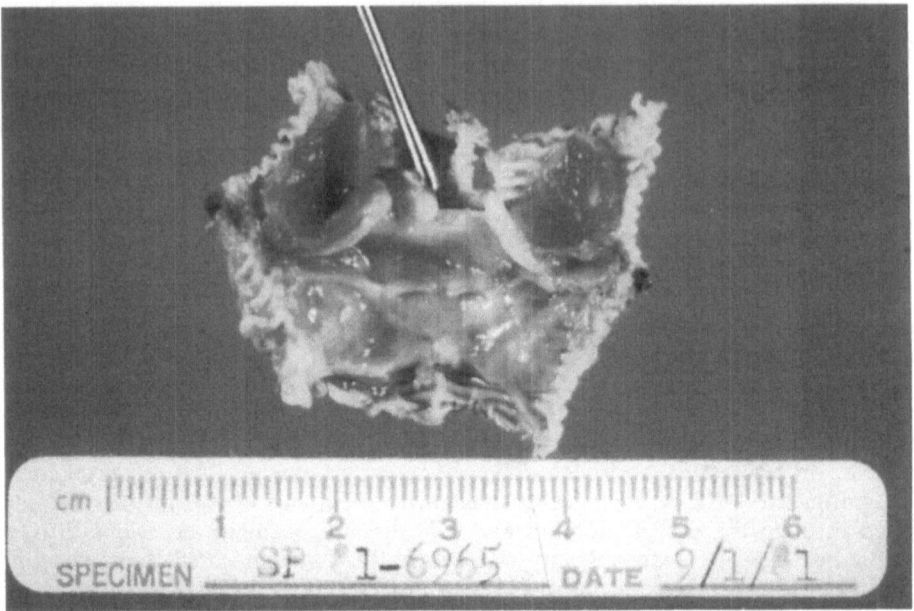

Fig. 1. Twelve-mm Dacron heterograft removed with dissection of the proximal intimal peel. Degeneration of the heterograft valve leaflets.

The reasons for the change are multiple, but not the least was the nature of an allograft repair (15). Experience with neonatal repair has resulted in a marked decrease in the problem of pulmonary vascular disease without increasing surgical mortality. In the neonate pulmonary vascular reactive episodes have been found to be much less frequent and more easily controlled. Allograft repairs then provided a more stable patient group, making pulmonary hypertensive crises rare. Bove, Beekman, Snider, et al. first reported these finding in 11 neonates in 1989 (2). Our discussion of that paper at the Society of Thoracic Surgeons meeting in 1989 noted the importance of small sized allograft availability in allowing for routine neonatal treatment. With this availability the University of Michigan in 1993 reported an 11% hospital mortality in 46 patients, 38 of whom were neonates. Actuarial survival was 81% with 3 non-cardiac late deaths. No factors including age accounted for increased mortality (3). Our own experience and that of UCLA (1991) and Boston Children's (1993), parallel these findings of lower mortality in uncomplicated truncus, while interrupted arch, truncal insufficiency, coronary anomalies, and most interestingly, age greater than 100 days are factors increasing the risk of repair (9, 11).

Thus, the era of allograft primary repair of truncus arteriosus has yielded the dividends we had hoped for at the last symposium. Neonatal repair, a valved conduit in the neonatal pulmonary bed and tissue-to-tissue anastomosis decrease hemorrhagic morbidity. To these are added a marked decrease in pulmonary hypertensive crises, increased conduit longevity over the small Dacron heterografts, and excellent survival in even complex patients.

Experience with small allografts, however, have not been consistently positive. In our initial report we noted the early calcification of 1 primary truncus aortic allograft. Further, concern was voiced as to ABO compatibility issue at the symposium (14).

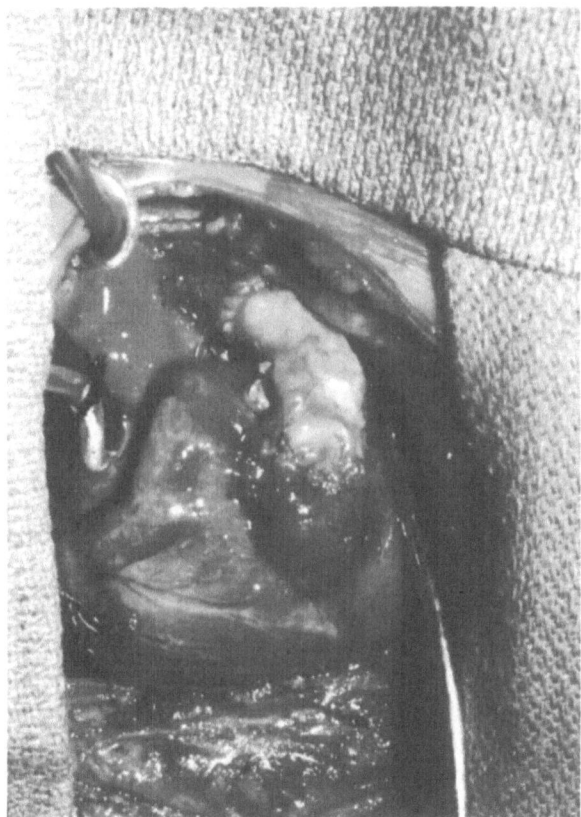

Fig. 2. Neonatal truncus repair with allograft right ventricular to pulmonary artery reconstruction.

Subsequently, we and other centers noted early calcification and valvar stenosis in a significant number of small aortic allografts. Albert et al. described this problem in multiple patient groups and our own experience with truncus patients confirm their findings (1). An immunologic source has been postulated and Clarke et al. and Yankah et al. have suggested the possibility of "minimal" immunosuppression (6, 18). Experience with pulmonary allografts in these small infants has now provided an alternative, which to date has yielded excellent neonatal repair with minimal morbidity. CryoLife, Inc. (which provides processing including sterile dissection, culturing, and cryopreservation of tissue) has followed 573 cases of truncus arteriosus from 1984 to 1995 in which allograft reconstruction was used. Two-hundred-eleven (56%) of the pediatric patients received aortic valves documented as used in the right heart and 166 (44%) received a pulmonary valve. Although overall more aortic valves were used, since 1986 an increasing number of pulmonary valves have been implanted. The number has increased from 25% in 1986 to 50% in 1993–95. Better long-term survival has been noted in this series. At 96 months, 73% of the pulmonary allografts versus 58% of the aortic allograft recipients survived. Although this is not statistically significant ($p = 0.1103$), the overall incidence of early replacement for calcification, stenosis, and regurgitation may be a factor since there was only a 65% actuarial freedom from structural deterioration in the aortic group versus a 93% freedom in the pulmonary group at 7 years. This does not include the morbidity associated with re-catheterizations and balloon arterioplasties performed in a significant number of our patients to extend the life of calcified aortic allografts (7). Thus, in our own experience and that of other centers the pulmonary allograft in small sizes appears to be the conduit of choice for repair of primary truncus arteriosus (10, 17).

This leads us to the second part of this update, the impact of allograft as replacement conduits. Our initial experience described at the 1987 symposium included only 16 patients. Nine of these underwent replacement of previous conduits for truncus arteriosus. Since that time allograft replacement has become a standard in both right heart conduit replacement and in autograft aortic replacement to reconstruct the autograft donor outflow tract. In large sizes, both the aortic and pulmonary allograft have been successful, although the relative availability of the latter has resulted in the preference for pulmonary allograft. Sharma et al. reported 15 replacements in 1992 with a O mortality, a 3-day ICU, and a 7-day hospital stay (13). In our most recent experience, 1-day ICU and 4–5-day hospitalization is standard. Thus, the allograft replacement results in low mortality and excellent functional results with low morbidity. However, a valve may not be needed in some patients in the pulmonary circuit at the time of replacement. Twenty-seven such patients have undergone opening of the previous allograft and Y-shape patch reconstruction of the right ventricular outflow tract. In each, bilateral pulmonary arterioplasties and proximal extension of the patch have been used to relieve the classic anastomotic stenosis found in allograft reconstruction using small sized conduits. This is a narrowing of both distal anastomoses with constriction and shortening as calcification occurs. An hour-glass configuration is seen in each pulmonary arterial branch and there is usually a fixed proximal anastomotic size. Patching of both of these critical areas, as well as the small-sized main conduit's section is necessary. In these patients with slow obstruction of the right-sided conduit, hypertrophy of the right ventricle is experienced. As long as significant prior regurgitation or right ventricular dysfunction have not occurred, regurgitation produced by the patch repair is well tolerated. Often in fact, residual leaflet tissue can provide a degree of competence. The use of allograft replacement has been restricted to patients in whom a right-sided valve is clearly beneficial. If regurgitation does subsequently result in sequelae, an allograft can be inserted. However, from our experience with tetralogy of Fallot in which right ventricular outflow patches have been used, the majority of patients tolerate the non-valve repair well and as in those patients, allograft replacement can be restricted to the patients in whom regurgitation is poorly tolerated or ventricular function deteriorates, avoiding the natural history of allograft calcification and degeneration in the majority of such patients. The long-term results of this type of repair are not clear. However, Cerfolio et al. have reported excellent results with patching of the pseudoadventitial tract of prosthetic conduits. Among 42 patients there were no early or late deaths and in no patient did an obstructive peel or valve obstruction occur. At 8 years the actuarial freedom from re-operation for conduit obstruction was 100% (5). This is a comparable approach and we believe with 10 years of follow-up, the same will be true in the allograft group. The allograft conduit replacement, however, remains the standard when valve right-sided reconstruction is necessary in the current era; prolonged conduit survival has been demonstrated, both in smaller sized and larger replacements, which can be commonly used, even in young children (16).

Since the symposium in 1987, much has been learned concerning allograft use and limitations. Much needs to be learned as to their biology and natural history (17, 18). They have, however, fulfilled the promise of the Berlin symposium and are currently the treatment of choice for primary repair of truncus arteriosus and valve conduit replacement.

References

1. Albert JD, Bishop DA, Fullerton DA, Campbell DN, Clarke DR (1993) Conduit reconstruction of the right ventricular outflow tract. J Thorac Cardiovasc Surg 106: 228–236
2. Bove EL, Beekman RH, Snider AR, Callow LB, Underhill DJ, Rocchini AP, Dick M II, Rosenthal A (1989) Repair of truncus arteriosus in the neonate and young infant. Ann Thorac Surg 47: 499–506
3. Bove EL, Lupinetti FM, Pridjian AK, Beekman RH, Callow LB, Snider AR, Rosenthal A (1993) Results of a policy of primary repair of truncus arteriosus in the neonate. J Thorac Cardiovasc Surg 105: 1057–1066
4. Castaneda AR, Jonas RA, Mayer JE, Hanley FL (1994) Cardiac surgery of the neonate and infant. Saunders, Philadelphia.
5. Cerfolio RJ, Danielson GK, Puga FJ, Schaff HV, Warnes CA (1995) Results of an autologous tissue reconstruction for replacement of obstructed extracardiac conduits. American Association for Thoracic Surgery, 75th Annual Meeting. Boston, Massachusetts.
6. Clarke DR (1994) Invited letter concerning: accelerated degeneration of aortic allografts in infants and young children. J Thorac Cardiovasc Surg 107: 1162–1164
7. CryoLife Inc. (1995) Analysis of valve type distribution trends for truncus arteriosus cases. Personal communication.
8. Ebert PA, Turley K, Stanger P, Hoffman JIE, Heymann MA, Rudolph AM (1984) Surgical treatment of truncus arteriosus in the first 6 months of life. Ann Surg 200: 451–456
9. Hanley FI, Heinemann MK, Jonas RA, Mayer JE, Cook NR, Wessel DL, Castaneda AR (1993) Repair of truncus arteriosus in the neonate. J Thorac Cardiovasc Surg 105: 1047–1056
10. Heinemann MK, Hanley FL, Fenton KN, Jonas RA, Mayer JE, Castaneda AR (1993) Fate of small homograft conduits after early repair of truncus arteriosus. Ann Thorac Surg 55: 1409–1412
11. Pearl JM, Laks H, Drinkwater DC, Milgalter E, Charas OR, Giacobetti F, George B, Williams R (1991) Repair of truncus arteriosus in infancy. Ann Thorac Surg 52: 780–786
12. Sharma AK, Brawn WJ, Mee RBB (1985) Truncus arteriosus: surgical approach. J Thorac Cardiovasc Surg 90: 45–49
13. Sharma S, Cobanoglu A, Dobbs J, Rice M (1993) Clinical results of cryopreserved valved conduits in the pulmonary ventricle-to-pulmonary artery position. Amer J Surg 165: 587–591
14. Turley K (1988) The use of aortic allografts in the primary repair of truncus arteriosus in early infancy and replacement of previous conduits. In: Yankah AC (ed.) Cardiac valve allografts. Steinkopff Verlag Darmstadt, Berlin, pp 223–227
15. Turley K (1989) Discussion: repair of truncus arteriosus in the neonate and young infant. Ann Thorac Surg 47: 506
16. Weipert J, Meisner H, Mendler N, Haehnel JC, Homann M, Paek SU, Sebening F (1995) Allograft implantation in pediatric cardiac surgery: surgical experience from 1982 to 1994. Ann Thorac Surg 60: S101–104
17. Yankah AC, Alexi-Meskhishvili V, Weng Y, Schorn K, Lange PE, Hetzer R (1995) Accelerated degeneration of allografts in the first two years of life. Ann Thorac Surg 60: S71–77
18. Yankah AC, Wottge HU, Muller-Ruchholtz W (1995) Short-course cyclosporin a therapy for definite allograft valve survival immunosuppression in allograft valve operations. Ann Thorac Surg 60: S146–150

Authors address:
K. Turley, MD
Chief, Pediatric Cardiac Surgery
California Pacific Medical Center
2100 Webster St., #332
San Francisco, CA 94115
U.S.A.

Orthotopic and heterotopic implantation of cryopreserved semilunar valves in the pulmonary circulation

A. C. Yankah, V. Alexi-Meskhishvili, Y. Weng, K. Schorn, F. Berger, P. Lange, R. Hetzer

German Heart Institute Berlin, Berlin, Germany

Introduction

Cryopreserved allografts were introduced in October 1986 at the German Heart Institute Berlin (19). Ever since, aortic and pulmonary homografts have been used for reconstruction of the right ventricular outflow tract in patients with obstructive lesions (1, 2, 5, 8, 9, 12, 16, 19, 21, 22). It was our aim to evaluate the durability of the two different valves in orthotopic and heterotopic positions and to establish the determinant factors for long-term valve performance by site of implantation, age of recipients and conduit size particularly in children.

Material and methods

Between October 1986 and March 1996, 297 patients with congenital valve lesions had homograft valve replacements (Fig. 1). Age distribution of the patients is shown in Fig. 2. 274 patients underwent homograft reconstructions of the right ventricular outflow tract obstruction. Of these 63 (40 males and 23 females) were operated within the first 2 years of life (27 infants and 36 small children with a mean body weight of 8.1 kg). The major diagnoses of the entire patients with right ventricular outflow tract obstructions are shown in Fig. 3. The allograft implantations were carried out with standard cardiopulmonary bypass technique. The implantation techniques are previously described (1, 2, 8, 9, 19). The internal diameter of the implanted allografts was between 9 and 29 mm (mean: 19.2 mm). The implanted allografts were obtained from our Institution- based bank in Berlin (DHZB), BioImplant service of EuroTransplant in Rotterdam (ET-BIS), European homograft bank in Brussels EHB), and homograft bank in Barcelona (HBB) with two different storage temperatures $-80\,°C$ (DHZB) and $-180\,°C$ (ET-BIS + EHB, HBB). The average storage time was 116 days which ranged from 14 to 442 days.

Follow-up: 104 patients were followed up between 4 months and 7 years, the end point was 30 September 1995. 47 (45%) had heart catheterization between 4 and 52 months at a mean of 12.5 months after the operation. They received routinely 3–5 mg/kg aspirin daily for 3 months. Of these 46 were operated within the first 2 years of life. All patients underwent routine postoperative evaluation of their allograft conduits and valves using M-mode and two-dimensional echocardiography with color flow Doppler imaging. Patients with x-ray identification of allograft wall

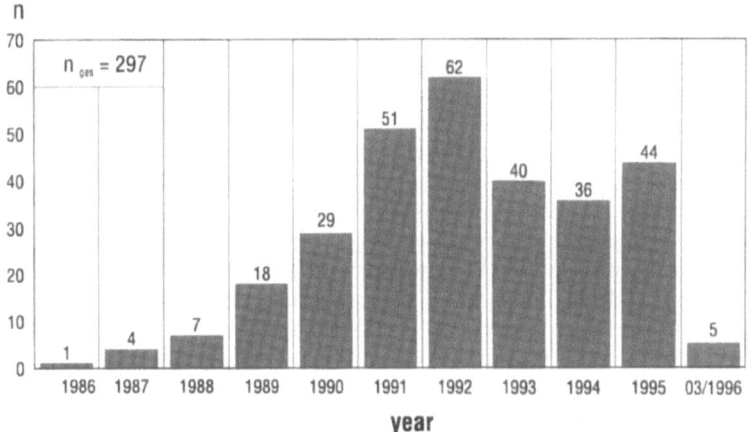

Fig. 1. Annual distribution of homograft valve operations for congenital obstructive valve and ventricular outflow lesions.

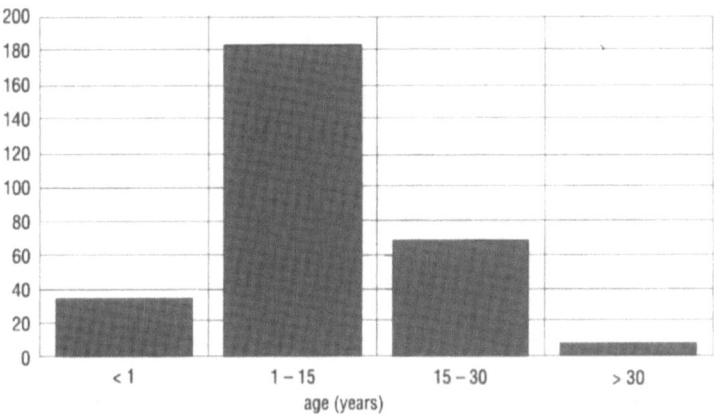

Fig. 2. Age distributions of patients undergoing homograft valve operations for congenital obstructive valve and ventricular outflow lesions.

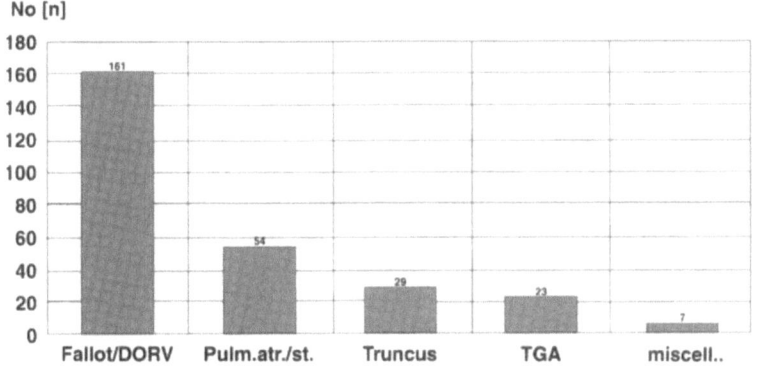

Fig. 3. Major diagnoses of patients undergoing homograft reconstruction of the right ventricular outflow tract.

calcification and valve dysfunction with suspicion of transconduit gradients were scheduled for cardiac recatheterization.

Indications for reoperation were established at the heart catheterization in 12 patients who required exchange of their allograft conduits 4–66 (mean: 17) months after operation. Findings at reoperation were considered typical pathological of allograft rejection if there was an inflammatory reaction on the valve surface, or of degeneration if there was a rigidity or calcification of the wall or valve and the valve is stenotic or incompetent, or a combination of valve stenosis and incompetence. Further, presence of mild to severe intimal hyperplasia with tubular stenosis or supravalvular stenosis and a general longitudinal and circumferencial shrinkage of the entire conduit including the annulus was also regarded as typical findings of allograft degeneration. Data analysis: Logistic analysis was performed with the following risk factors as independent variables to predict the occurences of structural deterioration and allograft failure: age of recipient, preservation technique, type of allograft, ABO-compatibility and -incompatibility. Valve survival analysis, actuarial estimates of freedom from reoperation and structural deterioration and calcification of allograft wall and valve dysfunction were calculated by Log rank test (4, 10). Intergroup differences of variables were analyzed using the Fisher test (4). Definition: Structural deterioration or dysfunction of allografts was established at the time at which calcific deposits in the allograft was first detected by x-ray or the time at which valve dysfunction was first observed at routine examination by echocardiography and confirmed at the time of heart catheterization or at reoperation.

Results

Allograft valve survival

Among the 104 patients with cryopreserved aortic and pulmonary allografts in the pulmonary circulation who were under observation 12 (11.5%) patients demonstrated early allograft structural degeneration during a follow-up period between 4 and 66 (mean: 17) months. Of the 47 patients who underwent heart catheterization 12 patients showed severe pulmonary stenosis with RV-PA pressure gradients between 30 and > 50 mmHg. Of these, four had supravalvular stenosis of the aortic conduits with RV-PA gradients between 30–49 mmHg and two others had with mild pulmonary insufficiencies (Fig. 4). All 12 patients needed their allografts exchanged. Allograft vascular wall calcification.

Calcification of allograft began in the wall as early as 4 months and was detected clinically by x-ray in 60% of the infants and 21% of children. Actuarial freedom of allograft wall calcification in children was 21% and in aortic and pulmonary allografts was 18% and 78% respectively at 48 months (Fig. 4).

Valve dysfunction

Actuarial freedom of transconduit gradient of ≥ 50 mmHg for the entire group was 60% and for aortic and pulmonary allografts 60% and 68% respectively at 60

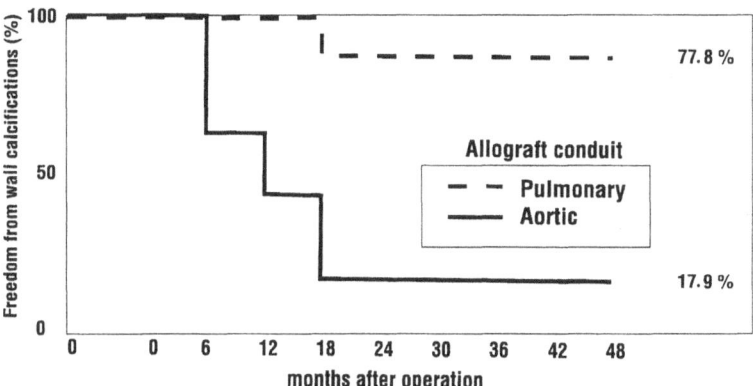

Fig. 4. Actuarial freedom from conduit wall calcification of cryopreserved, viable aortic and pulmonary homografts pulmonary circulation in children. Reproduction by permission (ref. 21).

months. The actuarial freedom of transconduit gradient of > 50 mmHg in infants was 37% and in 1–2 years age group was 73% at 48 months.

Reoperation

89% of the patients had their original allografts with satisfactory clinical performances, while 11% required reoperation for early structural degeneration between 4 and 66 (mean: 17) months after operation (Table 1) 20% (3/15) of the infants needed reoperation for exchange of their aortic allografts within 34 months after the first operation as compared to 6.2% (9/145) in patients beyond 1–2 years old ($p < 0.05$). Two patients died at the reoperation. Actuarial freedom of reoperation at 6 months was 99%, at 1 year was 98%, at 2 years was 91%, at 3 years was 88% and at 5 years was 81%. Actuarial freedom of reoperation for aortic and pulmonary allografts at 1 and 5 years was 96% and 78%, and 100% and 84% respectively (Fig. 5). Reoperation rate in infants was 74% and in 1–2 years old age group was 77% at 48 months.

Discussion

The medium-term hemodynamic and clinical results of homograft reconstruction of the RVOT in our series have been more gratifying and excellent than any other technique (16–18). Therefore, pulmonary homograft valves remain the preferential valves for repair of right ventricular outflow obstruction in children (1, 8, 9, 12). As compared to our previous studies the statistical trends were in favor of pulmonary homograft for reconstruction of the pulmonary circulation (5, 18, 21, 22). In the clinical observations early calcification of the vascular allograft did not represent dysfunction of the valve until at a time at which calcification developed in the valve to cause dysfunction. Interestingly, if one takes time as a factor for calcific degeneration of aortic and pulmonary allograft vascular wall and valve, reoperation for allograft valve failure was frequently observed in the aortic allografts (2, 8, 9).

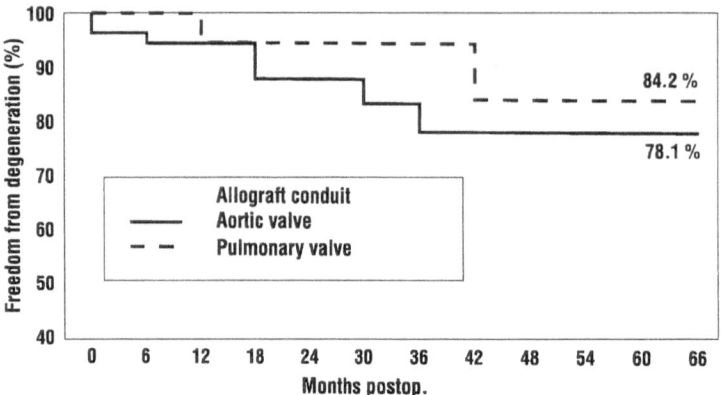

Fig. 5. Actuarial rates for freedom from reoperation due to valve degeneration and dysfunction of cryopreserved viable aortic and pulmonary allograft conduits in pulmonary circulation in children. Reproduction by permission (ref. 21).

Table 1. Determinant factors for early degeneration and reoperation of valved conduits in the pulmonary circulation

Risk factor	Homograft freedom from		
	dysfunction 48 mos. %	p-value	reoperation at 48 mos. %
Age			
< 1 yr	59	0.03	80
1–2 yrs	87	NS	90
Implant site			
Orthotopic (conduit)	77	NS	84
(valve)	93	NS	–
Heterotopic (conduit)	33	0.04	78
(valve)	62	0.02	
Size			
≤155 mm	74	0.0002	90
>16	79	NS	84
Storage temp.			
−80 C	80	NS	83
−180 C	74	NS	94
ABO			
Compatible	59	NS	76
Incompatible	*		*
Donor age			
≤40 yrs	73	NS	87
>41 yrs	*	*	*

* Few numbers available for evaluation

In 60% of the infants and 21% of the children fibroproliferative allograft vasculopathy was observed in the pulmonary circulation as early as 4 months by x-ray examination and at the cardiac catheterization. There was a correlation between valve dysfunction, transvalvular gradient and age at operation ($p = 0.048$). The risk of allograft wall calcification and valve dysfunction and reoperation was higher in infants than in small children with aortic homografts. In comparing with other variables no correlation was found between time after operation, preservation and storage techniques. While allograft valved conduit is antigenic, ABO blood group disparity was not identified as the only risk factor for early degeneration within individuals who received histoincompatible grafts (3, 6, 7, 11, 13).

The causes of early calcification of allografts, especially the aortic allografts in the pulmonary circulation in some unidentified group of young patients, is incompletely understood. The allograft failure in our series of patients might be explained in three ways. First, the aortic allografts demonstrated less durability than the pulmonary allografts because of greater ischemic damage to their thicker wall, that is, greater diffusion barrier to oxygen delivery. Second, we believe that the early homograft degeneration was associated with ongoing immune mediated anti-bodies against the endothelial cells – a form of humoral allograft rejection (14, 15, 20). Hereby abnormal synthesis and increase in elastin and type IV collagen might take place leading to medial and intimal fibrosis, stiffness and finally calcification (14). The ongoing rejection appears to be a factor for stimulating proliferative process in the allografts involving vascular smooth muscle cells and elastin for the subsequent development of allograft vasculopathy. Thirdly, infants in particular quickly outgrew their small valved conduits leading to high gradients across the valve leaflets, pathologic stress, structural deterioration causing traction, circumferential and longitudinal shrinkage of the conduit and annulus and leaflets inexpansibilty (21–23).

The immune pathogenesis is being supported by the findings in the isografts of inbred rat experiments, in which fibrocalcification did not develop (20). The aortic homograft in the pulmonary circulation is not implanted at a privileged site and therefore seemed to be victimized by immune response, on one hand leading to calcification resulting from a reparative fibroproliferative response in the vascular wall, and on the other hand by virtue of its heterotopic position. It is implanted in an environment of low oxygen saturation and low pressure system and it contains quantitatively more collagen and elastin which will favor early fibrocalcification due to pathologic tissue response.

We believe that modification of the preservation techniques of viable allografts by eliminating the endothelial cells and medication to minimize or arrest proliferation and migration of smooth muscle cells without interfering with the integrity of the extracellular matrix, might be a positive step to influence the fibroproliferative process in allografts. The use of anti-inflammatory drugs such as aspirin as we have been practicing in our patients might minimize inflammatory processes in the homografts, thus positively influencing the durability.

Conclusion

Pulmonary homograft demonstrated lower rate of wall calcification, valve dysfunction and early reoperation in comparison with aortic homografts in the pulmonary circulation, however there are some unidentified groups of infants and small children whose homografts underwent early structural deterioration. These groups of patients are our great concern. Our experience and the clinical results justify the continued use of pulmonary pulmonary homografts for reconstruction of the right ventricular outflow tract in combination with postoperative treatment with anti-inflammation drugs in young patients. The use of small size and short homograft conduits should be avoided in order to prevent infants from outgrowing their valves too early.

References

1. Ross DN, Somerville J (1966) Correction of pulmonary atresia with a homograft aortic valve. Lancet 2: 1446
2. Di Carlo D, de Leval M, Stark J (1984) "Fresh" antibiotic sterilized aortic homografts in ext extracardiac valved conduits: long-term results. Thorac Cardiovasc Surg 32: 10
3. Yankah AC, Wottge HU, Müller-Hermelink HK et al. (1987) Transplantation of aortic and pulmonary allografts, enhanced viability of endothelial cells by cryopreservation. Importance of histocompatibility. J Cardiac Surg 1 (suppl.): 209–220
4. Cambell MJ, Machin D (1993) Medical statistics, publishers, Wiley J and Son, New York, p 79
5. Clarke DR, Bishop DA (1993) Allograft degeneration in infant pulmonary valve allograft recipients. Eur J Cardio-thorac Surg 7: 365–370
6. Balch CM, Karp RB (1975) Blood group compatibility and aortic valve allotransplantation in man. J Thorac Cardiovasc Surg 70: 256–259
7. Lupinetti FM, Cobb S, Kioschos HC, Thompson SA, Walters KS, Moore KC (1992) Effect of immunological differences on rat aortic valve allograft calcification. J Cardiac Surg 7: 65–70
8. Monro JL, Salmon AP, Keeton BR (1993) The outcome of antibiotic sterilised aortic homografts used in the Fontan procedure. Eur Cardio-thorac Surg 7: 360–364
9. Cleveland DC, Williamsm WG, Razzouk AJ, Trusler GA, Rebeyka IM, Duffy L, Kan Z, Coles JG, Freedom RM (1992) Failure of cryopreserved homograft valved conduits in the pulmonary circulation. Circulation 86 (Suppl II): II-150–II-153
10. Grunkemeier GL, Starr A (1977) Actuarial analysis of surgical results: rationale and method. Ann Thorac Surg 24: 404
11. Yacoub MH (1987) Applications and limitations of histocompatibility in clinical cardiac valve allograft surgery. In: Cardiac valve allografts 1962–1987 (Yankah AC, Hetzer R, Miller DC, Ross DN, Somerville J, Yacoub MH eds.). Steinkopff Verlag, Darmstadt, Springer Verlag, New York, 95–102
12. Somerville J (1987) Late results of homograft function used for right ventricular outflow obstruction. In: Cardiac valve allografts 1962–1987 (Yankah AC, Hetzer R, Miller DC, Ross DN, Somerville J, Yacoub MH eds.). Steinkopff Verlag, Darmstadt, Springer Verlag, New York, 249–260
13. Müller-Hermelink HK, Yankah AC (1987) Immunohistopathology of cardiac allograft explant. In: Cardiac valve allografts 1962–1987 (Yankah AC, Hetzer R, Miller DC, Ross DN, Somerville J, Yacoub MH eds.). Steinkopff Verlag, Darmstadt, Springer Verlag, New York, 89–94
14. Gregory CR, Huie P, Billingham ME, Morris RE (1993) Rapamycin inhibits arterial intimal thickening caused by both alloimune and mechanical injury. Transplantation 55: 1409–1418
15. Schmitz-Rixen T, Megerman J, Colvin RB, Williams AM, Abbott WA (1988) Immunosuppressive treatment of aortic allografts. J Vasc Surg 7: 82–92
16. Yankah AC, Sievers HH, Lange PE, Regensburger D, Bernhard A (1982) Surgical repair of tetralogy of Fallot in adolescents and adults. Thorac Cardiovasc Surgeon 30: 69–74
17. Sievers HH, Lange PE, Regensburger D, Yankah CA et al. (1983) Short-term hemodynamic results after right ventricular outflow tract reconstruction using a cusp-bearing transannular patch. J Thorac Cardiovasc Surg 86: 777–83
18. Yankah AC, Lange PE, Sievers HH, Radtke W, Regensburger D, Heintzen PH, Bernhard A (1984) Late results of valve xenograft conduits between the right ventricle and the pulmonary arteries in patients with pulmonary atresia and extreme tetralogy of Fallot Thorac Cardiovasc Surgeon 32: 250–2
19. Yankah AC, Hetzer R (1987) Current and future trends in transplantation of heart valve allografts. Derzeitige und zukünftige Trends bei der Transplantation allogener Herzklappen. Z Herz-Thorax-Gefäßchir 1: 12–19
20. Yankah AC, Wottge HU, Müller-Ruchholtz W (1995) Short-course cyclosporin A therapy for definite allograft valve survival. Immunosuppression in allograft valve operations. Ann Thorac Surg 60: S146–50

21. Yankah AC, Alexi-Meskhishvili V, Weng Y, Berger F, Lange P, Hetzer R (1995) Performance of aortic and pulmonary homografts in the right ventricular outflow tract in children. J Heart Valve Dis 4: 392–395
22. Yankah AC, Alexi-Meskhishvili V, Weng Y, Schorn K, Lange P Lange, Hetzer R (1995) Accelerated degeneration of allografts in the first two years of life. Ann Thorac Surg 60: S71–77
23. Schorn K, Yankah AC, Alexi-Meskhishvili V, Weng Y, Lange PE, Hetzer R (1997) Risk factors for early degeneration of allografts in pulmonary circulation. Eur J Cardiothorac Surg 11: 62–69

Author's address:
A. Charles Yankah, MD, PhD
Consultant, Assistant Professor
Deutsches Herzzentrum Berlin and Humboldt University
Dept. Cardiothoracic and Vascular Surgery
Augustenburger Platz 1
D-13353 Berlin
Germany

Intermediate-term performance of CryoLife cryopreserved heart valve allografts

D. M. Fronk, S. B. Capps, R. T. McNally

CryoLife®, Inc., Marietta, GA, USA

Introduction

CryoLife, Inc., a tissue processing laboratory, specializes in ultra-low temperature preservation of human tissues for transplant, including aortic and pulmonary heart valve allografts. Since CryoLife's inception in 1984, the company has processed over 18 000 donated hearts, received from 150 Tissue Banks and Organ Procurement Organizations throughout the United States, and documented the implantation of more than 16 000 cryopreserved allograft heart valves from 450 institutions in the United States, Canada, and Europe (Fig. 1). The following chapter provides a summary of CryoLife's tissue processing methodology and documented clinical experience of allograft heart valves.

Tissue processing

Incoming tissue is accepted based on a comprehensive list of inclusion criteria including: age ranging from birth to 55 years, no history of rheumatic fever, absence of bacterial endocarditis, no significant murmurs, no history of hypertension, no significant chest wall injuries, and negative serologic cultures. On December 14, 1993, the United States Food and Drug Administration (FDA) issued Interim Rules regarding the screening and handling of donor tissue with the purpose of implementing standards to safeguard the public health (9). These Interim Rules require certain serological tests, donor screening, and record keeping to help prevent the transmission of AIDS and hepatitis through human allografts. Necessary serological screening tests include the following: HIV Type 1 antibody, HIV Type 2 antibody, Hepatitis B surface antigen, and Hepatitis C antibody. In addition, CryoLife performs a HTLV Type I antibody test and confirmation tests for the Hepatitis B surface antigen and Hepatitis C antibody.

In order to maintain sufficient tissue (fibroblast) viability, hearts must be recovered from qualified donors within 24 h of asystole and received by CryoLife within 52 h of asystole. Upon arrival, aortic and pulmonary valves are dissected from the heart by highly trained technicians with strict adherence to aseptic techniques. During the dissection process, the heart valves undergo minimal handling to assure low microbiological bioburden and preservation of the cellular and structural integrity of the valved tissue. Valves are inspected for competency, plaque, intimal disruptions, fenestrations, hemorrhagic areas, and other structural anomalies. Allograft tissues falling outside of established standards are rejected.

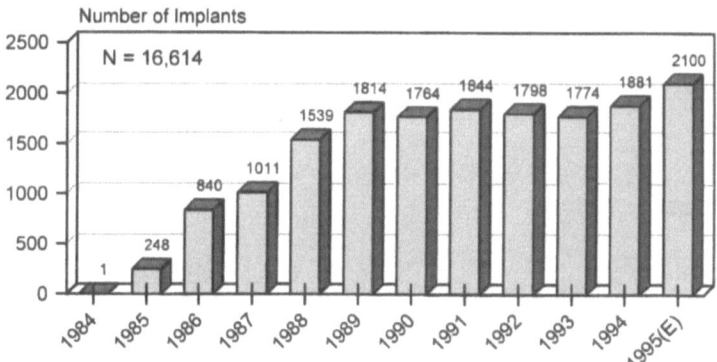

Fig. 1. Allograft valves implanted since December 1984. Total includes an estimate for 1995 implants (E = Estimate).

Early concerns over microbiologic bioburden and the transmission of infection led to aggressive sterilization techniques including ethylene oxide gas (2), chemical pre-treatment, i.e., β-propiolactone (24) and formaldehyde (20), gamma irradiation (15, 22), and highly concentrated antibiotic incubation (17). These initial sterilization methods, however, are believed to alter cellular viability which has been reported as one of the key elements influencing valve durability (7, 16, 19). Consequently, allograft valves prepared using these techniques often developed calcification and/or rupture of the valve leaflet, resulting in an unacceptable reoperation rate (3, 4, 12, 19). To address the problem of non-viable valve tissue, treatment with nontoxic, low-dose antibiotic sterilization along with valve storage by cryopreservation was introduced in the 1970s (17, 18). Numerous antibiotics and antibiotic mixtures have since been formulated in attempts to maximize decontamination and minimize cellular damage. CryoLife currently employs a 24 h, 37 °C antibiotic incubation utilizing a proprietary combination of antifungal and antibacterial agents within a nutrient media (U.S. patent pending). This cocktail yields tissue with high fibroblast survival, microbial decontamination, and minimal loss of structural properties.

Upon completion of the incubation in antibiotics, the tissue is packaged in a specially-designed, triple pouch packaging system (10). This packaging system provides superior tear and rupture strength which minimizes loss of pouch integrity during long-term storage in liquid nitrogen and shipping. The allograft is placed in the inner pouch along with a tissue cryoprotectant solution consisting of Dulbecco's Modified Eagles Medium (DMEM), 10% dimethylsulfoxide, and 10% fetal bovine serum. The allograft is cryopreserved using a microprocessor controlled rate freezer at a rate of approximately −1 °C per minute until the pouch contents reach −80 °C. Although a variety of freezing profiles have been developed and utilized by other researchers, CryoLife has found that the optimal profile allows for an initial equilibrium temperature of 4 °C, followed by a gradual freeze to −80 °C (14). The freezing rate is of vital importance to inhibit tissue damage secondary to ice crystal formation within the cells (5). Tissue is then stored at −135 °C or colder within a liquid nitrogen freezer. Previous researchers have theorized that tissue can be stored indefinitely at ultra-low temperatures due to the cessation of cellular activity and chemical interaction (5).

Prior to implantation, the cryopreserved allografts must undergo complete thawing and elution of the cryoprotectant following a patented process (6). Strict adherence to this protocol is critical to a successful outcome. Thawing and elution is a multi-step process designed to protect and maintain the cellular integrity of the tissue during its transition from the frozen state and to elute out the cryoprotectant.

Clinical experience

As indicated previously, CryoLife has documented the implantation of over 16 000 allograft heart valves since 1984. Despite the large number of recorded implants, incomplete follow-up data prohibits sufficient patient grouping and statistical analysis. Thus, the discussed clinical analysis was conducted from audited prospective and retrospective data collected from six primary centers. The selection criteria for primary centers included surgeon experience, a surgical practice specializing in adult or pediatric patients, a significant number of patients in each age group, and full access to patient records for monitoring.

One thousand two hundred twenty CryoValve® heart valve allografts were implanted at the six primary centers between February 1985 and August 1995. The population consisted of 817 males (67%) and 403 females (33%). The age of the patients at the time of implant ranged from newborn to 85 years, with 55% of patients between the ages of 0–14 years and 45% between 15–85 years. As shown in Fig. 2, children predominately received a pulmonary valve due to the prevalence of right heart congenital defects. Similarly, adults more frequently received an aortic valve to correct left heart degenerative disease of the aortic valve.

The study group was comprised of 640 aortic valves (52%) and 580 pulmonary valves (48%) used to correct a wide variety of congenital and acquired valvular diseases. Representative diagnoses included congenital defects such as tetralogy of Fallot, bicuspid valve, truncus arteriosus, myxomatous degeneration, pulmonary atresia, transposition of the great arteries, and hypoplastic left heart syndrome. Representative adult diagnoses were aortic stenosis/insufficiency, pulmonary stenosis/insufficiency, and endocarditis.

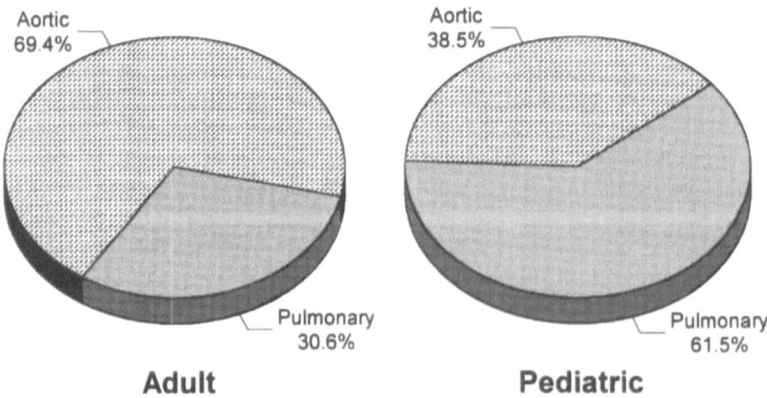

Fig. 2. Distribution of allograft valve type by recipient group. The population consisted of 552 adult and 668 pediatric valve recipients. A total of 640 aortic valves and 580 pulmonary valves were implanted in the total group.

The operative procedures performed to correct the associated valvular disorders were aortic valve replacement (freehand technique), aortic root replacement, extended aortic root replacement, aortoventriculoplasty (Konno procedure), Rastelli procedure, pulmonary autograft (Ross Switch procedure), pulmonary valve replacement, and right ventricular outflow tract reconstruction. Figure 3 illustrates the overall percentage distribution of documented surgical procedures and further demonstrates the individual breakdown between adult and pediatric recipients. Concomitantly, 82 patients had replacement of a malfunctioning prosthetic valve and 45 patients had replacement of a malfunctioning allograft valve.

Data collection for all patients included demographic information, surgical details, and postoperative follow-up data. Comprehensive follow-up data were obtained on 89% of the 1220 valve recipients. The range of follow-up was 1 day to 9.3 years, with a mean follow-up time of 1.9 years. For purposes of actuarial analysis, study endpoints were patient death or reoperation for allograft explant.

Data from the six investigational centers were pooled and analyzed by overall population, pediatric and adult groups, adult aortic and pulmonary valve replacement, and pediatric aortic and pulmonary valve replacement. Due to the wide use of aortic and pulmonary allografts for pediatric right ventricular outflow tract reconstruction, this group was further subdivided by the allograft type, i.e., aortic and pulmonary valve comparisons. Statistical methods included Cox regression analysis for the calculation of overall freedom from adverse events and complications and a Wilcoxon test for statistical comparisons between groups. A dotted line was used on all actuarial curves to signify the point at which the standard error (SE) exceeded 10% (21). Actuarial results (%) plotted and discussed in the text have a SE less than 10% as data beyond these points are statistically invalid due to low patient populations. The

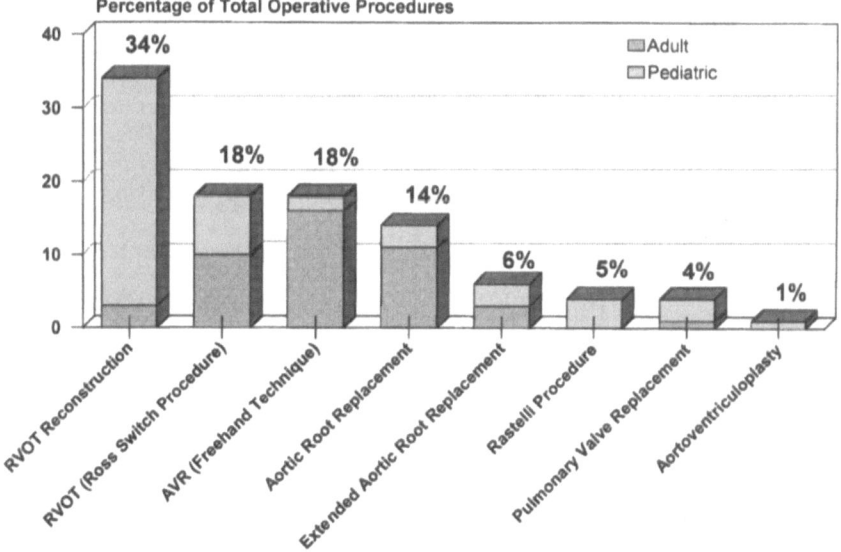

Fig. 3. Percentage distribution of documented operative procedures used in the adult and pediatric groups. The adult group consisted of valve recipients ≥15 years of age. Pediatric valve recipients predominantly underwent right heart procedures while the majority of adult cases underwent left heart procedures.

number at risk and the number of events are included for all outcome data presented. Statistical data analyses were conducted using SPSS statistical software (SPSS Inc., Chicago, IL).

All allograft removals and patient deaths were categorized based on the type and consequences of the specified event. The classification codes used were based on the guidelines for reporting morbidity and mortality after cardiac valvular operations established by the Ad Hoc Liaison Committee for standardizing definitions of prosthetic heart valve morbidity of The American Association of Thoracic Surgery and The Society of Thoracic Surgeons (8).

Of the 1220 valve recipients enrolled in the study, 271 events occurred that resulted in either patient death or allograft removal (Table 1). Operative mortality, predominately in the pediatric population, accounted for 133 of the 172 patient deaths. No operative mortality was attributed to valve dysfunction. Overall patient survival at 7 years for the adult and pediatric groups was 85% and 74%, respectively (Fig. 4).

Structural deterioration of the allograft heart valve, typically involving the valve leaflets and/or conduit, resulted in the removal of 57 valves (Table 1). Twenty-six of these were associated with normal pediatric outgrowth of the allograft valve. An additional 11 valves experienced non-structural dysfunction identified by valve dehiscence, suture entrapment, or stenosis of the annulus not intrinsic to the valve. Seventeen patients had their allografts removed because of endocarditis, nine of whom had pre-existing endocarditis. Five allografts were removed due to valve insufficiency attributed to surgical technique. Seven patients returned to the operating room to have the allograft valve repaired or resuspended due to implant technique-related complications. There were two unrelated valve removals in which the allograft had to be explanted. The first was due to pseudoaneurysm development in the pericardial patch used to supplement the allograft. The second removal occurred in a patient who underwent cardiac transplant secondary to cardiomyopathy 48 h postoperative to initial valve implantation. There was no incidence of thromboembolism-related complications or patient death attributed to the valve. Table 2 provides a detailed breakdown of failure modes for allograft heart valves removed due to structural deterioration.

Table 1. Adverse events resulting in either allograft removal or patient death. Classification codes follow guidelines suggested by The American Association of Thoracic Surgery and The Society of Thoracic Surgeons (see text for description).

Classification[1]	Number of events	% of total events	% of total implants
Operative mortality	133	49.1	10.9
Structural deterioration	57	21.0	4.7
Non-valve related patient death	39	14.4	3.2
Endocarditis[2]	17	6.3	1.4
Non-structural dysfunction	11	4.1	0.9
Reoperation: repair allograft	7	2.6	0.6
Technique related removal	5	1.8	0.4
Non-valve related valve removal	2	0.7	0.2
Thromboembolism	0	0.0	0.0
Anticoagulant related complications	0	0.0	0.0
Total	271	100.0	22.3

[1] As defined by: JTCVS 96: 351–353, 1988.
[2] No incidence of endocarditis was attributed to the allograft valve.

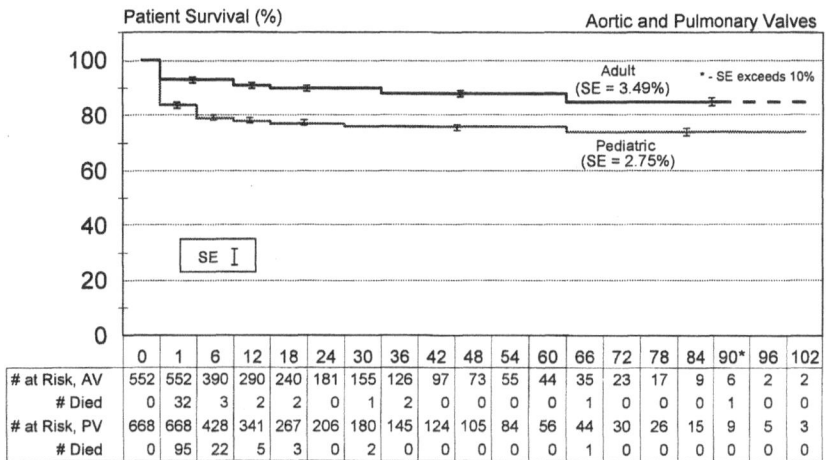

Fig. 4. Overall patient survival in the adult and pediatric population. The adult group was comprised of 552 valve recipients with the pediatric group totaling 668 valve recipients. The patient survival for the adult and pediatric groups at 7 years follow-up was 85% and 74%, respectively. A dotted line signifies the time point at which standard error exceeds 10% (SE = ± 1 Standard Error). The standard error SE listed was assessed at the last plotted time point.

Table 2. Reason for removal related to structural deterioration of the allograft valve. Structural deterioration refers to changes intrinsic to the valve which cause stenosis or regurgitation.

Reason	Number removed	% of total removals	% of total implants	Mean implant time (years)
Pulmonary stenosis	24	42.1	2.0	4.4
Cusp degeneration	8	14.0	0.7	4.5
PS/PI	7	12.3	0.6	3.6
Calcification	5	8.8	0.4	3.0
Pulmonary insufficiency	3	5.3	0.2	3.9
AS/AI	8	14.0	0.7	3.8
Leaflet tear	2	3.5	0.2	4.9
Total	57	100.0	4.8	

In the adult population, actuarial freedom from reoperation (all causes) was 95% at 1 year, 90% at 3 years, 81% at 5 years, and 73% at 8 years. Structural deterioration, defined as any abnormality causing stenosis or regurgitation, was used as a direct measurement of allograft performance. Within the adult population, 96% of all aortic valves (AV) were implanted in the aortic position with 92% of the pulmonary valves (PV) being implanted in the pulmonary position. There were seven reported occurrences of structural deterioration within the adult group. Five occurred in the sub-group with aortic valves and two in the sub-group with pulmonary valves. As shown in Figs. 5(a) and 5(b), the actuarial freedom from structural deterioration for the AV sub-group was 99% at 1 year, 98% at 4 years, and 96% at 6 years. Similarly, freedom from structural deterioration for the PV sub-group was 100% at 1 year and 98% at 4 years.

In the pediatric population, actuarial freedom from reoperation (all causes) at 5.5 years was 60% for aortic allografts and 83% for pulmonary allografts. This difference was statistically significant ($p = 0.025$). A total of 45 cases of structural deterioration were

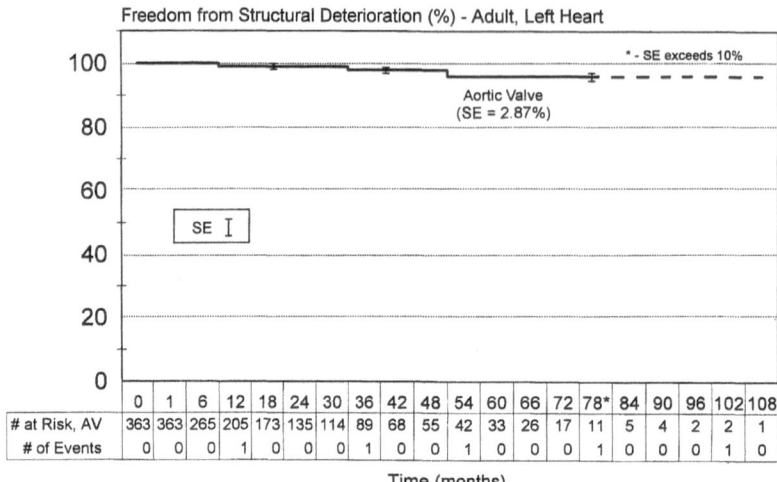

Fig. 5(a). Actuarial freedom from structural deterioration in the adult population for left heart procedures. The adult freedom from structural deterioration was 96% at 6 years follow-up. A dotted line signifies the time point at which standard error exceeds 10% (SE = ± 1 Standard Error). The standard error (SE) listed was assessed at the last plotted time point.

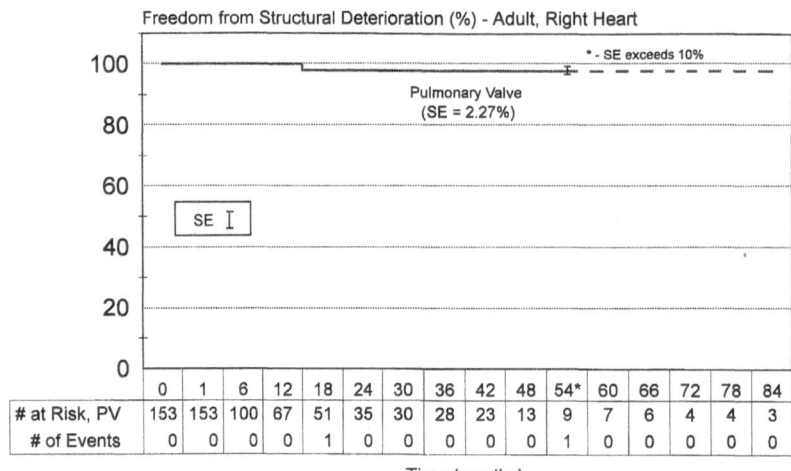

Fig. 5(b). Actuarial freedom from structural deterioration in the adult population for right heart procedures. The adult freedom from structural deterioration was 98% at 4 years follow-up. A dotted line signifies the time point at which standard error exceeds 10% (SE = ± 1 Standard Error). The standard error (SE) listed was assessed at the last plotted time point.

reported in the pediatric group for right and left heart procedures. Of these reported cases, 26 were attributed to normal pediatric outgrowth. At 5.5 years, the actuarial freedom from structural deterioration was 57% for the aortic valves and 84% for the pulmonary valves when used in right ventricular outflow tract reconstruction. These results demonstrate a statistically significant difference ($p = 0.019$) in the performance of aortic and pulmonary allografts used on the right side of the heart, illustrating the better long-term performance of the pulmonary allograft valve, see Fig. 6(a). The observed results agree favorably with other researchers who have reported similar outcome for pulmonary allografts used in right heart procedures (1, 11, 13, 23, 25). Theories explaining this effect include lower calcium content, less elastic tissue, and abnormal metabolism of the structures (10, 13, 26). Similarly, 102 allograft aortic valves were used in the pediatric group for left heart procedures. As shown in Fig. 6(b), the actuarial freedom from structural deterioration in the left side at 4.5 years was 83%. Seventeen pulmonary valves were also used in the left side, but were not analyzed due to the small sample size.

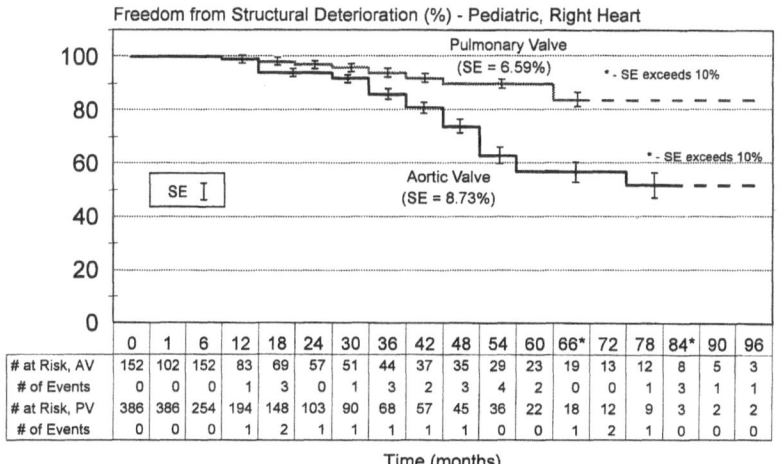

Fig. 6(a). Actuarial freedom from structural deterioration comparing pulmonary valves (PV) versus aortic valves (AV) used in right ventricular outflow tract reconstruction for pediatric cases. The pediatric freedom from structural deterioration for pulmonary and aortic valves was 84% and 57%, respectively, at 5.5 years follow-up. This difference was statistically significant ($p = 0.19$). A dotted line signifies the time points at which standard error exceeds 10% (SE = $\pm$ 1 Standard Error). The standard errors (SE) listed were assessed at the last plotted time points.

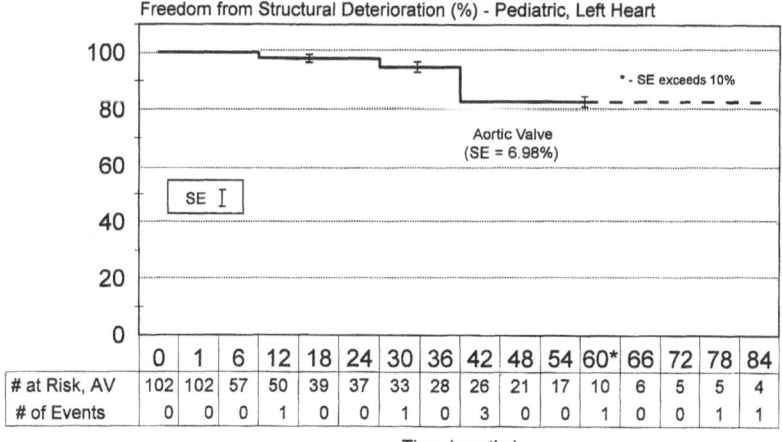

Fig. 6(b). Actuarial freedom from structural deterioration in the pediatric population for left heart procedures. The pediatric freedom from structural deterioration was 83% at 4.5 years follow-up. A dotted line signifies the time point at which standard error exceeds 10% (SE = $\pm$ 1 Standard Error). The standard error (SE) listed was assessed at the last plotted time point.

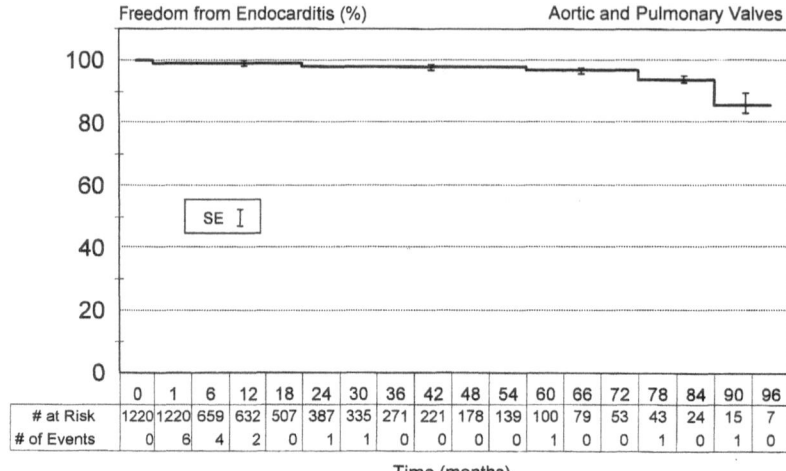

Fig. 7. Actuarial freedom from endocarditis in the combined 1220 population. The freedom from endocarditis in the aortic and pulmonary valves was 86% at 8 years follow-up (SE = ± 1 Standard Error).

Due to the low rate of endocarditis in both groups, the data were pooled to determine the rate within the entire population. The presence of endocarditis necessitated the removal of a total of 17 allografts, 12 of these removals occurring within the first postoperative year. Of the 17 total removals, 12 were the result of the endocarditis, while the remaining five were due to severe valvular insufficiency that developed following the endocarditis. Nine allograft removals were in patients having pre-existing endocarditis. No reported incidence of endocarditis was attributed to the heart valve allograft. Actuarial freedom from endocarditis was 99% at 1 year, 98% at 4 years, and 86% at 8 years. These actuarial estimates compare favorably with previously reported endocarditis levels (18).

Conclusions

Based on the described clinical outcome analysis of 1220 CryoValve heart valve allograft recipients, the following conclusions can be made:

- No occurrences of thromboembolic or anticoagulant-related complications were observed in recipients of cryopreserved heart valve allografts.
- While the cardiac reoperation rate in the adult population was 27% at 8 years, less than one-third of these were for removal of the valve due to structural deterioration. Thus, long-term survival of allograft heart valves in the adult population is indicated.
- Pulmonary valve allografts have better intermediate-term performance than aortic valve allografts when used for right ventricular outflow tract reconstruction in the pediatric patient population.
- Patients receiving cryopreserved heart valve allografts had a low incidence of endocarditis. These data support the opinion that cryopreserved allograft heart valves are the valve of choice for patients with pre-existing endocarditis (15, 18).

References

1. Bailey WW (1987) Cryopreserved pulmonary homografts valved external conduits: early results. J Cardiac Surg 2: 199–204
2. Barratt-Boyes B (1964) Homograft aortic valve replacement in aortic incompetence and stenosis. Thorax 19: 131
3. Barratt-Boyes B (1971) Longterm follow-up of valve grafts. Br Heart J 33
4. Barratt-Boyes B, Roche A, Whitlock R (1977) Six year review of the results of freehand aortic valve replacement using an antibiotic sterilized homograft valve. Circulation 55: 353–61
5. Brockbank KG (1995) Essentials of cryobiology. In: Brockbank K (eds) Principles of Autologous, Allogeneic, and Cryopreserved Venous Transplantation. R.G. Landes Company, Austin, pp 91–100
6. Carpentier JF, Brockbank KG (1992) United States patent #5,160,313
7. Crescenzo DG, Hibert SL, Barrick MK, Corcoran PC, St. Louis JD, Messier RH, Ferrans VJ, Wallace RB, Hopkins RA (1992) Donor heart valves: electron microscopic and morphometric assessment of cellular injury induced by warm ischemia. J Thorac & Cardiovasc Surg 103: 253–7
8. Edmunds HL, Clark RE, Lawrence CH, Miller CD, Weisel RD (1988) Guidelines for reporting morbidity and mortality after cardiac valvular operations. J Thorac Cardiovasc Surg 96: 351–3
9. Food and Drug Administration (1993) Human Tissue Intended for Transplantation – Interim Rule. Federal Register – Part V. Washington, pp 65514–21
10. Heacox A (1993) United States patent #5,257,692
11. Livi U, Abdulla A, Parker R, Olsen EJ, Ross DN (1987) Viability and morphology of aortic and pulmonary homografts. J Thorac Cardiovasc Surg 93: 755–60
12. Manhas D, Mohri H, Merendino K (1973) Late results of beta-propiolactone sterilized aortic homograft valves. Am J Surg 126: 255–62
13. McGrath LB, Lavin-Gonzalez L, Graft D (1988) Pulmonary homograft implantation for ventricular outflow tract reconstruction: early phase results. Ann Thorac Surg 45: 273–7
14. McNally RT, Kelvin KG, Heacox A, Bank HL (1990) United States patent #4,890,457
15. Mitchell RN, Jonas RA, Schoen FJ (1995) Structure-function correlations in cryopreserved allograft cardiac valves. Ann Thorac Surg 60: 108–13
16. Niwaya K, Sakaguchi H, Kawachi K, Kitamura S (1995) Effect of warm ischemia and cryopreservation on cell viability of human allograft valves. Ann Thorac Surg 60: 114–7
17. O'Brien MF, Gardner M, McGiffin D, Brosnan A (1987) The viable cryopreserved allograft aortic valve. J Cardiac Surg 2: 153–67
18. O'Brien M, Stafford E, Gardner M, McGiffin DC, Pohlner PF, McLachlan GJ, Gall K, Susan S, Murphy E (1991) Allograft aortic valve replacement: long-term comparative clinical analysis of the viable cryopreserved and antibiotic 4 °C stored valves. J Card Surg 6: 534–43
19. O'Brien M, Stafford E, Gardner M, Pohlner PG, McGiffin DC (1987) A comparison of aortic valve replacement with viable cryopreserved and fresh allograft valves, with a note on chromosomal studies. J Thorac Cardiovasc Surg 94: 812–23
20. Paneth M, O'Brien M (1966) Transplantation of human homograft aortic valve. Thorax 21: 115
21. Rutherford RB, Flanigan DP, Gupta SK, Johnston KW, Allastair K, Whittemore AD, Baker JD, Ernst CB (1986) Suggested standards for reports dealing with lower extremity ischemia. J Vasc Surg 4: 80–94
22. Smith J (1967) The pathology of human aortic valve homografts. Thorax 22: 114–38
23. Stelzer P, Elkins RC (1989) Homograft valves and conduits: applications in cardiac surgery. In: Wells SA (eds) Current Problems in Surgery. Years Book Medical Publ. Chicago, pp 381–452
24. Wallace R, Giuliani E, Titus J (1971) Use of aortic valve homografts for aortic valve replacement. Circulation 43: 365
25. Yankah AC, Alex-Meskhishvili V, Weng Y, Schorn K, Lange PE (1995) Accelerated degeneration of allografts in the first two years of life. Ann Thorac Surg 60: 71–77

Author's address:
Robert T. McNally, PhD
CryoLife, Inc.
2211 New Market Pkwy., #142
Marietta, GA 30067,
U.S.A.

Replacement of the mitral and tricuspid valves with aortic and pulmonary valve allografts

F. Robicsek

The Sanger Clinic, Charlotte, North Carolina, USA

"Again, with homograft aortic valves, nothing fundamental has changed in the design principle since it has been introduced several million years ago, but there has been a little bit of juggling with the preparation and storage media." Donald N Ross, 1972

Implantation of fresh aortic unstented homografts into the mitral position was initially championed by the Toronto group. Their first report was that of the great Gordon Murray who in 1956, after having experimented extensively with "pericardial slings," proposed the replacement of the mitral valve with an aortic allograft. Using the closed technique in a canine model, he removed the mitral leaflets and replaced them with an allograft aortic valve with extended strips of aortic wall attached. After the graft was pulled into the mitral orifice, its upper portion was sutured to the mitral annulus under the control of the index finger, and the aortic wall-strips were attached to the ventricular wall. In spite of the technical difficulties, the study of surviving animals of 8–9 months after insertion showed well functioning and mobile valve cusps and good hemodynamic results. Post-mortem microscopic examination disclosed only slight thicknening of the transplanted valve (9). He also gave a report on a clinical case:

"The procedure as described in the experimental work was then applied to mitral regurgitation.
The chief problem here was to make sure that the mitral orifice was large enough to accommodate the transplanted valve. With Bailey knives, the commissures and the valve cusps were lacerated widely to divide the valve curtains as well as the chordae tendineae and in that way a satisfactory opening was obtained. The sutures were then passed as described, with a long curved needle and all this was accomplished quite satisfactorily. There was massive regurgitation through the mitral valve on palpation through the atrium. After transplantation of the valve, there was no regurgitation. The procedure was carried out quite satisfactorily. The effect postoperatively was quite satisfactorily" (10).

In 1961, Willman et al. replaced canine mitral valves with aortic valve alografts in the manner suggested by Murray et al., but under direct vision. Of 23 dogs, 16 died within 2 weeks due to technical problems, and four dogs were lost within 1 month because of development of mitral regurgitation due to separation of the suture line at the mitral annulus. Survivors for 1, 2, and 5 months all died due to mitral regurgitation (18). In contrast to Murray et al. (9, 10) who attached the aortic valve graft with strips of the aortic wall to the interior of the left ventricle, in his experiments, Heimbecker sutured the commissures directly to the ventricular wall while replacing the tricuspid and mitral valve with aortic allografts. He also reported a patient who

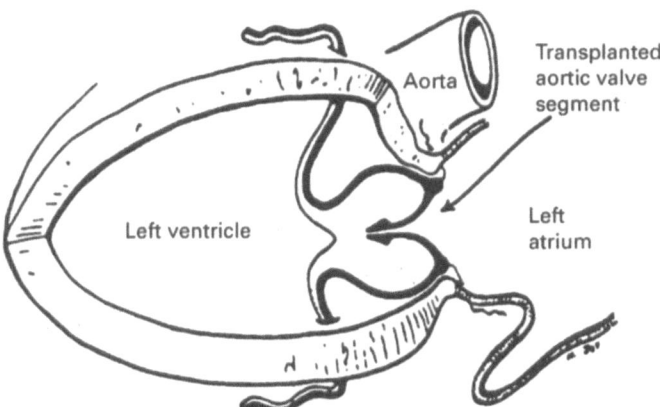

Fig. 1. Transplantation of a homograft aortic valve into the mitral position. The annulus of the aortic valve is sutured to the mitral orifice and further held in position by strips of the aortic wall attached to the left ventricular myocardium serving as chordae tendineae. (From Murray et al., *Angiology* 1969, 7:446. Reprinted with permission.)

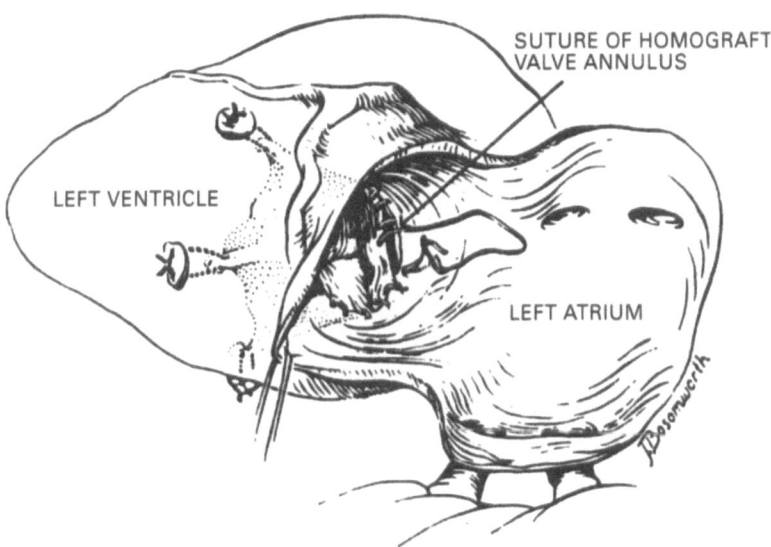

Fig. 2. Aortic homograft valve replacement of the mitral valve. (From Heimbercker et al., *Canad Med Ass J*, May 5, 1962, Vol 86. Reprinted with permission.)

did well initially but died 1 month later of infection (2). This might have been the same patient to whom Murray was referring (10).

A respectable series of 35 patients in whom freeze-dried aortic homografts were implanted into the mitral position with good short-term results was reported by Cornish in 1965 (1).

McKenzie et al. in 1966 made extensive experimental studies on the different methods of preservation of mitral allografts. They found comparable survival rates among dogs regardless of the method, but better anatomical results with fresh rather

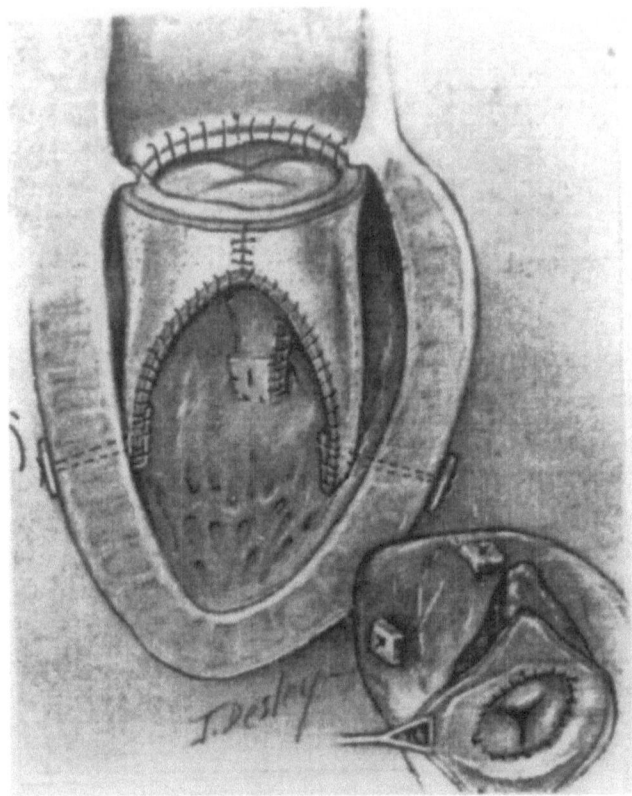

Fig. 3. Aortic allograft in the mitral position (From McKenzie et al., *J Thorac and CV Surg*, 51, No 21, February 1966. Reprinted with permission.)

than with preserved valves. Their technique included reinforcement of the aortic wall with Teflon. With the passing of time, significant degenerative changes were noted in the transplanted valves; however, in periods exceeding 1 year, the central core of the valvular tissues remained thin, pliable and functional. Late hemodynamic and cineangiographic studies showed evidence of increasing mitral stenosis due to contraction of the aortic cuff of the grafted valve (7).

Suzuki and Kay used fresh as well as preserved aortic allografts as mitral valve replacements in their experiments. After excision of the host valve, the donor valve was turned inside-out and placed into the left ventricular cavity. After its edge was attached to the host's mitral annulus with a continuous suture, the graft was turned right side out again and brought back into the left atrial cavity and attached to its wall with a continuous suture. Hemodynamic and angiographic studies in three of the nine survivors showed competency of the transplanted valve and systolic bulging of the aortic cusps into the left atrium without regurgitation. The same authors also reported the case of a 47-year-old woman who underwent a similar procedure in 1966 for calcified mitral stenosis with good short-term results (17).

The matter of mitral valvular tissue grafts was "revisited" in the experiments of Rastelli and Titus in 1968. Their conclusion was that, in dogs, homograft replacement of the entire mitral valve with fresh viable orthotopic grafts can lead to long-term survival and normally functioning valve-apparatus (13).

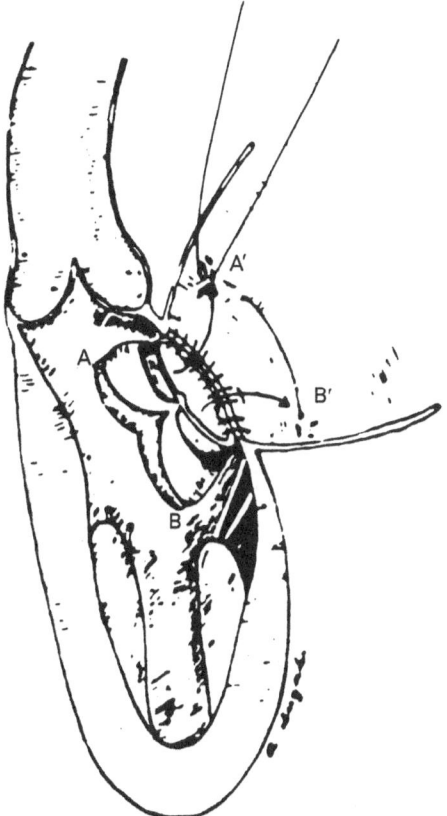

Fig. 4. Technique of insertion of homologous aortic valve to mitral area. The graft is turned right side out and brought back into left atrium. (From Suzuki et al., *Japanese Circ J*, Vol 30, Sept 1956. Reprinted with permission.)

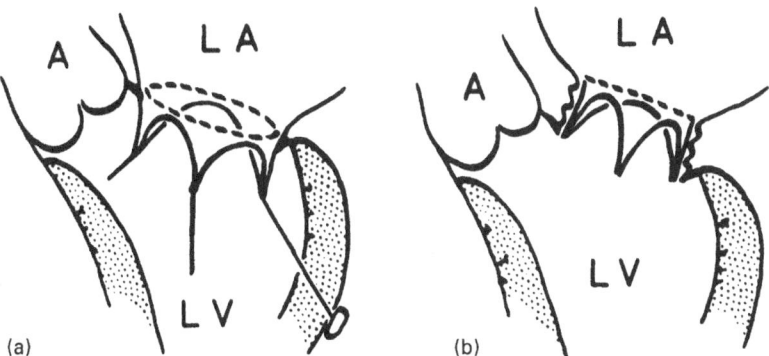

Fig. 5. Diagrammatic representation of aortic to mitral valve transplantation a) intraventricular placement with fixation of the commissures to the ventricular wall and b) intra-atrial placement with plication of the atrial wall to support the base of the valve cusps. (From Baird et al., *The Canadian J of Surg*, Vol 12, Jan 1969. Reprinted with permission.)

Yacoub introduced his technique in 1969 to replace the mitral valve with fresh aortic allograft. The method included suturing the graft into a Dacron tube and reinforcing the annulus with a collar of autogenous pericardium. This "top-hat" graft was sterilized with electron beam energy and stored for not more than 7 days before implantation. Good long-range clinical results in 16 patients have been reported. Yacoub et al. followed up their initial paper 3 years later with a report of 191 patients, mostly with rheumatic mitral valve disease, with similarly satisfactory long-term results (20). Their clinical observations were accompanied with simultaneous scholarly studies on the properties of valve allograft with the conclusion that long-term results depend on the preservation of the physical properties and anatomical integrity of the valve graft (19). One may wonder why the procedure was not applied any longer.

Pappas in 1972, presented a small number of patients in whom the mitral valve was replaced with unstented aortic fresh grafts. In the follow-up period he found moderate residual stenosis and some degree of mitral insufficiency in most of the patients (12). Allograft replacement of the tricuspid valve for Ebstein's disease was carried out in 1976 by Senoo (16) using an unstented aortic allograft and applying the technique à la Yacoub et al. (19, 20)

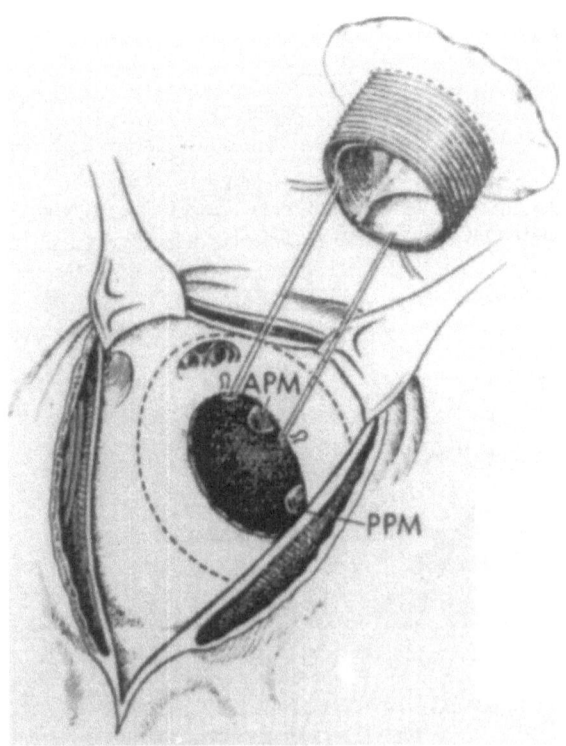

Fig. 6. Diagram illustrating fixation of the aortic end of the graft to the mitral "annulus" by a series of everting mattress sutures. The *dotted line* shows the position of the second suture line. (From Yacoub et al., *J Thorac and Cardiov Surg*, Vol 58, No 6, Dec 1969. Reprinted with permission.)

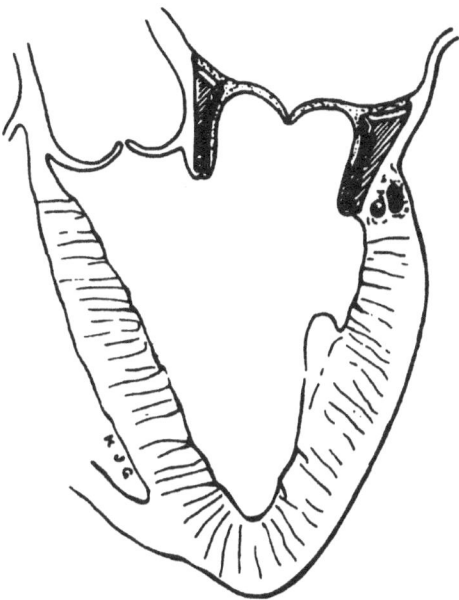

Fig. 7. Diagram illustrating position of aortic allograft used for mitral valve replacement. (From Yacoub M, *Singapore Med J*, Vol 14, No 3, Sep 1973. Reprinted with permission.)

Pulmonary allografts

In 1961, Lower et al. described the technique of inserting autologous pulmonic valves into the mitral valve area in such a fashion that the valve ring itself was anchored to the left atrial wall, and the distal border of the grafted valve was sutured to the mitral annulus. In about half of the animals the grafted valve was incompetent due to either disruption of the suture line or inadequate coaptation of the cusps (6).

In 1967, Ross (14) reported two patients in whom pulmonary valve autograft was used to replace the mitral valve. Both patients did well in the reported follow-up period of 3 and 2 months respectively.

In 1988, McKay (11) used an unstented pulmonary allograft enclosed in a Dacron tube. Recently, Kumar et al. (3–5) reported on three children in whom allograft pulmonary valves were used to reconstruct the tricuspid orifice using the same technique.

Aortic and pulmonary valves in the atrioventricular position played an important role in the very early history of heart valve transplantation. While stented aortic xerografts were and are still used extensively in the mitral and tricuspid positions, the replacement of atrioventricular valves with unstented, aortic or pulmonary auto and allografts is an issue which is, if not dead, then is at least dormant. For that reason this chapter was written as a historical perspective and not as a practical guide.*

---

* *Author's Note*

Nota Bene: Mitral or tricuspid allografts were not even mentioned in the book by Metras (8) published but a few years ago. The predecessor of this book published in 1987 (21) also omitted the subject of the use of mitral and tricuspid allografts. Now they are making a comeback, a proof that nobody knows for sure when a "sleeper" will awaken. FR

References

1. Cornish CB (1964) Use of freeze-dried aortic valve homografts in aural surgery. Lancet i, 1133
2. Heimbecker RO, Baird RJ, Lajos TZ, Varga AT, Greenwood WF (1962) Homograft replacement of the human mitral valve. J Canad Med Ass 86: 805–9
3. Kumar AS, Chander H, Trehan H (1995) Surgical technique of multiple valve replacement with biological valves: A new option. J Heart Valve Dis 4:
4. Kumar N, Gallo R, Al-Halees Z, Al-Fadley F, Duran CMG (1995) Unstented semilunar homograft replacement of tricuspid valve in Ebstein's malformation. Ann Thorac Surg 59: 320–2
5. Kumar AS, Trehan H (1994) Homograft mitral valve replacement. A case report. J Heart Valve Dis 3: 473–5
6. Lower RR, Stofer RC, Shumway NE (1961) Total excision of the mitral valve and replacement with autologous pulmonic valve. J Thorac and CV Surg 42(5): 696–702
7. McKenzie MB, Pappas G, Titus JL, Ellis FH (1966) Replacement of canine mitral valve with preserved homologous aortic valves. J Thorac Cardiovasc Surg 52: 855–62
8. Metras D (1995) Allogreffes et autogreffes valvulaire cardiagues. Conservation et Chirurgie, Masson, Paris
9. Murray G, Roschau W (1956) Homologous aortic valve segment transplants as surgical treatment for aortic and mitral insufficiency. Angiology 7: 466–71
10. Murray G (1960) Aortic valve transplants. Angiology 11: 99–102
11. McKay R, Sono J, Arnold RM (1988) Tricuspid valve replacement using an unstented pulmonary homograft. Ann Thor Surg 46: 58–62
12. Pappas G, Titus JL, Berchuis J, McKenzie MB, Ellis FH Jr (1966) Dog mitral valve homografts and heterografts. Surg Forum 17: 175–6
13. Rastelli GC, Titus JL (1968) Pulmonary and mitral heterografts. Int'l Coll of Angiology, Geneva Switzerland 23–8
14. Ross DN (1967) Replacement of aortic and mitral valves with a pulmonary autograft. Lancet 2: 956–8
15. Ross DN (1972) Biologic valves. Their performance and prospects. Circulation 45: 1259–72
16. Senoo A, Ohishi K, Nawa S, Teramoto S, Sunada T (1976) Total correction of Ebstein's anomaly by replacement with a biological aortic valve without plication of the atrialized ventricle. J Thorac Cardiovasc Surg 72: 243–8
17. Suzuki A, Kay EB (1966) A new technique of mitral valve replacement with a homologous aortic valve. Japanese Circulation J 30: 1193–1203
18. Willman VL, Zafiracopoulos P, Hanlon CR (1961) Replacement of the mitral valve with homograft aortic valve. In: Merendino KA (ed) Prosthetic Valve for Cardiac Surgery. Springfield, Ill. Charles C. Thomas, Publisher, pp 142–8
19. Yacoub MH, Kittle CF (1970) Measurement of the physical properties of valve homografts. Proc Roy Soc Med 63: 994–5
20. Yacoub M, Towers M, Sommerville W (1972) Results of mitral valve replacement using unstented fresh semilunar valve homografts. Circulation 14(Suppl I): 44–50
21. Yankah AC, Hetzer R, Miller DC, Ross DN, Somerville J, Yacoub MH (eds) (1988) Cardiac Valve Allografts 1962–1987: Current Concepts on the Use of Aortic and Pulmonary Allografts for Heart Valve Substitutes. Springer-Verlag, New York

Author's address:
F. Robicsek MD
Surgeon-in-Chief
The Sanger Clinic, PA
1001 Blythe Boulevard,
Suite 300
Charlotte, NC 28203
U.S.A.

Mitral valve homograft

C. Acar

Department of Cardiovascular Surgery, Hopital Bichat, Paris, France

Introduction

The replacement of the mitral valve with a homograft was one of the first operations conceived in the development of valvular surgery. The use of a semilunar valve homograft in mitral position did not provide satisfactory results (24, 31). The theoretical advantages of the mitral valve homograft are multiple (7): homologous tissue has been shown to remain viable and its longevity is probably superior to that of heterologous glutaraldehyde treated tissue. It is a biological material and does not require anticoagulation. In this method of mitral valve replacement the subvalvular apparatus is preserved, thus retaining its important role in ventricular function. Hence, mitral homograft constitutes the logical limit of mitral valve reconstruction (11).

Experimental studies

The first experiments with orthotopic heart valve transplantation were done in 1951 by Robicsek who transferred the tricuspid valve apparatus from the heart of one dog into another (23).

In the early 1960s, the transplantation of the mitral valve was the subject of a number of animal studies (Bernhard (6), Cachera (8), Hubka (14), O'Brien (19), Rasteli (21) and Van Vliet (30)). The technique of implantation was variable. In most cases, the recipient papillary muscles were divided at their base and the graft papillary muscle was inserted end-to-end using pledgets. In a recent study by Vetter (28), the suture was reinforced with Goretex or pericardium.

Most authors recommended to perform papillary muscle fixation as a first step. Nervertheless, Berghuis et al. advised to initially attach the leaflet tissue to the annulus in order to allow determination of the appropriate site of implantation of the papillary muscles on the ventricular wall (5).

None of these technique of mitral homograft implantation appeared to be safe and reproducible. Early valve failure was demonstrated in a large number of cases. However, some animals survived with a good valvular function and were followed for a period of up to 3 years (19, 30). Histological studies in survivors allowed to assess the healing process of the mitral homograft with time (Fig. 1).

It has been interesting to observe the rapidity with which the papillary muscle remained strongly attached to the ventricular myocardium (5, 22). The papillary muscles of the homograft were unavoidably subjected to several hours of ischaemia immediately after retrieval, and subsequently underwent significant stress during the preservation process. It would have been delusive to expect any viability of the grafted papillary muscle.

Histological studies in transplanted valves in animals showed that the muscular portion of the graft promptly suffered ischemic necrosis and replacement by fibrotic tissue derived from adjacent host tissue (5, 14, 22). Papillary muscle attachment was reasonably advanced at 3 weeks (5, 14). Dense scar tissue was present 6 months following implantation and sporadic areas of viable myocardium most likely corresponded to remnants of the native papillary muscle (Fig. 1).

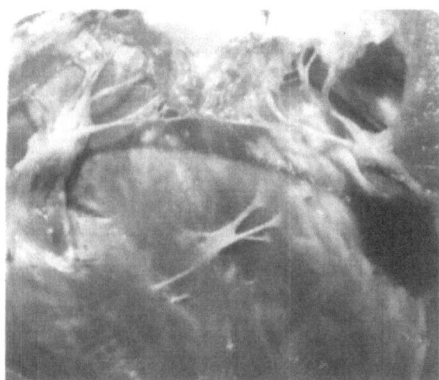

Fig. 1. Mitral homograft 12 months after implantation in a goat. Note normal leaflet tissue and cordae with partial fibrosis of papillary muscles.

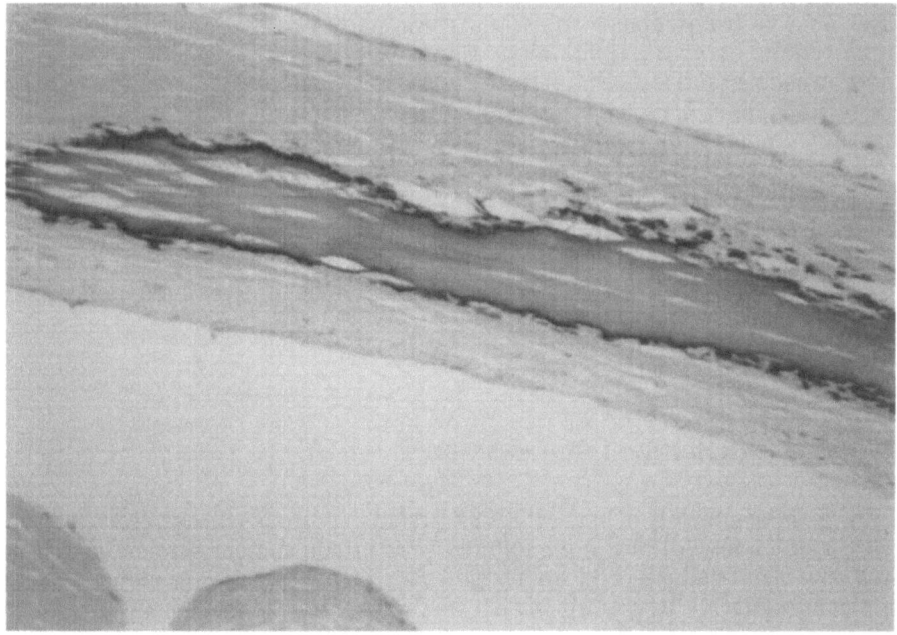

Fig. 2. Calcification of a chordae tendinae fixed with glutaraldehyde 8 months after implantation.

The appearance of the leaflets and chordae varied according to the mode of preservation. Tamura et al. showed that fixation with formaldehyde as well as glutaraldehyde resulted in early valve calcification (27).

This observation was confirmed by our finding in an experimental study in which eight goats underwent a homograft replacement of the mitral valve. The papillary muscles of the graft were selectively treated by immersion into glutaraldehyde for 40 min with the aim to facilitate their insertion. After 6 months, calcifications involving the chordae at their attachment on the papillary muscle were noted (Fig. 2). Consequently, glutaraldehyde fixation of the papillary muscles which had been used in the clinical series for the first patients was subsequently abandoned.

In contrast, antibiotic preservation as well as cryopreservation allowed structural integrity of the valve (22). Interestingly, mitral homografts explanted early were completely acellular. After 1 year, viable endothelial cells and connective tissue fibroblasts were observed (22). As for aortic homografts, cryopreservation, which permits a better availability, appears to be the preservation method of choice for mitral homografts.

Clinical background

In 1965, Senning performed the first mitral homograft in a patient (25). Mitral homografts were used to replace either the mitral or the tricuspid valve in 11 cases. The papillary muscles were buried in a trench created in the recipient muscles. Early valve failure occurred and all patients were reoperated within 3 years.

A few years later at the University of Kiel, Bernhard used an antibiotic preserved mitral homograft in three cases for mitral valve replacement. The technique of papillary muscle insertion was modified using a transmural suture through the ventricular wall (transpapillary muscle extracardiac epicardial fixation (26)). Early chordal rupture occurred within the first postoperative year due either to technical error or to endocarditis (32). One patient had a stable result for 4 years until rupture of the scarred papillary muscle occurred, requiring reoperation (32).

Recently, Pomar et al. reported their experience with the use of mitral homograft for tricuspid valve endocarditis in three drug addict patients (20). Stimulated by this experience, we decided to apply general principles established by Carpentier for mitral valve reconstruction (9) to the use of homograft for mitral valve replacement. In 1992, a cryopreserved mitral homograft was successfully inserted in a patient with calcified rheumatic stenosis (1). Since then, we have reevaluated the use of either partial or total mitral homograft replacement in 45 patients (2–4).

Homograft procurement and storage

In France, the availability of homografts harvested in postmortem donors is poor due to legal restrictions. All mitral homografts were obtained from beating hearts: the valves were harvested either in brain-dead patients considered unsuitable as heart donor or in recipient's hearts explanted at the time of transplantation (4). The mitral valve of transplant recipients was collected as a homograft provided that it was anatomically normal. Ischemic heart disease was not considered as a contraindication for valve storage even in case of associated mitral valve regurgitation secondary to annular dilatation. The presence of a fibrotic papillary muscle due to previous infarction would even facilitate graft insertion.

The entire mitral valve apparatus was dissected free including both the attachment of the papillary muscles onto the ventricular wall and the myocardium surrounding the mitral annulus. Care was taken in dissection of the aorto-mitral triangular area to ensure that an aortic homograft could also be harvested. This dissection was performed in a sterile theatre. Cryopreservation was performed within 18 h of retrieval of the homograft in the Tissue Bank of Hospital St. Louis. A preservative solution containing 5% dimethyl sulfoxide without antibiotics was used and the temperature was gradually decreased using vapourised nitrogen to $-150\,^{\circ}$C. The homograft was stored in nitrogen until its use.

Categorization of the papillary muscles

The shape of the papillary muscles is highly variable and has been described by Victor in figurative language as conical, grooved, wavy, saucerized, stepped, interlinked, two-tiered, arched, v-shaped and so-on (29). At first glance, they appear as random formations escaping any categorization. However, close intra-operative observations have revealed the existence of anatomical patterns as well as insertional modalities that reappear regularly.

Careful examination of the anatomy of the papillary muscles in 68 hearts confirmed our clinical perception of the existence of a correspondence between the papillary muscle division and the chordae's mode of attachment to the leaflets. We thus established a classification irrespective of the shape which takes only into account the existence of a dividing plane and the relationship between the papillary muscle and the leaflets (14). Four types of increasing complexity were distinguished (Fig. 3):

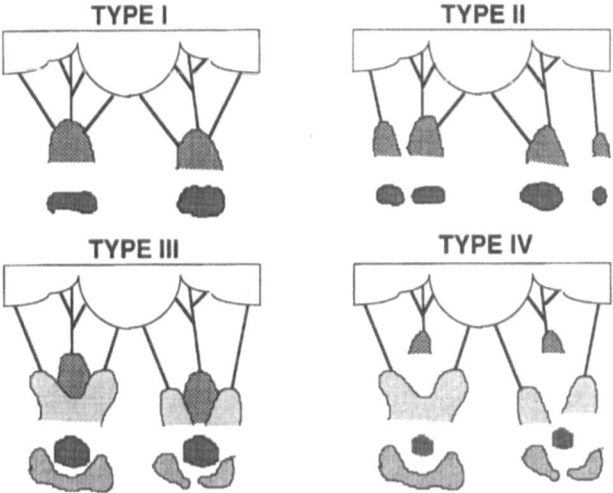

Fig. 3. Morphological classification of papillary muscles (cross-sectional views are shown below the main diagram).

Type I – The P.M. is undivided. It gives rise to all chordae tendineae which fan out to the corresponding hemivalves. Type I is the most common presentation and accounts for 63% of the antero-lateral and 41% of the postero-medial muscle (Fig. 4A).

Type II – The P.M. is divided in a sagittal plane into two heads. One head supports exclusively the posterior leaflet. The other is related to commissural region and to the anterior leaflet. This type is observed in 7% of the antero-lateral and in 39% of the posteromedial P.M. (Fig. 4B).

Type III – The P.M. is divided in a coronal plane into two or more heads. A single head relates exclusively to the commissural zone. The remaining heads support the chordae to the anterior and to the posterior leaflets. The different heads originate from the same level on the ventricular wall. The proportions are 15% for the anterolateral and 7% for the posteromedial P.M. (Fig. 4C).

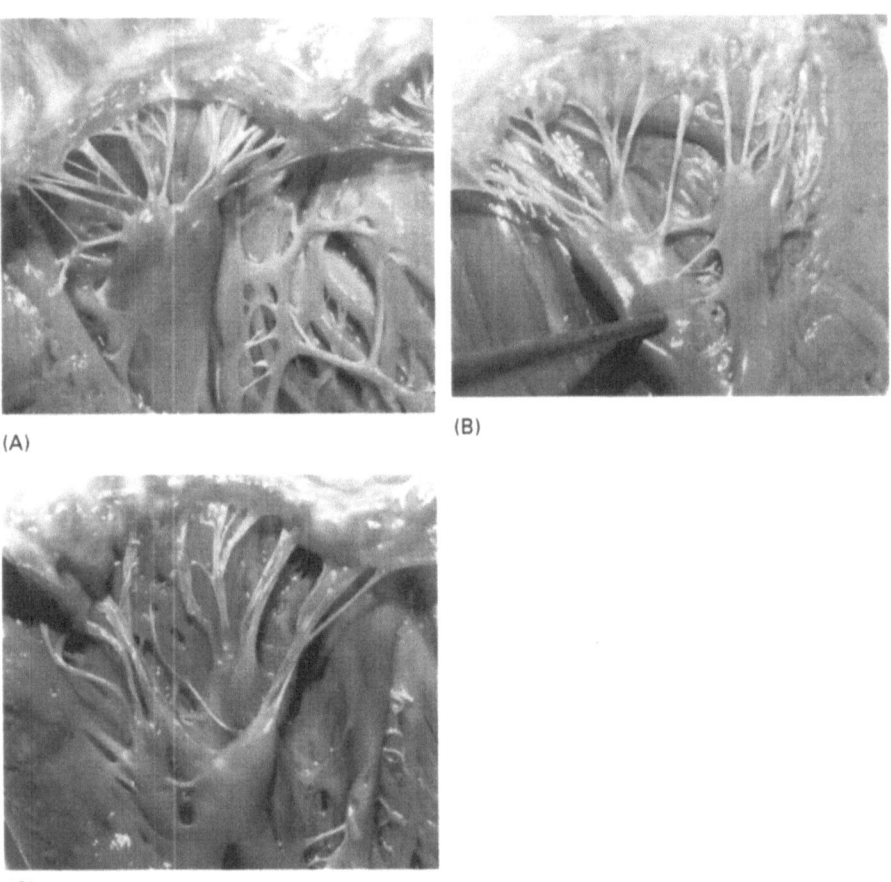

(A)

(B)

(C)

Fig. 4. A) Type I: Simple, single muscle. B) Type II: Division in the sagittal plane forming an individual head supporting the posterior leaflet (arrow). C) Type III: Division in the coronal plane forming an individual head supporting a commissure (arrow). D) and E) Type IV: Divisions with multiple levels of origin from the ventricular wall. Short commisssural cordae inserted on an isolated muscular band, the remaining head originates at a lower level on the ventricle (arrow).

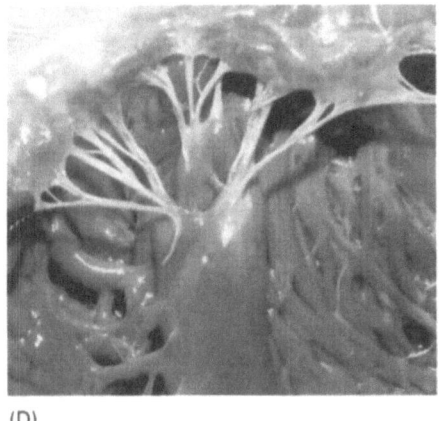

(D)

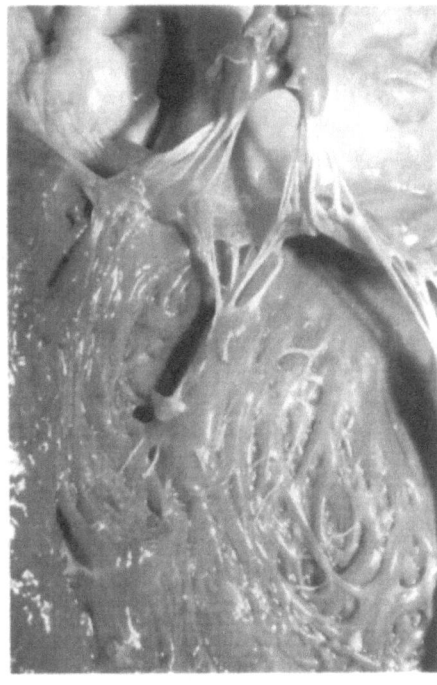

Fig. 4(D) and (E).   (E)

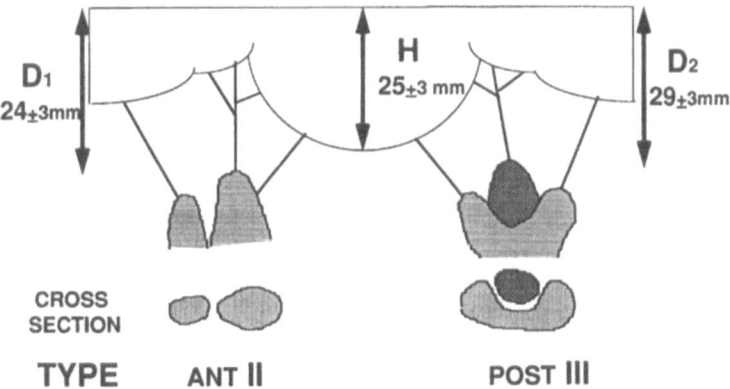

Fig. 5. Identification card with mean dimensions of 68 mitral homografts: height of the anterior leaflet: 25 mm distance between annulus and papillary muscle (anterior 24 mm: and posterior: 29 mm), schematic representation of papillary muscles cross-section and morphological type of papillary muscles.

Type IV – The P.M. is complex and is characterized by division in a coronal plane and by staged origin of the different heads. One tiny muscular band close to the annulus gives insertion to commissural chordae. As a result, the latter are invariably short. The rest of the P.M., which may be single or divided, is located at a lower level on the ventricular wall and supports the rest of the leaflet. This type represents 15% of the anterolateral and in 13% of the posteromedial P.M. (Fig. 4D and E).

Intermediate cases exist, of course, in which one may hesitate between types II and III or between III and IV. However, by following the guidelines described, one can always classify an apparently ambiguous form.

Type I is easy to handle as well as types II and III, as long as the orientation of the separate heads are preserved. Type IV, however, raises important technical difficulties and should be discarded. The morphological type of each papillary muscle should be indicated on the homograft identification card in order to help the surgeon to be more specific about his choice (Fig. 5).

Valve sizing and graft selection

Whereas the cylindrical form of the aortic valve allows its size to be measured by the transverse diameter of the orifice as the sole measurement, the evaluation of the dimensions of the mitral valve is more difficult. Both the extent of valvular leaflet tissue and that of the subvalvular apparatus must be taken into consideration.

In our series the measurement chosen to size the leaflet tissue of the valve was the height of the anterior leaflet tissue in its mid-portion (Fig. 2). This measurement was obtained in the recipient by transoesophageal echocardiography using a sagittal section of the mitral orifice passing through the papillary muscles and aortic orifice (10, 17) (Fig. 6). The height of the leaflet was measured in the open position (diastole) so as to clearly identify the free edge of the valve. The same parameter was obtained for the homograft by direct measurement of the valve (Fig. 5).

Assessment of the dimensions of the subvalvular apparatus raised a difficult issue. At first, it was thought that easily identifiable cordae, as commissural or main cordae, would serve as a reference. However, due to the pathological process, the cordae might have lengthened as in degenerative processes or shortened as in rheumatic disease. For these reasons, it did not seem appropriate to evaluate the subvalvular apparatus with a view to homograft implantation using length of the cordae as a standard.

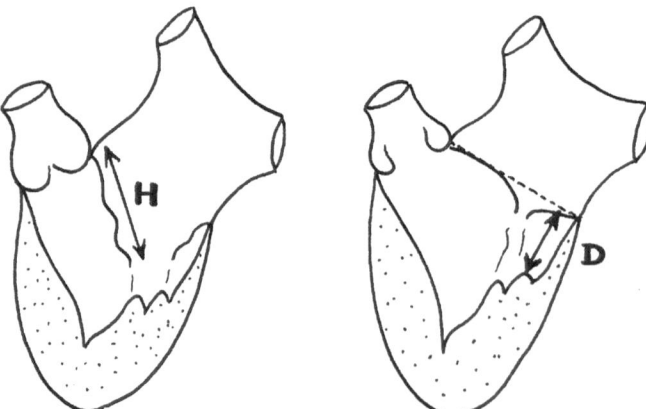

Fig. 6. Echocardiographic measurements of the valve using a sagittal view (aortic valve and papillary muscle were visible). Height of the anterior leaflet (H) was measured in diastole. In systole, the distance (D) between annulus and papillary muscle was measured.

A good estimate of the size of the subvalvular apparatus could be obtained by measuring the distance between the annulus and the apex of the papillary muscle (Fig. 6). This parameter is not directly affected by any pathological process involving the valve. It has the advantage of taking into consideration ventricular dilatation if present, which would indicate the need for a larger homograft. This parameter can be obtained using both direct measurement of the homograft and echocardiographic study of the patient's valve (Figs. 5 and 6).

The identification card of the mitral homograft included the different measurements (height of the anterior leaflet, distance between papillary muscles and annulus) whose mean values are shown in Fig. 5. In order to obtain an optimal sizing, echocardiographic measurements of the valve were matched with those of the identification card of the homograft. A homograft 3 millimeters larger than the valve was selected to provide slight excess tissue and offer a large surface of coaptation.

Surgical technique

Preparation of the graft

The homograft was prepared before cardiopulmonary bypass was instituted. The homograft was thawed in the operating room at 40 °C and then rinsed in successive baths of saline containing decreasing concentrations of DMSO (Fig. 7). Firstly, the ventricular muscle inserted to the annulus of the valve was dissected off without traumatising the valve tissue, particularly the commissural areas. Then the wall of the left atrium attached to the annulus was excised. The connective tissue of the right and left trigones which were frequently the site of a fibrocalcareous nodule was trimmed. Finally, the fatty tissue in the atrio-ventricular junction was removed.

Before preparing the papillary muscles their morphology was examined and noted to ensure that the orientation would be maintained at the time of implantation. In cases of divided papillary muscles, sutures were placed in order to preserve the respective positions of the different heads. Each papillary muscle was detached from its insertion into the ventricular wall leaving approximately 15 mm of muscular tissue beyond the origin of the cordae. The valve was then placed in a container of saline until its use (Fig. 8).

Myocardial protection was achieved using cold cardioplegia injected into the aortic root. The left atrium was approached via the classical parallel incision in the inter-atrial sulcus. The mitral valve was inspected to assess the pathological process and to decide which operative technique would be necessary. In the presence of an isolated lesion affecting less than half of the valve (calcification or valvular abscess) a partial homograft was inserted provided that the remainder of the valve was normal. On the other hand, in the presence of extensive lesions involving the entire valve, total homograft replacement was performed.

Fixation of the papillary muscles

Firstly, the pathological valve tissue was excised and the relevant cordae divided at their insertion. Contrary to various methods described in the literature (20, 25, 26) which use an end-to-end fixation of homograft to native papillary muscles, we have

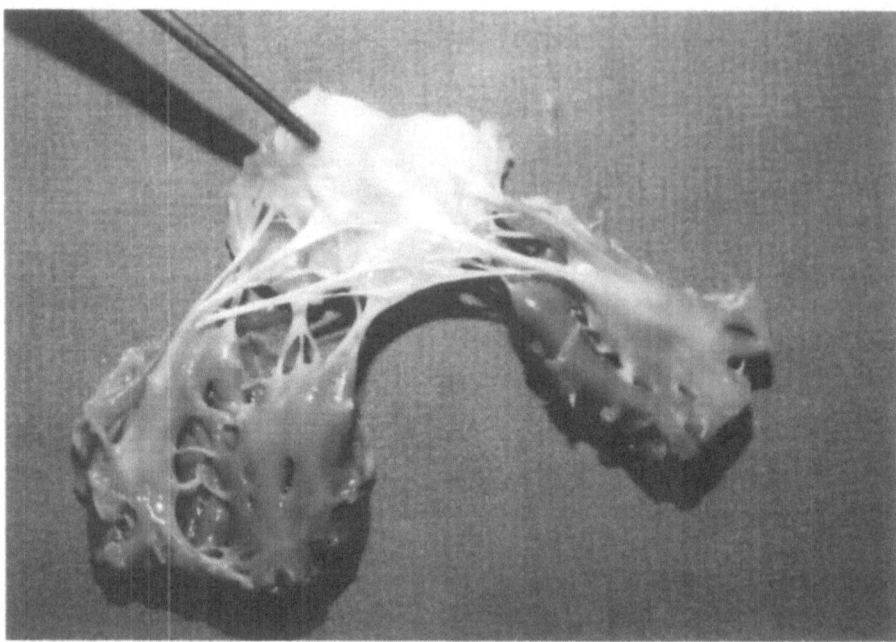

Fig. 7. Mitral homograft following retrieval including myocardium attached to the annulus and to the papillary muscles.

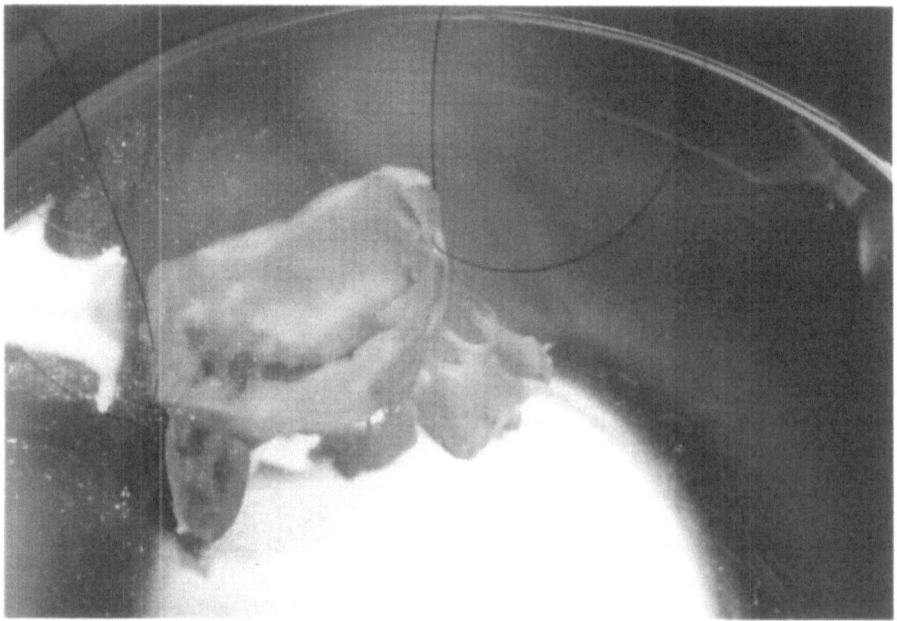

Fig. 8. Mitral homograft immediately before implantation.

adopted a different approach using a side-to-side suture of the papillary muscles (1, 4). The papillary muscle of the recipient was not amputated so that the maximum amount of viable myocardium remained to support the homograft. These were mobilised by dividing the muscular bands attaching them to the ventricular wall. The homograft implantation was then commenced by fixation of the papillary muscles starting with the posterior one. The exposure of the recipient papillary muscle was optimised by applying gentle traction on a stay-suture placed at this level. Each homograft papillary muscle was inserted into the slit between the native papillary muscle and the wall of the left ventricle. Great care was taken to maintain the respective positions of the different heads to obtain an even distribution of traction on the leaflet tissue. The head supporting the commissure was used as a reference point and was positioned at the corresponding site on the native papillary muscle. This site was easily identified since the commissural cordae invariably originate from the apex of the papillary muscle.

As a general rule the papillary muscle of the homograft was sutured side-to-side at a slightly lower level on the recipient. A double row of sutures was used to implant the papillary muscle. Firstly, several mattress sutures were placed at the base of the graft papillary muscle; secondly, multiple interrupted sutures around the margins of the graft and then the apex were used to attach it firmly to the native papillary muscle. The sutures were placed so as not to interfere with the origin of the cordae as this could eventually lead to cordal erosion. At the level of emergence of the cords the problem was avoided by using sutures in a vertical mattress pattern.

No material was used to reinforce the suture whether prosthetic (Teflon or PTFE) (15, 16, 26, 28) or biological (pericardium) (28). Based on experience acquired through the technique of cordal shortening described by Carpentier (9), it is our belief that the use of foreign material at the point of origin of the cords can weaken their insertion and induces an appreciable risk of cordal erosion and rupture. This opinion is further corroborated by the experience with Biocor mitral bioprostheses in which papillary muscles were carefully prepared using prosthetic material and occasionally underwent early chordal rupture at their site of insertion on the papillary muscle (18).

The reliability of the technique of implantation used in this study relies on the healing process of the papillary muscles with progressive replacement with fibrotic tissue (Fig. 1). This method contrasts with a purely mechanical approach using interposition of prosthetic material and/or transfixing stitches through the ventricular wall to counteract the physical stress.

Fixation of the leaflet tissue and ring annuloplasty

The homograft leaflet tissue was then sutured circumferentially to the mitral annulus using continuous 5/0 prolene. The various portions of the valve were attached in the following order: 1) posteromedial commissure, 2) anterior leaflet, 3) anterolateral commissure and 4) posterior leaflet. Particular attention was taken in positioning the commissures and the suture was effected without tension in the areas of the anterior leaflet and commissures. In cases of excess or deficient homograft leaflet tissue with respect to the mitral annulus the suturing style was modified to achieve equilibration while attaching the posterior leaflet.

Ring annuloplasty was systematically performed in all cases of mitral homograft (4). The sutures for the annuloplasty ring were placed before the valve leaflet tissue was attached. The size of annuloplasty ring was chosen according to the size of the anterior leaflet of the homograft measured with an obturator. The use of an annuloplasty ring provides many advantages: 1) it permits precise adaptation of the size of the annulus to that of the homograft, 2) the semi-rigid structure of the ring absorbs some of the mechanical stress exerted by ventricular contraction and alleviates traction that would otherwise be directly applied on the valvular suture line, and 3) ring annuloplasty allows a greater surface of leaflet coaptation thereby lowering the tension on the subvalvular apparatus. The slight overcorrection achieved by annuloplasty may compensate for imperfections in the regulation of tension of the cordae.

After completion of the placement of the homograft the final result was evaluated by infusion of saline under pressure into the ventricle.

Partial mitral homograft

The idea to partially replace the mitral valve with a portion of homograft is not new. In 1964, Cachera introduced the concept of partial homograft replacement (8). He studied varied techniques of mitral valvuloplasty: 1) grafting of a patch of homologous leaflet tissue, 2) replacement of the entire anterior leaflet with its subvalvular apparatus using the corresponding portion of a homograft, and 3) total homograft replacement (8). More recently, Revuelta, in a study using an animal model and scanning electron microscopy, has demonstrated the perfect integration of a partial homograft when placed amidst native mitral tissue (22).

Use of a partial mitral homograft should be considered as part of the wide range of techniques of mitral valve repair. It is technically feasible to reconstitute a portion of mitral valve leaflet tissue using biological material (autologous pericardium), and it is also possible to replace several cordae either using cordal transposition or prosthetic cordae (9, 12). However, the presence of a voluminous pathological process which

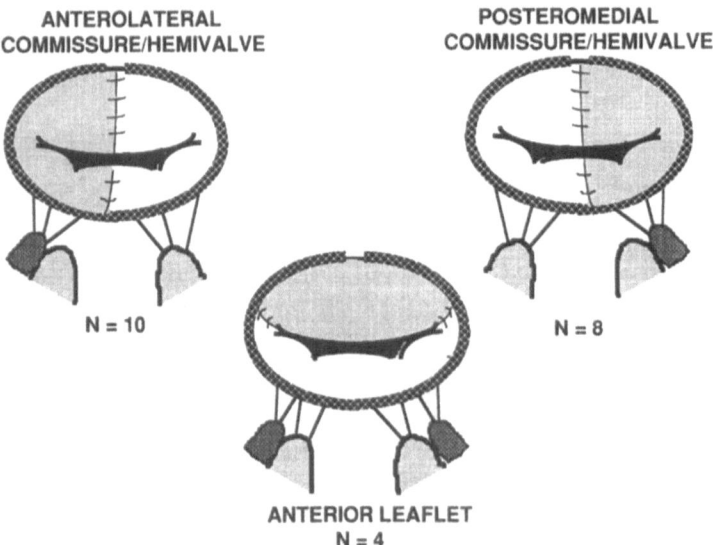

Fig. 9. Sites of partial homograft

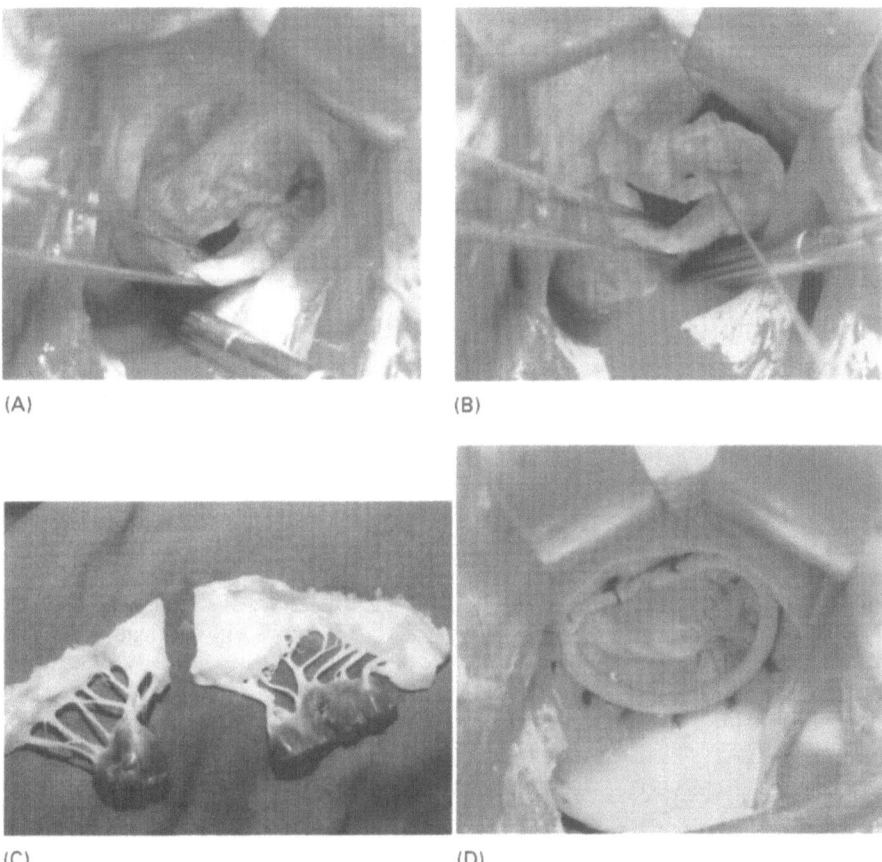

Fig. 10. Partial mitral homograft implantation for calcific mitral stenosis: A) Localised calcification affecting the posterior commisure. B) Resection of the calcification with the underlying cordae. C) Partial mitral homograft showing the commissure with adjacent portions of leaflets and subvalvular apparatus (arrow). D) Result following reconstruction with partial homograft and annuloplasty.

affects both leaflet tissue and cordae, especially when involving a commissural region, represents a serious limitation to valve reconstruction. This situation is met most frequently in two conditions, mitral stenosis with calcification and acute bacterial endocarditis with localised abscess formation and vegetations. The remainder of the valve must be normal since a pathological remnant may lead to a mediocre result (4).

Technically, it seems preferable to divide the valve vertically with the aim of replacing a commissural region or a hemi-valve (Figs. 9 and 10), rather than dividing the valve along the horizontal axis and achieving replacement of an entire leaflet. A vertical division allows selective replacement of 25 to 50% of the valve according to the extent of the lesion. A distinct advantage is that only one papillary muscle needs to be reimplanted (Fig. 9). Also, valvular closure results from coaptation between two leaflets of the same origin belonging either to the homograft or to the native valve.

Transplantation of an entire leaflet does not appear to be a fully satisfactory procedure and presents certain drawbacks. Both papillary muscles must be reimplanted and exposure is made more difficult by the presence of the opposing leaflet and its cords. Afterwards, the presence of a suture line in the region of the commissures can potentially impair the opening of the valve. Furthermore, valve closure results from apposition between the homograft and the opposite native leaflet and the mildest asymmetry in cordal tension may lead to relative prolapse (Fig. 9). Although none of the patients having undergone this type of repair have required reoperation, we no longer recommend its use. In the presence of lesions invading a whole leaflet, total replacement of the mitral valve is accomplished.

Patient population

Indications

Since 1992, forty-five patients aged 10 to 69 years (mean age 34 ± 5) underwent partial ($n = 22$), or total ($n = 23$) mitral valve replacement with a cryopreserved homograft. The indications for operation were either rheumatic mitral stenosis on acute infective endocarditis.

In the cases of acute bacterial endocarditis, the indication for surgery was haemodynamic instability with severe mitral insufficiency, systemic emboli, large mobile vegetations viewed at echocardiography, and persistent septicaemia despite maximal antibiotic therapy. Operations were performed within 1 week of antibiotic therapy. Most patients were in sinus rhythm and half of the patients undergoing total homograft insertion were repeat operations.

Results

There were two early deaths due to severe biventricular failure despite normally functioning homografts. These patients had severe preoperative contractile dysfunction and had undergone multiple reoperations.

One elderly patient required an early reoperation at 10 days. This patient had a staphylococcal bacterial endocarditis on a Starr Edwards mitral prosthesis. Initial echocardiography was satisfactory, but a rapid deterioration occurred at 10 days, requiring reoperation. There was a dehiscence of the homograft at the suture-line attaching the leaflet tissue to the annulus in the region of the anterior commissure, probably due to excess traction on the cords. Following reoperation, the patient made a subsequent uneventful recovery. In general, the insertion of a mitral homograft for replacement of a prosthetic valve has not been satisfactory (one death and one early reoperation). All other patients had uneventful postoperative courses.

All patients were reviewed after a follow-up of up to 3 years. One patient who had undergone partial homograft replacement for an aseptic endocarditis with an inflammatory syndrome that appeared to be related to advanced lung carcinoma died 5 months later.

One patient with partial homograft replacement required reoperation at 22 months. Echocardiography demonstrated residual mitral stenosis. At reoperation the native valve leaflet and cords were found to be fibrotic and the valve was replaced. All 40 remaining patients had normal functional status, NYHA I or II and most of them were in sinus rhythm with no medical treatment.

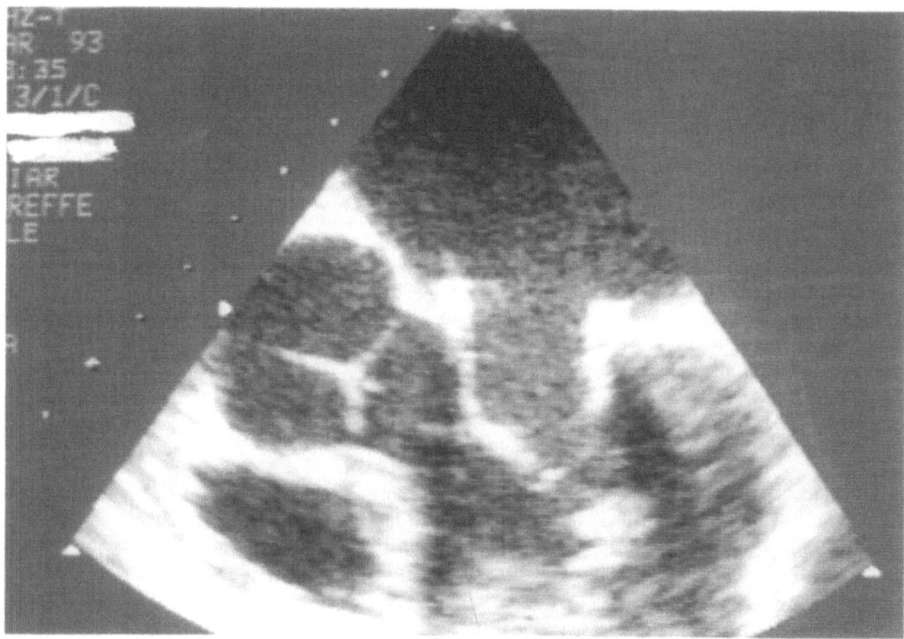

Fig. 11. Transoesophageal echocardiography at 12 months: satisfactory opening of the mitral homograft in diastole.

Echocardiography at a mean follow-up of 17 months revealed stable results when compared to intraoperative echocardiography (Fig. 11). There was no case with moderate or severe insufficiency. The transvalvular gradient was 3 ± 4 mmHg and the surface valve area measured by planimetry was 2.5 cm^2.

References

1. Acar C, Farge A, Ramsheyi A, Chachques JC, Mihaileanu S, Gouezo R, Gerota J, Carpentier A (1994) Mitral valve replacement using a cryopreserved mitral homograft. Ann Thor Surg 57: 746–8
2. Acar C, Gaer J, Chauvaud S, Carpentier A (1995) Technique of homograft replacement of the mitral valve. J Heart Valve Dis 4: 31–4
3. Acar C, Iung B, Cormier B, Grare P, Berrebi A, D'Attelis N, Acar J, Carpentier A (1994) Double mitral homograft for recurrent bacterial endocarditis of the tricuspid and mitral valves. J Heart Valve Dis 3: 470–2
4. Acar C, Tolan M, Berrebi A, Gaer J, Gouezo R, Marchix T, Gerota J, Chauvaud S, Fabiani JN, Deloche A, Carpentier A (1996) Homograft replacement of the mitral valve: graft selection, technique of implantation and results in forty-three patients. J Thorac Cardiovasc Surg 111: 367–80
5. Berghuis J, Rastelli GC, Van Vliet PD, Titus JL, Swan HJ, Henry Ellis F (1964) Homotransplantation of the canine mitral valve. 29: 47–53
6. Bernhard VA, Ringdal R, Babotai I, Linder E, Krayenbuhl HP, Senning A (1965) Zur Homotransplantation der Mitralklappe technik und postoperative funktionelle Resultate Thoraxchirurgie 13: 89–95
7. Bodnar E (1994) Editorial. Clinical use of homologous and heterologous mitral valves. J Heart Valve Dis 3: 468–69
8. Cachera JP, Salvatore L, Hermant J, Herbinet B (1964) Reconstructions plastiques de l'appareil mitral chez le chien au moyen de valves mitrales homologues conservées. Ann Chir Thorac Cardiovasc 3: 459–74

9. Carpentier A, Mitral Valve Repair: The French "Correction" (1983) J Thorac Cardiovasc Surg 86: 323– 37
10. Come PC, Riley MF (1966) M-Mode and cross-sectional echocardiography recognition of fibrosis and calcifications of the mitral valve chordae and left ventricular papillary muscle. Am J Cardiol 1982: 49: 461–85
11. Duran CMG (1995) Editorial. Mitral valve allograft. An opportunity. J Heart Valve Dis 4: 29–30
12. Frater RWM, Vetter HO, Zussa C, Dahm M (1992) Chordal replacement in mitral valve repair. Circulation 82: IV: 125–30
13. Fuzellier JF, Acar C, Jebara V, Grare P, Mihaileanu S, Slama M, Carpentier A (1993) Plasties mitrales au cours de la phase aiguë de l'endocardite. Arch Mal Coeur 86: 197–201
14. Hubka M, Siska K, Brozman M, Holec V (1966) Replacement of mitral and tricuspid valves by mitral homograft. J Thorac Cardiovasc Surg 51: 195–204
15. Kumar AS, Chander H, Trehan H (1995) Surgical technique of multiple valve replacement with biological valves: a new option. J Heart Valve Dis 4: 45–6
16. Kumar AS, Trehan H (1994) Homograft mitral valve replacement – A case report. J Heart Valve Dis 3: 473–5
17. Mihaileanu S, El Asmar B, Lamberti A, Carpentier A (1991) Intraoperative transoesophageal echocardiography after mitral repair-specific conditions and pitfalls. Eur Heart J 12 (Suppl. B): 26–9
18. Morea M, de Paulis R, Galtoni M, Gastaldi L, di Summa M (1994) Mitral Valve Replacement with the Biocor stentless mitral valve: Early results. J Heart Valve Dis 3: 476–82
19. O'Brien MF, Gerbode F (1964) Homotransplantation of the mitral valve: Preliminary experimental report and review of the literature. Austr New Zealand J Surg 34: 81–8
20. Pomar JL, Mestres CA (1993) Tricuspid valve replacement using a mitral homograft: Surgical technique and initial results. J Heart Valve Dis 2: 125–28
21. Rastelli GC, Berghuis J, Swan HJC (1965) Evaluation of function of mitral valve after homotransplantation in the dog. J Thorac Cardiovasc Surg 49: 459–74
22. Revuelta JM, Cagigas JC, Bernal JM, Vaf F, Rabasa JM, Requerica MA (1992) Partial replacement of the mitral valve by homografts: An experimental study. J Thorac Cardiovasc Surg 104: 1274–9
23. Robicsek F, Sanger PW, Taylor FH, Robicsek L (1962) Transplantability of heart valves. Arch Surg 84: 141–8
24. Ross DN (1967) Replacement of the aortic and mitral valves with a pulmonary autograft. Lancet 2: 956
25. Senning A (1968) Rekonstruktion der Mitralklappe: Homoioplastik Thoraxchir Vask Chir 16: 601–5
26. Sievers HH, Lange PE, Yankah AC et al. (1986) Allogeneous transplantation of the mitral valve. An open question. Thorac Cardiovasc Surg 33: 227–29
27. Tamura K, Jones M, Yamada I, Ferrans VJ (1994) A comparison of failure modes of glutaraldehyde-treated versus antibiotic-preserved mitral valve allografts implanted in sheep. J Thorac Cardiovasc Surg 110: 224–38
28. Vetter HO, Dagge A, Liao K, Erhorn A, Chryssagis K, Strenkert C, Reichart B (1995) Mitral allograft with chordal support: Echocardiographic evaluation in sheep. J Heart Valve Dis 4: 35–9
29. Victor S, Nayak VM (1995) Variations in the papillary muscles of the normal mitral valve and their surgical relevance. J Heart Valve Dis 10: 597–607
30. Van Vliet PD, Titus JL, Berghuis J et al. (1965) Morphologic features of homotransplanted canine mitral valves. J Thorac Cardiovasc Surg 49: 504–10
31. Yacoub MH, Kittle C (1969) A new technique for replacement of the mitral valve by a semilunar valve homograft. J Thorac Cardiovasc Surg 58: 859–69
32. Yankah AC, Sievers HH, Lange PE, Bernhard A (1995) Clinical report on stentless mitral allografts. J Heart Valve Dis 4: 40–4

Author's address:
C. Acar, MD
Department of Cardiovascular Surgery
Hopital Bichat
46 rue Henri-Huchard
75018 Paris, France

Mitral valve allografts in the mitral position

J. M. Revuelta, J. M. Bernal

Hospital Universitario Marqués de Valdecilla, Universidad de Cantabria, Santander, Spain

Introduction

Heart transplantation programs have increased the availability of valve allografts, resulting in a resurgence in their use to replace or repair severely diseased valves. Mitral valve allograft was first transplanted in the dog by Robicsek and colleagues (14) in 1962. Two years later, the mitral allograft was experimentally implanted in the mitral position by Cachera et al. (4). However, experimental results with mitral allografts to substitute mitral valves were not satisfactory, as Rastelli et al. (10) demonstrated at the Mayo Clinic. By that time, Hubka et al. (6) trying to replace the atrioventricular valves with mitral allografts obtained unpredictable results. Methods of sterilization and preservation were the main limitations to the use of mitral allografts with this technically demanding operation for valve replacement. Advances on the methods of harvesting, sterilization, preservation and storage of heart valves, for more than three decades, were determinants for the satisfactory clinical results with aortic allografts. Cryopreservation of valve allografts was introduced by O'Brien in Australia, 20 years ago (8, 9), and later with minor modification by Kirklin (7) at the University of Alabama; since then, institutions worldwide have organized heart tissue banks. Most of them have preserved aortic and pulmonary valves, and only a few have experience with mitral allografts.

Experimental study

Since 1988, mitral valve allograft have been used at our University in Santander, in the chronic animal model (12) to repair or replace mitral and tricuspid valves. In order to evaluate the viability and behavior of the mitral allograft, an experimental study was carried out. Mitral allografts were harvested within the first 30 min after death of donor sheep. Twenty-five mitral allografts were prepared by washing them in distilled water and in a modified Hanks solutions, before being introduced in an antibiotic solution (Table 1) at 4 °C, during 24 h. Ten fresh allografts were immersed in a TC-199 culture medium for another 24 h, before surgical implantation. Fifteen allografts were cryopreserved in a controlled-rate liquid nitrogen freezer at -1 °C per min up to -40 °C, and then faster to reach the -196 °C, using 10% dimethylsulfoxide (DMS) as cryoprotectant. After the appropriate sterilization control system the fresh and cryopreserved mitral allografts were ready to be implanted in the recipient animal.

Twenty-five sheep with an average age of 12 months and mean weight of 23.4 kg were used for this study. The heart was exposed through the fourth left intercostal space. Cardiopulmonary bypass was established by cannulation of the femoral artery and a single cannula in the right atrium, the aorta was not crossclamped, no cardioplegic solution was perfused and normothermia was maintained.

The mitral valve was exposed via a wide left atriotomy from the left lower pulmonary vein to the atrial appendage. Partial resection of the anterior leaflet in 20 animals and posterior leaflet in 5, with the subvalvular apparatus was performed. The corresponding portion of the anterior and posterior leaflets and subvalvular apparatus of the mitral allograft was inserted in order to repair the resected valves.

The main technical steps of the mitral valve repair with partial mitral allografts are:

1) The amount of tissue obtained from the allograft should be at least 5 mm wider than the resected leaflet, in order to have enough material to allow adequate suture lines overlapping the native leaflet (Fig. 1). Redundant leaflet should be easily

Table 1. Composition of the antibiotic solution

Cefoxitin	240 mg/ml
Lincomycin	120 mg/ml
Polymyxin B	100 mg/ml
Amphotericin B	25 mg/ml
Vancomycin	50 mg/ml
Modified Hanks solution	
pH	6.8–7.0

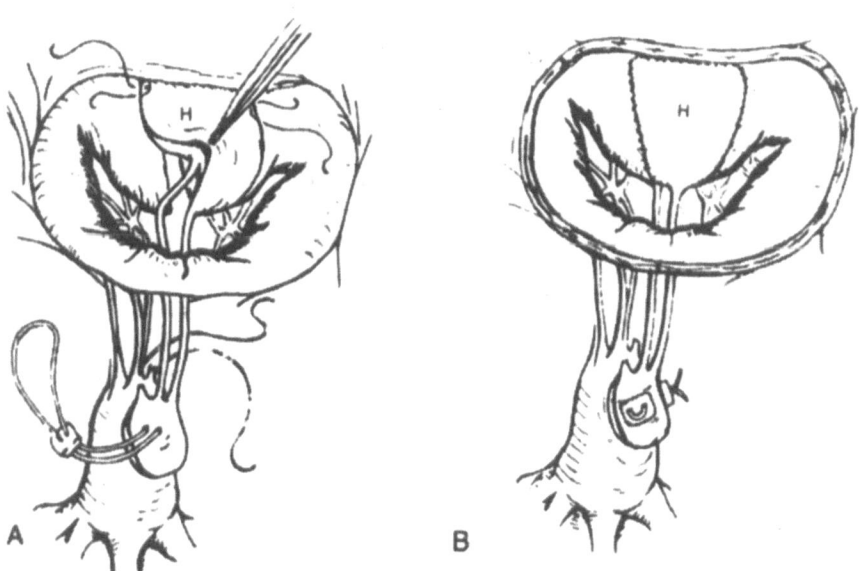

Fig. 1. Partial mitral allograft implanted in the anatomic position. A, A segment of the anterior leaflet and subvalvular apparatus of the mitral valve has been resected and replaced by the corresponding partial allograft (H). B, Implanted mitral allograft (H) with a flexible annuloplasty ring. (By permission of The Journal of Thoracic and Cardiovascular Surgery, Revuelta JM et al., Partial replacement of mitral valve by homograft. 1992; 104: 1274–9).

corrected with an annuloplasty ring, but deficient allograft leaflet resulted in a non-correctable mitral incompetence.

2) The tip of the donor papillary muscle, site of insertion of the chordae tendineae, which is the anatomical area of the greatest strength to support the tension of sutures, is used for the insertion. Lateral areas of papillary muscles are weaker and, consequently, could be the cause of dehiscence of the reimplanted subvalvular apparatus. A doubled armed 3-0 pledget Ticron suture is passed through the tip of the allograft papillary muscle and then through the recipient papillary muscle, with a termino-lateral implantation (Fig. 1). The site of implantation is determined by the appropriate measurement of the adjacent native marginal chordae tendineae.

3) Four 5-0 polypropylene stay sutures are placed on each side of the leaflet at annular and marginal levels, so that maneuvers with the partial mitral allograft are simplified and maintained in the correct position during surgery.

4) The two 5-0 polypropylene stay sutures placed at the free edges of the partial mitral allograft are tied to the corresponding portion of the native leaflet and then run to reach the annulus, and the suture of the annular portion of the allograft is run to complete the allograft implantation.

All cultures obtained at the time of implantation were negative for infection. There have been no instances of late infection in this series. Residual severe mitral insufficiency due to malposition of the subvalvular apparatus of the allograft was the cause of death in three animals during the first 3 months after surgery. Twenty-four animals survived the operation and were electively killed. Mean follow-up was 8 months, ranging 3 to 12 months. Mild to moderate residual mitral incompetence was detected in three animals.

No intracardiac thrombi, signs of endocarditis or degenerative failure were found at macroscopic examination. The mitral allografts were totally incorporated into the recipient leaflet and subvalvular apparatus retaining their original length and flexibility. The tip of donor papillary muscle was completely healed. Chordae tendineae were intact in all specimens (Fig. 2).

Microscopic evaluation revealed the presence of superficial cells from the recipient invading the mitral allograft and connective tissue fibroblasts. These findings were first detected in the mitral allograft, 3 months after implantation, and never described before in "in vivo" studies with the atrioventricular allografts. A sheath of connective tissue around the chordae tendineae in all allografts was observed. Organized dense collagen tissue was detected in all implanted allografts without signs of degeneration. Mitral allograft was completely acellular within the ground substance, with no sign of infiltration of mononuclear cells or of fibroblast necrosis. Fresh and cryopreserved mitral allografts explanted early after implantation were almost acellular. Hematoxylin and eosin stained sections of the cryopreserved allograft showed acid mucopolysaccharide, which appeared to be the precursor of microcalcifications, as Gonzalez-Lavin et al. (5) have already reported.

Transmission electron microscopy showed dense organized collagen fibers with a uniform distribution with rest of fibroblasts. Scanning electron microscopy showed the allograft denuded of endothelial cells, with an ingrowth tissue of superficial cells trying to cover the surface of the allograft (Fig. 3), with organized collagen fibers without cellular infiltration and chordae tendineae re-endothelization in fresh and cryopreserved allografts, 6 months after operation. No cellular component of inflammatory reaction demonstrating evidence of cellular immunologic allograft rejection was found in this experience.

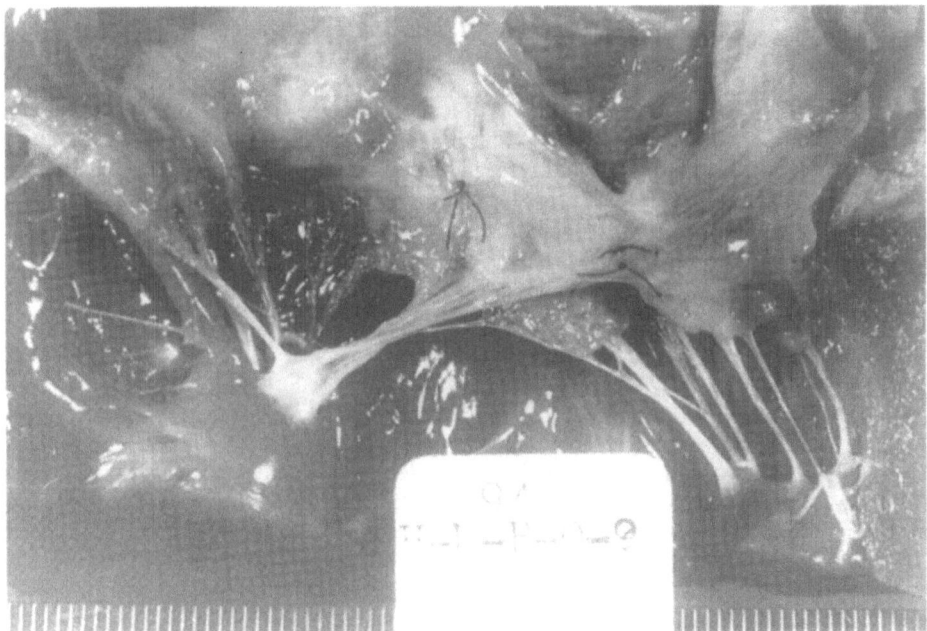

Fig. 2. Specimen of an animal, 9 months after cryopreserved mitral allograft implantation. The graft appears almost like the native mitral valve. (By permission of The Journal of Thoracic and Cardiovascular Surgery, Revuelta JM et al., Partial replacement of mitral valve by homograft. 1992; 104: 1274–9).

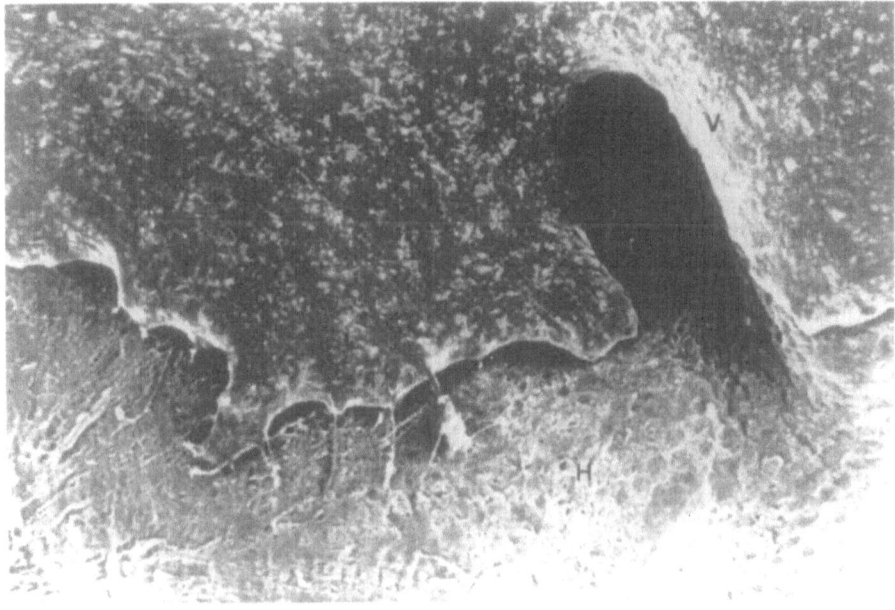

Fig. 3. Scanning electron mircoscopy shows a cryopreserved mitral allograft denuded of endothelial cells with an ingrowth tissue of the viable superficial cells from the recipient. Original magnification 160 × 1.1. (By permission of The Journal of Thoracic and Cardiovascular Surgery, Revuelta JM et al., Partial replacement of mitral valve by homograft. 1992: 104: 1274–9).

Clinical experience

The first successful human implantation of a partial mitral allograft was performed at our institution on May 22, 1992 (11). Since then, mitral allograft has been used either to repair or replace the mitral valve (13). This preliminary experience has resulted in two early failures due to technical errors, 2 and 7 days after partial mitral allograft implantation, requiring prosthetic valve replacement.

Mid-term follow-up

From our clinical experience, three patients have been followed-up a minimum of 24 months (24, 25 and 43 months).

Case 1. A 70-year old man with the diagnosis of bacterial endocarditis 5 years earlier, affected by progressive dyspnea, cardiac failure and mitral valve dysfunction, was studied with echocardiography and cardiac catheterization demonstrating severe mitral regurgitation due to rupture of chordae tendineae of the entire posterior leaflet with giant left atrium and dilated left ventricle. A 15-mm diameter perforation of the posterior leaflet close to the posteromedial commissure with rupture of the contiguous marginal chordae was found at operation. The remaining marginal chordae of the central portion of this leaflet were severely elongated causing massive mitral insufficiency. A cryopreserved mitral allograft was used for partial mitral valve repair. A 5-cm segment of the posterior leaflet was replaced by the corresponding mitral allograft. The papillary muscle of the allograft was sutured to the posterior papillary muscle of the recipient, taking into account the correct length of the native marginal chordae tendineae (Fig. 4). A 31-mm Duran flexible annuloplasty ring was implanted to support this extensive repair. Intraoperative transesophageal echo-Doppler confirmed a satisfactory mitral valve function. Forty-three months after surgery, the patient remains asymptomatic with a mild mitral regurgitation and a normal functioning mitral valve with flexible and intact subvalvular apparatus.

Case 2. A 61-year old woman with the diagnosis of degenerative mitral valve incompetence due to massive rupture of marginal chordae tendineae of the posterior leaflet involving the anterior commissural area. A cryopreserved partial mitral allograft was used to repair the diseased valve. The corresponding segment of the allograft, including the anterior commissure and most of the posterior leaflet, was implanted, suturing the tip of the two papillary muscles (Fig. 5). The repaired valve was supported with a 29 mm Duran flexible annuloplasty ring. Twenty-five months after surgery the patient is symptom-free. Clinical and echocardiographic evaluation shows a competent and normal functioning mitral valve.

Case 3. A 64-year old man with a progressive dyspnea and pulmonary edema, was diagnosed with severe mitral regurgitation with massive prolapse of the posterior leaflet caused by rupture of the marginal chordae tendineae, with left ventricular dilation. At surgery, extensive prolapse of the anterior and posterior leaflets with rupture of the marginal chordae of the posterior leaflet and elongation of marginal chordae of the anterior leaflet, and annular dilatation were found. A cryopreserved mitral allograft, 31 mm in diameter, was used to replace the valve. Each papillary muscle was fixed to the recipient with termino-lateral sutures using 3-0 polypropylene

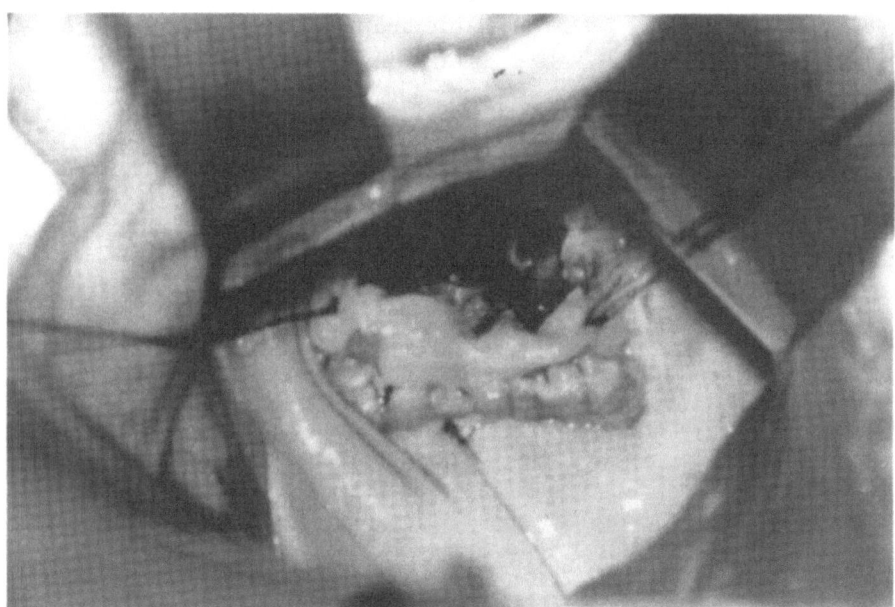

Fig. 4. Operative view of the repaired mitral valve with a partial allograft replacing the posterior leaflet (Case 1).

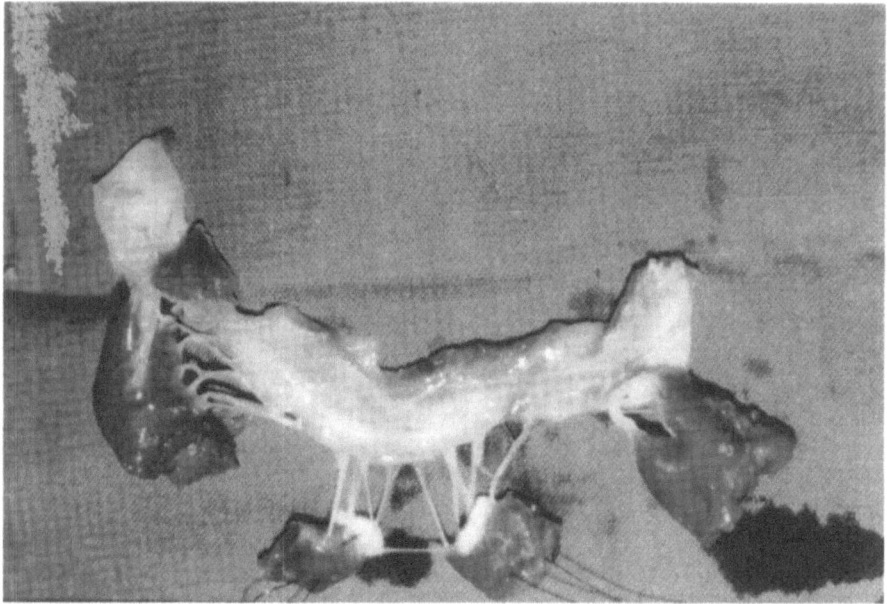

Fig. 5. Partial mitral allograft with both papillary muscles prepared to be implanted (Case 2).

pletged supported stitches. A transvalvular technique for allograft implantation was used, in order to preserve the native subvalvular apparatus (13). A 31-mm flexible annuloplasty ring was implanted. Echocardiographic evaluation 24 months after surgery showed a normal functioning mitral allograft with minimal insufficiency due to anterior leaflet prolapse.

Comments

Soon after cardiopulmonary bypass was available, mitral allograft was experimentally evaluated (4, 10, 14). While aortic allograft is considered to be the best substitute for aortic disease, mitral allograft implantation was eventually abandoned due to unsatisfactory results (8, 15). Encouraged by the results obtained with cryopreserved aortic allografts, a second chance was given at our institution to the mitral allografts for repairing or replacing the atrioventricular valves (3, 11, 12, 13). Recently, the largest clinical experience of partial and total allograft replacement of the mitral valve has been reported by Acar et al. (1, 2) from the Broussais Hospital, with excellent early results.

After these stimulating preliminary experience, a report by Yankah et al. (15) demonstrating a sudden rupture of the scarred graft papillary muscle, 44 months after implantation requiring emergency reoperation, cooled the initial enthusiasm since the stability of the technique is still to be proved. This valuable report has contributed to the necessity of being cautious in the clinical use of the mitral allografts, since the long-term behavior of the implanted subvalvular apparatus currently represents the Achilles heel of this exciting surgery.

References

1. Acar C, Farge A, Ramsheyi A, Chachques JC, Mihaileanu S, Gouezo R, Gerota J, Carpentier A (1994) Mitral valve replacement using a cryopreseved mitral homograft. Ann Thorac Surg 57: 746–748
2. Acar C, Gaer J, Chauvaud S, Carpentier A (1995) Technique of homograft replacement of the mitral valve. J Heart Valve Dis 4: 31–34
3. Bernal JM, Revuelta JM (1995) Mitral valve homografts. J Heart Valve Dis 4: 47–48
4. Cachera JP, Salvatore L, Herbinet B (1964) Reconstructions plastiques de l'appareil mitral chez le chien au moyen de valves mitrales homologues conservees: rapport preliminaire. Ann Chir Thorac Cardiovasc 3: 494–501
5. Gonzalez-Lavin L, Bianchi J, Graf D, Amini S, Gordon CI (1987) Homograft valve calcification: evidence for an immunological influence. In: Yankah AC, Hetzer R, Miller DC, Ross DN, Somerville J, Yocoub MH (eds) Cardiac Valve Allografts 1962–1987. New York: Springer-Verlag, pp 69–75
6. Hubka M, Siska K, Brozman M, Holec V (1966) Replacement of mitral and tricuspid valves by mitral homograft. J Thorac Cardiovasc Surg 51: 195–204.
7. Kirklin JK, Kirklin JW, Pacifico AD, Phillips SJ (1987) Cryopreserved of aortic valve homografts. In: Yankah AC, Hetzer R, Miller DC, Ross DN, Somerville J, Yacoub MH (eds) Cardiac Valve Allografts 1962–1987. New York: Springer Verlag, pp 35–6
8. O'Brien MF, Stafford G, Gardner M, Pohlner P, McGiffin D (1987) A comparison of aortic valve replacement with viable cryopreserved and fresh allograft valves, with a note on chromosomal studies. J Thorac Cardiovasc Surg 94: 812
9. O'Brien MF, Stafford G, Gardner M, Pohlner P, McGiffin D, Johnston N, Brosnan A, Duffy P (1987) The viable cryoperserved allograft aortic valve. J Cardiac Surg 2(Suppl): 153–67

10. Rastelli GC, Berguis J, Swan HJC (1965) Evaluation of the function of the mitral valve after homotransplantation in the dog. J Thorac Cardiovasc Surg 49: 459–462
11. Revuelta JM, Bernal JM, Rabasa JM (1994) Partial homograft replacement of mitral valve. Lancet 334: 514
12. Revuelta JM, Bernal JM, Rabasa JM (1996) Transvalvular technique for implantation of a mitral valve homograft. J Thorac Cardiovasc Surg 11: 281–282.
13. Revuelta JM, Cagigas JC, Bernal JM, Val F, Rabasa JM, Lequerica MA (1992) Partial replacement of mitral valve by homograft. J Thorac Cardiovasc Surg 104: 1274–9
14. Robicsek F, Sanger PW, Taylor FH et al. (1962) Transplantability of heart valves. Arch Surg 84: 150–158
15. Yankah AC, Sievers HH, Lange PE, Bernhard A (1995) Clinical report on stentless mitral allografts. J Heart Valve Dis 4: 40–44

Author's address:
J. M. Revuelta, MD, PhD
Cardiovascular Surgery
Hospital Universitario Valdecilla
39008-Santander, Spain

Immunology and fate of mitral allografts. What are the operative technical options and prerequisites for durability?

A. C. Yankah*, H. H. Sievers**, A. Bernhard

German Heart Institute Berlin*, Depts. of Cardiovasc. Surg., University of Lübeck** and Kiel, Germany

Introduction

There is a renewed interest in the use of mitral allograft for mitral valve replacement in view of achieving better results in patients with destructive endocarditis and avoiding use of anticoagulants and related hemorrhage and thromboembolic complications (1, 2). For a variety of reasons, it appears that there is a controversy on the implantation technique (1, 7) regarding the inevitable incidence of immunologic related complications such as tissue degradation leading to an early or late valve dysfunction (3). Mitral and tricuspid homograft implantation has not been popular because of 1) the complexed implantation technique, 2) the problem of proper valve sizing, and 3) the undefined durability. The third problem and that which seems to be the major concern of cardiac surgeons is how to improve the implantation technique. This report will highlight some factors related to the appearance of postoperative valve dysfunction and how to influence them.

Patients and methods

Our experience is based on immunological studies (3) and clinical implantation of aortic and pulmonary valve allografts, mitral reconstruction, and laboratory experimental work. Three clinical patients aged 43, 64 and 54 years (two females and one male) with mitral stenosis without associated coronary heart or other valvular diseases underwent replacement of mitral valve and its subvalvular apparatus at the Dept. of Cardiovascular Surgery, University of Kiel in 1984 (4, 6, 7).

Valve sizing and selection

After excision of the diseased mitral leaflets and chordae the papillary muscles are left intact in place and the native annulus is measured. The measured annulus size was used as the reference size number for selecting the mitral allograft which will be 2 mm smaller than that of the measured native annulus diameter (Fig. 1). The implantation technique has been described elsewhere (4, 7).

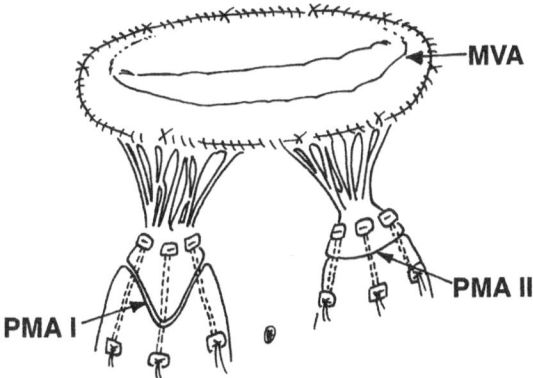

Fig. 1. Different techniques for anastomosing the allograft-recipient papillary muscles to achieve proper chordae-papillary muscle length. In case of malalignment the technique of side-to-side anastomosis described by Acar (3) is useful. (MVA: mitral valve allograft, PM I and PM II: Papillary muscle anastomosis technique I and II). Reproduction by permission (ref. 7).

Results

After uneventful postoperative course acute mitral allograft valve failure developed from chordal rupture which led to reoperation and prosthetic valve replacement of the grafts in two patients 2 and 9 months after the operation while a late graft failure occurred after rupture of a scarred graft papillary muscle 44 months (64 years old) after the operation. All three patients are alive with prosthetic valves.

The histology of the explant at 2 months postoperatively showed signs of immune response by the host. The viable mitral allograft became completely devoid of viable donor cells. Mononuclear cellular infiltrations were seen in the graft (Fig. 2) and were identified by immunohistochemistry to be mainly inflammatory cells in particular macrophages and minority of T-cell of CD-3 subtypes of host origin (Fig. 3). The methods for immunohistochemistry have been described previously (3). On the mitral valve which was explanted 44 months postoperatively re-endothelization by the host was observed which appeared to be ongrowth of host cells per continuitatem from the left atrium. At the graft-host papillary muscle union site fibrocalcification and retraction of the chordae were observed.

Comments

Proper sizing of viable mitral valve allograft, alignment of allograft chordae with the host papillary muscles (5, 7) and the use of HLA-compatible allografts alone or immunosuppression to maintain cellular viability might be the essential factors for

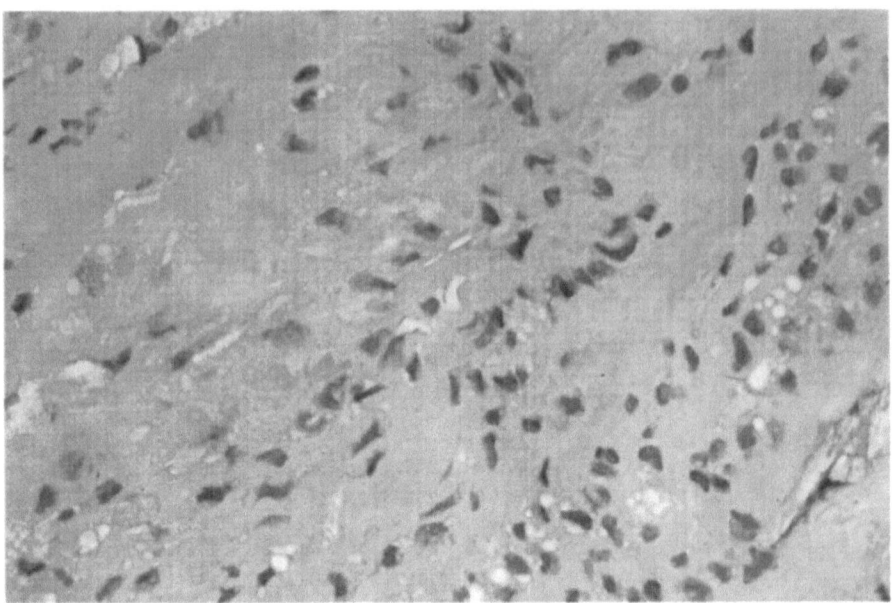

Fig. 2. Granuloma-like dense infiltration of valve tissue with focal collections of inflammatory cells (HE, × 200).

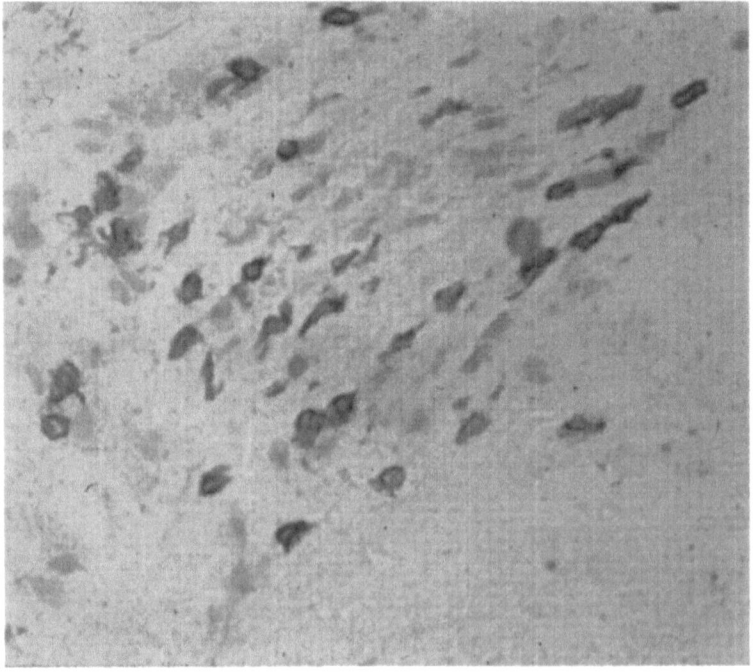

Fig. 3. Demonstration of Pan T-cell antigen CD3, showing a minority of T-lymphocytes (indirect immunoperoxidase, × 200).

improving the long-term durability of mitral valve allografts. The observation of re-endothelization of mitral allograft is encouraging and makes this valve interesting as an alternative valve substitute in a selected group of patients. It needs to be proven whether reinforcement of the chordae might be useful as well as an effective approach for long-term durability.

Conclusion

The results and the findings suggest that intermediate-term performance and durability of mitral homograft can be achieved when the valves are properly sized and positioned to avoide unduly traction, redundancy and malalignment of the chordae. Implantation of an additional supportive annular prosthetic ring to regulate and counterbalance tractional force of the subvalvular apparatus and if necessary reinforcement of the chordae might stabilize the sophisticated functional unit of the mitral valve apparatus. We believe that the durability and performance of non-viable mitral homograft is limited and can only be improved with the above additional procedures including the union site of the graft-host papillary muscles are considered. Maintenance of graft viability will demand immunosuppression of the host but it needs to be proven whether the use of immunosuppression for allovital mitral homografts might improve the durability and performance of mitral homografts.

References

1. Acar C, Farge A, Ramsheyi A, Chachques J-C, Mihaileanu S, Gouezo R, Gerota J, Carpentier A (1994) Mitral valve replacement using a cryopreserved mitral homograft. Ann Thorac Surg 57: 746–48
2. Duran CG (1995) Mitral valve allografts. An opportunity. J Heart Valve Dis 4: 29–30
3. Müller-Hermelink HK, Yankah AC (1987) Immunohistopathology of cardiac valve allograft explants. In: Cardiac valve allografts 1962–1987 (Yankah AC, Hetzer R, Miller DC, Ross DN, Somerville J, Yacoub MH eds.). Steinkopff Verlag, Darmstadt, Springer Verlag, New York, pp 89–94
4. Sievers HH, Lange PE, Yankah AC, Wessel A, Bernhard A (1985) Allogenous transplantation of the mitral valve. An open question. Thorac Cardiovasc Surgeon 33: 227–29
5. Vetter HO, Dagge A, Nerlich A, Liao K, Erhorn A, Brenner P, Chryssagis K, Yoganathan AP, Reichart B (1994) In vitro and in vivo examination of a new design of a stentless chordally supported allograft mitral valve: Preliminary results. In: New horizons and the future of heart bioprostheses. (S. Gabbay, RWM Frater eds.) Silent partners, Inc. Austin, 92–102
6. Yankah AC, Wottge HU, Müller-Hermelink HK, Feller AC, Lange P, Wessel U, Dreyer H, Bernhard A, Müller-Ruchholtz W (1987) Transplantation of aortic and pulmonary allografts, enhanced viability of endothelial cells by cryopreservation. Importance of histocompatibility. J Cardiac Surg 1 (Suppl.): 209–20
7. Yankah AC, Sievers HH, Lange PE, Bernhard A (1995) Clinical report on stentless mitral allografts. J Heart Valve Dis 4: 40–44

Author's address:
A. Charles Yankah, MD, PhD
Consultant, Assistant Professor
Deutsches Herzzentrum Berlin and Humboldt University
Dept. Cardiothoracic and Vascular Surgery
Augustenburger Platz 1
D-13353 Berlin
Germany

Unstented live tricuspid and mitral valve allografts

F. Robicsek

The Sanger Clinic, Charlotte, North Carolina, USA

"Fiascos should not serve as deterrent – only previous experience from which lessons may be learned." Endre Bodnar, 1994

"Durability represents the crux of this procedure."
Carlos M G Duran, 1995

The advantages of mechanical and bioprosthetic atrioventricular valves are well known. It is also recognized, however, that they are in many respects biologically and hemodynamically inferior to the patient's own valvular apparatus.

In vitro results in pulsatile flow chamber show greater effective orifice areas and lower transvalvular pressure gradients in mitral allografts than with commercial bioprostheses of the same diameter (46, 47). Also, even if prosthetic replacement of the tricuspid or mitral valve is done in a "chordae-sparing" fashion, the coordination between the valve apparatus and the ventricular wall is disrupted; thus, the functional entity composed of the annulus, valve and ventricular wall is destroyed (43). Contrary to this, unstented allografts, unlike the other devices, do not only replace the valve but also preserve the function of the subvalvular apparatus – an important factor in preserving left ventricular function following valve replacement (19).

Mitral and tricuspid allografts are also intended to overcome the disadvantage of limited lifespan of stented pericardial and porcine bioprostheses, Stent-mounted tri-leaflet valves are prone to cusp-tearing, and often develop calcium deposits (46, 47). Because of this, bioprostheses are used mostly when the life expectancy of the patient matches that of the valve. The medical profession is now looking at allografts as potentially more promising valve substitutes.

Another reason the idea to replace diseased valves with allografts has been resuscitated is the recent upsurge in the number of drug-habit induced endocarditis which brought the issue, especially the matter of tricuspid valve transplantation, into the foreground again. At some institutions right-sided endocarditis now constitutes more than half of all infectious cases managed (34). While medical treatment is effective in most patients, a considerable number of them still require removal and replacement of the infected valve. Allografts are supposed to be more resistant to infection than mechanical valves or bioprostheses.

Because of the above, within the past few years several important events occurred in the ongoing saga of atrio-ventricular unstented fresh allograft transplantation: 1) The report of Pomar et al. from Barcelona of tricuspid valve replacement in septic tricuspid endocarditis, 2) Kumar et al. and Acar et al. published experience with allograft mitral valve replacement (1–5, 24–26), and 3) The report of Acar et al. on combined tricuspid and mitral valve replacements using fresh allograft (1).

While the definition of allo (homo)-graft is very easy, the definition of unstented fresh allograft is not as easy as it sounds. To tell what is a "live" or "fresh" valve graft is complex, and in this regard, we refer the reader to appropriate chapters of this book.

In general, under "stent" we understand a device with prongs which maintains the shape of the grafted valve in a desired position. There are, however, several papers in which "unstented" valves are presented which contain Teflon or Dacron reinforcement. A number of authors who investigate "free" or "unstented" grafts, also support the leaflet edge of donor valves with pericardium or Teflon, reinforce the chordae with PTEE sutures, cover the tip of the papillary muscle with a PTEE patch, and then on top of everything, insert an annuloplasty ring – a picture which is certainly not that of a "natural" valve. While it is still called "unstented" or "free," in reality it should be defined as "supported." Naturally where the "support" ends and the "stent" begins is also anybody's guess.

The history of live, unstented tricuspid and mitral valve allografts reaches back into the 1950s and 1960s, when they were already transplanted both experimentally and clinically. Because of technical difficulties and poor late results, however, these attempts were abandoned and there was a nearly 20-year hiatus before the concept of mitral and tricuspid allo-transplantation was rejuvenated.

Now, we seem to have made a "full" historical circle, from our own modest animal experiments in 1952, when in temporary inflow occlusion, we transferred the atrio-ventricular valve apparatus from one animal into the other (36) to the present impressive clinical results in allo-grafting the tricuspid[6] and the mitral valves (1). It is interesting to note the many difficulties encountered *en route* which different authors tried to overcome with modifications of the technique and preservation which now seem to have been resolved merely by passage of progress in general cardiac surgery and improved understanding in repair of atrioventricular valves (51).

Replacement of the tricuspid valve with tricuspid and mitral allografts

Tricuspid allografts

The first experiments in orthotopic heart valve transplantation were done by us in 1952 (36, 37, 38). These studies involved the removal of the atrio-ventricular (tricuspid) valve and its replacement with a freshly obtained tricuspid allograft. The surviving 25 animals were observed for 1 month to 3.5 years. The allografts consisting of the valve leaflet, chordae tendineae and papillary muscle showed good hemodynamic function in 18 of the 25 animals. In the sacrificed dogs, some degree of scarring and thickening was found in all grafts. In three cases, the scarring was extensive and the valve was grossly distorted. In most of the animals, however, besides some degree of thickening and scar formation, the valves appeared to be good on visual inspection and were found to be hemodynamically well functioning Notably, the transplanted papillary muscle obtained from several long-term survivors appeared anatomically and histologically viable. Ideal conditions; no murmurs, right atrial pressure less than 5 mm/Hg, lack of calcification and only moderate scar tissue formation at the line of attachment and pliable valve leaflets were present in six animals, three of them observed for a period exceeding 3 years. (Figs. 1, 2).

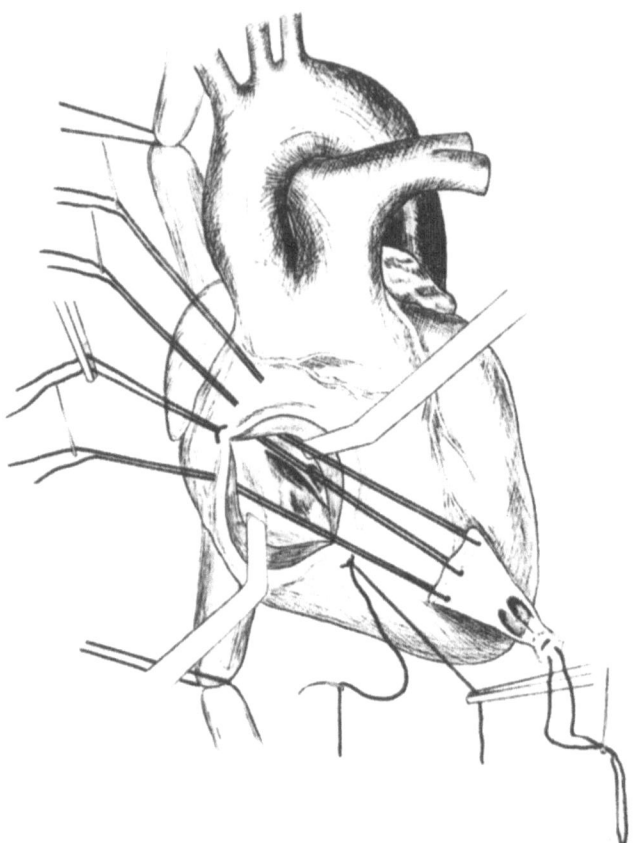

Fig. 1. Transplantation of the tricuspid valve (annulus fibrosus, leaflet, chordae tendineae and papillary muscle) into the right ventricle. (From Robicsek, *Orvosi Hetilap* 1953; 25: 1–8. Reprinted with permission.)

These experiments did not only prove that orthotopic allograft repflacement of atrio-ventricular valves was technically possible, but also laid down the principles which seem valid even today:

1) The allograft should contain all elements of the valvular apparatus, annulus, leaflet, chordae tendineae and papillary muscle.

2) It should be transplanted as early as possible following removal.

3) The transplantation should follow strict anatomical principles. The leaflets should be sutured meticulously to the host's annulus, the papillary muscle should be sutured to the stump of the host resected papillary muscle and this attachment should be assured by transmural fixation.

These studies also proved, in some cases anyhow, that the transplanted valves remain viable and properly functioning and that the transplanted myocardium (papillary muscle) as well as connective tissue (leaflets and chordae) may maintain viability for prolonged periods (36–40).

Experiments similar to ours were performed 4 years later by Pollock and Thomas. In the 10 animals observed for 6 to 7 months, they found healing of the host tissue to

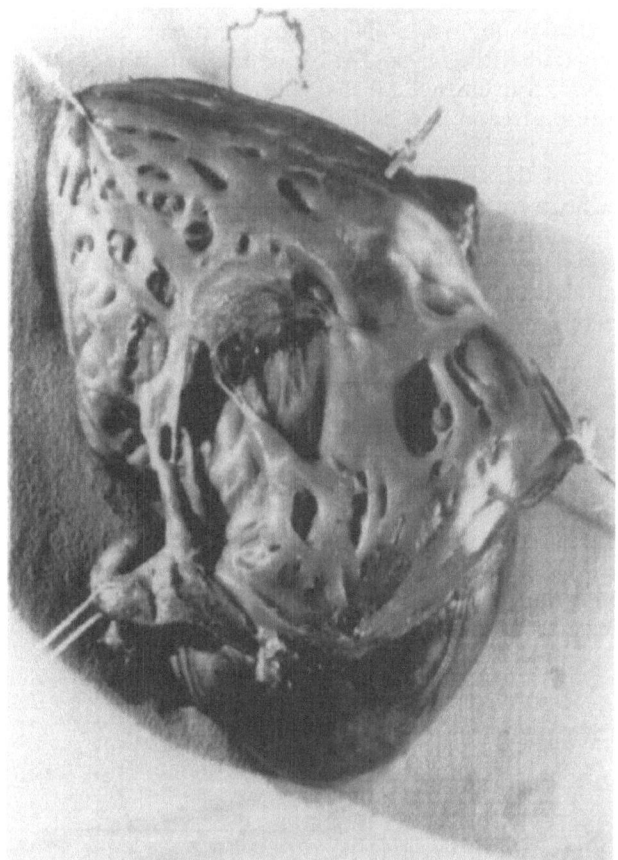

Fig. 2. The appearance of the transplanted tricuspid valve 3 years later. (From Robicsek, *Oroosi Hetilap* 1953; 25:8. Reprinted with permission.)

the grafted heart, but also considerable scarring of the leaflets (32). Transplantation of the tricuspid (as well as mitral) valves was performed by Hubka et al. in 1965 in 30 dogs using extracorporeal circulation. In the course of the experiments, the entire mitral valve was excised and transplanted into either mitral or tricuspid orifice, and fresh allograft mitral valves were put in the tricuspid and the mitral position in 12 animals, respectively. Tricuspid valve allografts were placed in the tricuspid position and mitral allografts into the mitral position in three dogs each. The survival of the animals varied from a few days to 2 years. Good healing of the allograft was found in several animals. They found that no immunobiological reactions were induced. Hubka et al. reiterated that "The homograft of the mitral valve must be thought of as an important functional unit; hence, homotransplantation included not only the leaflet of the valve, but also part of the fibrous annulus, chordae tendineae and part of the papillary muscle" (21, 22, 23).

In 1993, the tricuspid valve was successfully replaced in a 16-year old patient with infectious tricuspid endocarditis by Summa et al. using a fresh tricuspid allograft. The patient did well and showed satisfactory valvular function during the 6-month reported observation period (44).

Mitral allografts in tricuspid position

While some authors believe that *similis simile gaudet* (similar prefers similar) (10), tricuspid valves should be replaced with tricuspid valve homografts, based on anatomical considerations (48) and convenience (33, 34), mitral allografts have been recommended as better substitutes to replace both the mitral and tricuspid valves (Figs. 3, 4).

Pomar et al. in 1993 replaced the tricuspid valve with a cryopreserved mitral allograft in three patients who were HIV positive and had right-sided infective endocarditis, massive tricuspid insufficiency and uncontrollable bacterial or fungal infections (33). The report encompasses a 20-month follow-up period in the course of which two of the three transplanted valves showed "trivial" and one "moderate" incompetence. All the patients returned to active life without further evidence of endocarditis (34).

Replacement of the mitral valve

The mitral valve may be replaced either in part or entirely. Besides Hubka et al. (21–23), pioneering work in mitral valve allotransplantation was performed by Cachera et al (12) who in 1964 experimented with all types of mitral allografts including valve "patches", the replacement of anterior leaflets with the papillary muscle and chordae tendineae, as well as total mitral allograft transplants. While

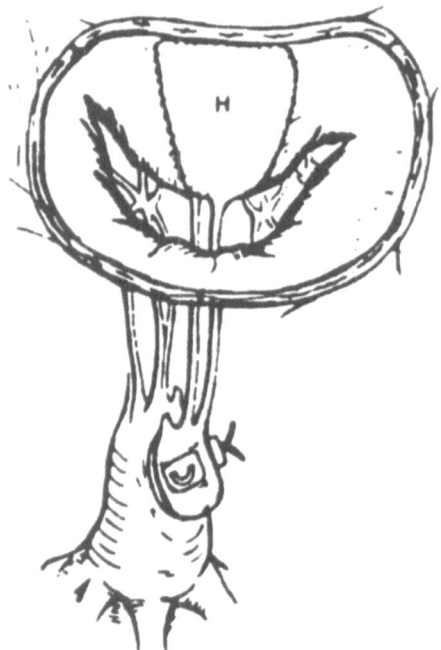

Fig. 3. Mitral allograft prepared for insertion. The posterior part of the annulus is reinforced with a strip of the recipient's pericardium. (From Pomar JL et al., *J. Heart Valve Dis.* Vol. 2, No. 2, March 1993. Reprinted with permission.)

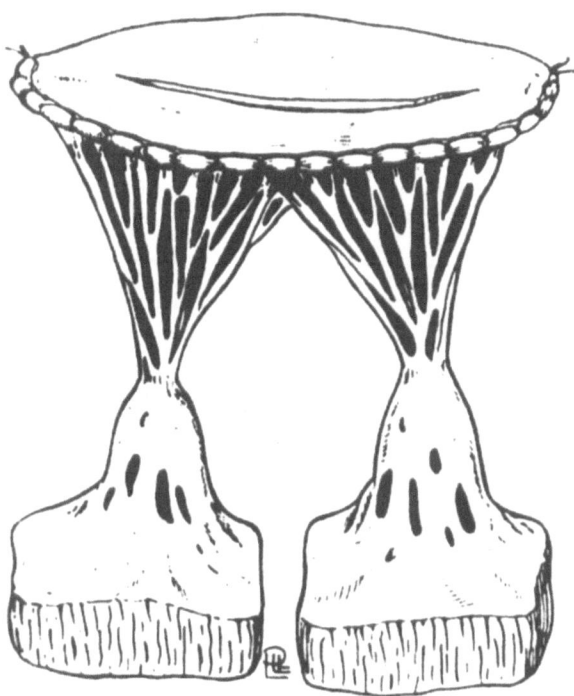

Fig. 4. Partial replacement of the posterior leaflet of the mitral valve allograft. (From Revuelta et al., *J. Thorac. Cardiovasc. Surg.*; Vol. 104, No. 8: 1974–8. Reprinted with permission.)

being somewhat reserved on the efficiency of complete mitral valve transplantation, Cachera et al. expressed the view that the method may be applicable clinically in the future (12) (Fig. 5).

In the late 1960s, there was an upsurge of experiments concerning allogenous mitral valve transplantation. O'Brien et al. (29), Van Vliet et al. (45) and Bernhard et al. (9) reported relatively good short-term results with mitral valve allografts. In 1969, Baird et al. (7) from the Toronto group presented extensive experiments which included mitral valve allograft replacements in dogs as well as in calves. The observation period of the animals was relatively short, and the late results discouraging; however, in a few cases they achieved good, long-term results with pliable valves and unruptured subvalvular apparatus (7).

In 1964, Berghuis and Rastelli using cardiopulmonary bypass transplanted the entire mitral valve apparatus in 17 dogs using fresh allografts. First, the valves were sutured to the donor's annulus in an inverted position, then the chordae and papillary muscles were reverted into the cavity of the left ventricle, to perform an end-to-end anastomosis between the donor and the host papillary muscle-stumps. The experiments were plagued with technical complications, but nine animals survived from 3 to 12 months with competent allografts. Bacterial endocarditis was the major cause of failure in the rest of the dogs. Their conclusions were that "homotransplantation of the mitral valve in the dog is feasible with low operative mortality and long-time survival...." and that morphologically the "death" of the graft and replacement of tissues of the host seemed to proceed slowly, resulting in a viable structure which preserved its shape and function of the valve for prolonged periods (8) (Fig. 6).

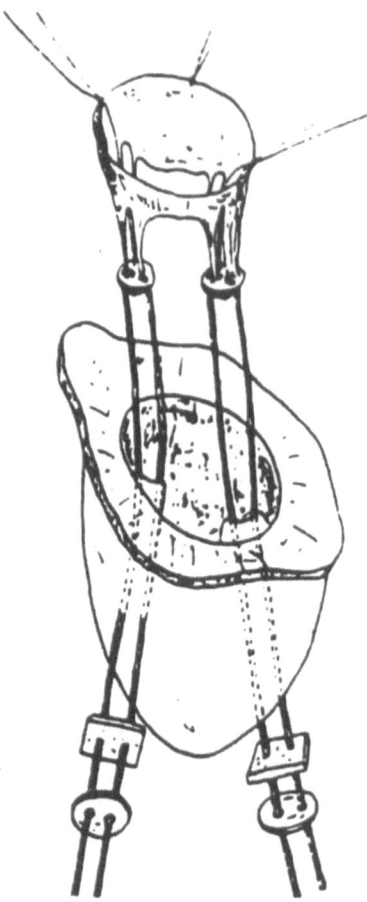

Fig. 5. Mitral homograft inserted in the tricuspid position. (From Pomar JL et al., *J. Heart Valve Dis.* Vol. 2, March 1993. Reprinted with permission.)

Pappas et al. from the Mayo Clinic also demonstrated excellent function extending as long as 6 years of experimentally transplanted mitral valve allograft. While in several animals the transplanted valve developed severe degenerative changes, in most of the dogs the graft functioned well and had close to normal anatomical appearance at autopsy. Their results were significantly better if the grafts were implanted fresh and the dogs were not treated with immunosuppressive drugs (31). The feasibility of partial transplantation of the mitral valve was also studied recently by Revuelta et al. in the sheep model. They excised a portion of the posterior mitral leaflet and replaced it with a fresh, anatomically identical donor structure in one group and with a cryopreserved allograft in another. During the follow-up of an average of 8 months, grafts of both groups showed equally good structural integrity but better cellular viability in the fresh valves (35).

Experiments emphasizing the advantages of stentless mitral allografts were also recently published by Vetter et al. They used cold stored valves implanted into weanling sheep. The grafts were anatomically considerably modified by sewing

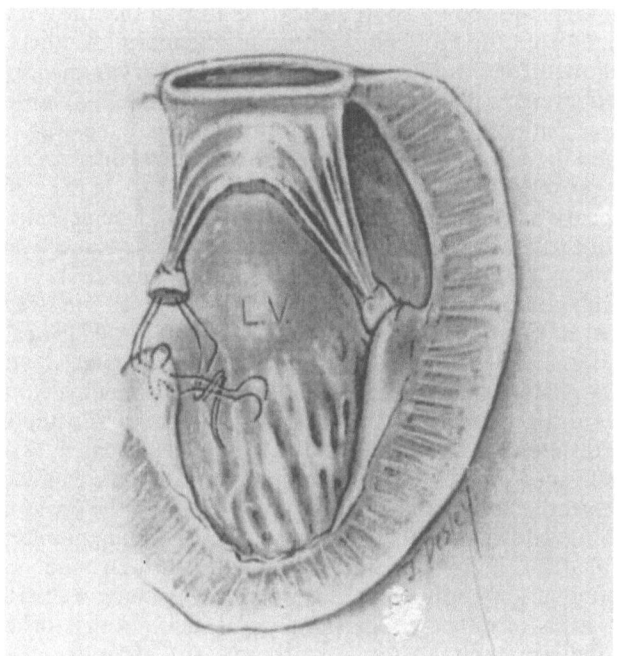

Fig. 6. Transplantation of the mitral valve apparatus with the papillary muscle-attachment is accomplished with the enhancing sutures tied on the epicardial surface. (From Bernhard et al., *Thoraxchirurgie*, 1965; 13: 89–95. Reprinted with permission.)

pericardium over the annulus margin, applying a PTFE patch over the papillary muscle and by reinforcing the native chordae tendineae with PTFE sutures. They documented reasonably good hemodynamic function in the seven survivors and concluded that "this new design of mitral allograft shows excellent *in vivo* echocardiographic behavior after 5 months of implantation; therefore, human allografts of this type could be recommended for clinical application" (46, 47).

While the study of Vetter et al. is quite valuable, their conclusions may have gone too far, considering the relatively short time of their follow-up. Also, it needs to be emphasized that the authors suggest "allograft of this type," which specifically refers to their technique. Considering that the chordae are the most vulnerable part of the graft valve apparatus, one may wonder if they were testing the durability of the transplanted chordae or the PTFE sutures.

The first clinical report of mitral allograft transplantation is that of Senning et al. (9, 42) in 1967 with good short-term results.

Additional clinical experience and late results of the Zurich group were reported in 1975 by Huber et al. Between 1966 and 1969 mitral valve allographs were inserted in 11 patients into mitral and in two patients in the tricuspid position. Three patients died in the perioperative period, eight allografts in the mitral and one in the tricuspid position functioned well. Four allografts had to be replaced later because of progressive deterioration of the allografts and four continued to function well 4 to 6 years after the implantation (20). The discouraged Senning concluded his second report: "*Because of the poor durability of the results, this method of mitral valve replacement is not used any more*" (20).

The work of Senning et al. was followed by sporadic articles during the late 1960s and early 1970s. In 1973, Ohta, from the Hokkaido University School of Medicine, reported two patients with follow-up of 18 and 26 months respectively in whom viable unstented mitral vlve allografts were implanted (30). Sievers et al. in Kiel implanted allograft mitral valves in three patients with isolated mitral stenosis. One was re-operated 2 months after surgery because of sudden onset of severe mitral insufficiency thought to be due to technical error (43). The later report of Yankah et al. of the same patients mentions that the other two eventually had to be reoperated as an emergency, because of acute valve failure due to chordae rupture, 9 and 44 months later respectively due to endocarditis in one and papillary muscle detachment in the other (51).

Mitral allograft valve transplantation has been revived by Vrandecic et al. in Brazil (49) in 1992 and by Kumar et al. in New Delhi in 1994 (24). The latter reported the case of a patient with recurrent mitral stenosis whose valve was excised and replaced with a fresh mitral allograft. The papillary muscles were treated with glutaraldehyde and anchored to the myocardium using pericardial "slings." Six week follow-up report showed good postoperative results (24–26). Partial mitral valve replacement with a mitral allograft was also performed on a 42-year-old man with intractable endocarditis by Dossche et al. in 1994. At the time of the operation, two-thirds of the posterior leaflet of the donor valve with its chordae and the tip of the corresponding papillary muscle was removed and replaced. The post-operative follow-up showed moderate mitral regurgitation 1 year after surgery; otherwise, this patient was doing well (18).

The largest contemporary series of mitral allograft transplantation is that of the present leading propagators of this method, Acar et al. working with Carpentier at the Hôpital Broussais (1–5). Their present technique includes cryopreservation of the donor mitral valve or storage in a solution containing dimethyl-sulphoxide and the insertion of an annuloplasty ring. The latter thought is essential because it permits molding of the native mitral annulus to the size of the donor valve and also reduces the traction on the donor mitral annulus in position and increases the area of the surface of coaptation of the mitral leaflets, thereby reducing the tension on the subvalvular apparatus.

The recent report of Acar et al. includes a total of 32 patients. Fourteen have received total homograft replacement of the mitral valve while 18 have undergone partial replacement. One patient died as a result of intractable left ventricular failure and one patient required re-operation on the 10th postoperative day for partial dehiscence of the annular suture line. The remaining 30 patients had good functional results. At a mean follow-up of 12 months, they showed stable clinical and echocardiographic results remain stable (1) (Fig. 7).

Acar et al. also reported the first "double" (mitral and tricuspid) transplantation using mitral allograft in both the mitral and the tricuspid position in the same patient in 1994 (1–5). The unique experience of using a heterograft mitral valve instead of a valve of human origin was discussed by Morea et al. (28). His studies using stentless, porcine mitral valve, by and large, presented unsatisfactory function and failed early.

Storage and handling

As we see today, the main question regarding allotransplantation of atrio-ventricular valves remains durability which probably has to do less with technical aspects than

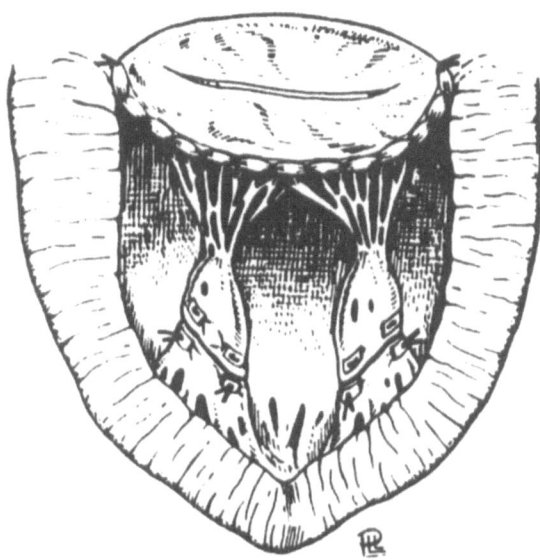

Fig. 7. Double mitral homograft in mitral and tricuspid positions. Note the rotated mitral homograft in the tricuspid position. Carpentier ring annuloplasty has been performed using a rotated prosthetic ring of the mitral type. (From Acar et al., *J. Heart Valve Dis.*, Vol. 3, No. 5, September 1994. Reprinted with permission.) Different methods of fixation of the papillary muscles.

with the way we handle the allografts. The clinical superiority of one method of storage against the other is still lacking.

We have yet to define what is a "fresh," allograft and how many days can it be regarded as "fresh?" Probably not more than a week! Different materials intended to preserve the graft, such as nutrients or antibiotics, may also influence the concept of "freshness," too. Also, is a cryopreserved graft really "fresh?" A frozen then thawed apple could not be sold as "fresh" in the grocery store! Does antigenicity play a role? (29, 31, 50) Do "life" homografts benefit by immuno-suppressive therapy? These questions still await answers.

In the early 1950s, we studied (36–40) the long-term viability of freshly transplanted tricuspid allografts and found some of them, including the papillary muscle, "live" after several years of follow-up. Similar studies on mitral allografts have also been carried out recently by Revuelta et al. (35) who observed good incorporation of the implanted mitral homograft in the recipient valve and noted that the subvalvular apparatus also retained its original flexibility and length. In histo-biological studies they demonstrated that viable cells from the recipient valve grow into both fresh and cryopreserved mitral homografts and are later covered with new endothelium. Just as Berghuis et al. (8), Revuelta et al. also observed organized dense collagen tissue in the implanted homograft, but no signs of degeneration (35).

At present, the question of best storage method remains unsettled. Acar et al. (1–5) use cryopreserved valves while Kumar et al. (24–26) and Yankah et al. (50, 51) prefer fresh allograft stored at 4 °C. Past studies strongly discourage the usage of im-munosuppressive agents and, as far as we know, nobody applies them today in conjunction with mitral and tricuspid allografts (31). At the present time, with the exception of Yankah et al. (50, 51), no other authors consisder ABO compati-bility.

It took two decades to give half-acceptable answers to the above questions with raortic allografts. It might take some time to do the same with atrioventricular valves.

Technique

It is evident that before we can determine the expected long-term freedom of structural deterioration of the different components of mitral and tricuspid allografts, we have to be sure that we have already eliminated valve-related failure due to surgical technical mishaps (51).

The technique of implantation of a valve homograft into the atrioventricular position is more difficult than a similar procedure in an aortic or pulmonary position. Duran's recommendation that only surgeons well versed in mitral valve repair should undertake tricuspid and mitral valve allotransplantation is certainly well taken (19).

The process of implantation may involve the entire valve or part of it. Success of the operation will grately depend on appropriate recognition of leaflet geometry, proper matching of the annulus size, and the establishment of the appropriate tension (not too much, not too little) of the chordae tendineae. The limited clinical experience available already highlights some very important technical features: 1) The necessity of accurate sizing of the annulus and proper orientation of the graft; 2) The secure attachment of the edge of the donor valve-leaflets to the host's annulus; 3) Decide the necessity and if it appears to be advisable, modify the shape and/or mechanically stabilize the allograft in its new position; 4) Establishment of the proper length and appropriate alignments of the subvalvular apparatus; and 5) Secure papillary muscle anastomosis.

The selection of the proper size allograft could be difficult even in the aortic position (50), but while in semilunar allografts, one may be inclined to select a somewhat smaller size than the aortic annulus, in cases of atrioventricular allografts, it is advisable to choose one which is somewhat larger than that of the host to assure appropriate leaflet adaptation (1–5). This increases the problem of graft availability because most of the time large sizes (30–36 mm) are required, and also grafts with multiple papillary muscle heads must be discarded (10).

If one implants tricuspid or mitral allografts the orientation should mimic the original anatomy as much as possible. If, however, we place a mitral valve into the tricuspid orifice, the matter is different, because the architecture of the valves is comparable but not identical.

In the tricuspid position, Pomar et al. (33, 34) place the mitral allograft according to its previous orientation in the left ventricle. The Carpentier school rotates it so that anterior leaflet faces the septum so as not to occlude right ventricular outflow tract (1–5). They also argue that because in most cases, mitral allograft implantation are being done for mitral regurgitation induced by annular dilatation; one may expect the same process to continue even after implantation of the allograft and recurrence of mitral incompetence may easily recur. To prevent this in both tricuspid and mitral position as final stage of the procedure, a mitral annuloplasty ring of appropriate size should be utilized (naturally, of the Carpentier design) (1). The data of Kunzelman et al. (27) also suggests that ring-reinforced atrioventricular homografts may last longer. The presence of the annuloplasty ring, however, may not fit the definition of "free" allograft, but according to Munich terminology, it may more properly be called a "supported" valve. Also, one may certainly argue whether the ring supports the annulus or supports the valve.

This view regarding the annuloplasty ring is not generally accepted (24–25, 26, 33, 34) and some even believe that it defies one of the purposes of unstented allograft transplantation, i.e., to preserve the physiologic motion of the annulus (52). Yankah et al. recommend (52) that in some cases "ringless" annuloplasty should be used in connection with allograft implantation. One may rightly argue, however, that if the mitral orifice is so distorted, if such an intervention appears to be necessary; the patient may fare better with a mechanical prosthesis or a bioprosthetic valve rather than with an allograft. In 1974, Dalichau et al. from Hannover presented an annuloplasty ring with arms extended in the cavity of the left ventricle designed to "hold" the valve in position and make the fixation to the papillary muscles unnecessary. One could really call it a "stent" (16).

The limited experience suggests that while dehiscence of the donor leaflets of the hosts' annulus is a frequent occurrence in the early experiments, it does not represent a major problem anymore (19). It still remains a matter of some concern, however, because the free edges of the allograft leaflets are quite flimsy and the suture which attaches it to the host annulus may cut through and could lead to leaflet detachment. To prevent this, Vetter et al. (46, 47) and Kumar et al. (24–26) recommend that for reinforcement a strip of pericardium should be sewn around the annulus margin. Duran also suggests that the same may be accomplished by leaving a "skirt" of atrium on the donor annulus to buttress the suture-line (19).

In the rearrangement of the subvalvular apparatus the primary concern is how to measure the proper chordal length to avoid both the leaflet prolapse and abnormal leaflet retraction. There is disagreement among authors as to exactly how to select the leaflet and papillary muscle attachment (1–4, 28, 49) to assure proper position of the allograft. As Cosgrove recently called attention to it, surgeons so far have failed to develop a systemic method for locating the proper points of implantation to be widely adopted, and "unless researchers refocus their attention to this point, the results will be less than acceptable" (15).

Durability

The main problem of replacement of atrioventricular valves with fresh allografts is their durability, which in contrast to glutaraldehyde preserved biografts, probably depends on the continued tissue viability. The Achilles heel of the procedure appears to be the behavior of the choradae tendineae which may rupture causing late failure of the transferred homograft (51).

The reason why the chordae are the "trouble spots" of mitral allograft transplantation have been shown by all Al-Janabi et al. in 1973. Working in Donald Ross' laboratory with mitral valves presesrved in nutrient and antibiotic solution, they found that the viability of the chordae tendineae decreases much faster than that of the leaflets and papillary muscles, and they lose most of their vital functions after 24 h storage (6). Vetter et al. recommended that the chordae tendineae be reinforced with 5-0 PTFE sutures to prevent rupture, or serve as "stand-ins" to replace them if they indeed do (46, 47) (Figs. 8, 9).

In handling and anchoring the allograft valve, one must also realize that it must support the load of approximately 75 tons per day (7, 11). Also, with the beating of the heart, in every systole the size of the mitral orifice is reduced by 20 to 15% (7, 17). This combined stress requires that the grafted valve should be resilient as well as that the

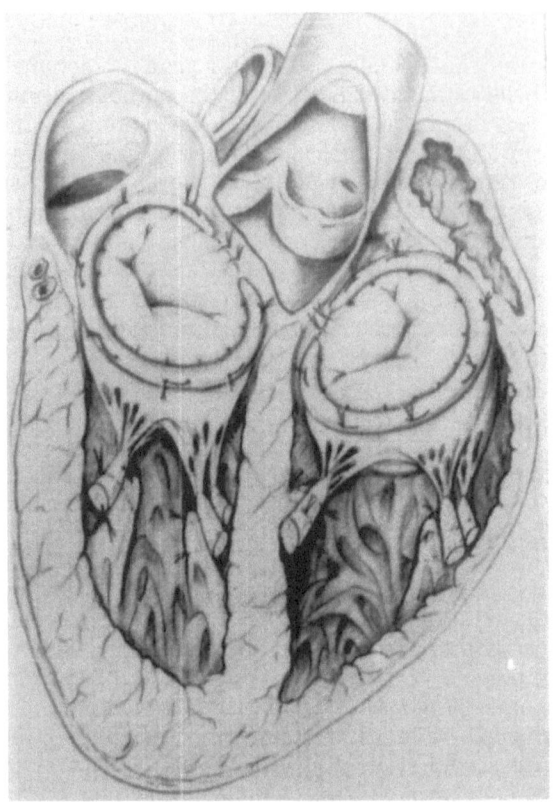

Fig. 8. Final securing of the papillary muscle. One papillary muscle has been attached. LV, *Left ventricle*. (From Beghuis et al., *Supplement to Circulation*. Vol. 29, April 64, Reprinted with permission.)

suture lines both at the annular and at the papillary muscle level should be strong. Compared to the annulus of the aortic valve which is formed of a thick layer of collagen, a much flimsier tricuspid and mitral annuli contain only a thin strand of collagen; thus, they are much less resistant.

As Baird et al. have emphasized, the papillary muscles, by supporting the mitral valve, transfer the force applied to the valve through the lateral ventricular wall; thus, secure attachment and preservation of papillary muscle function is already an important objective (7). Yankah et al. believe that the graft papillary muscle which is of dubious viability at the time of the insertion is incorporated into the host papillary where it becomes fibrotic, and with all probability eventually calcifies. Therefore, the shock-absorbing capacity of the subvalvular apparatus decreases while the load of tension remains constant" (51). To some degree, we disagree with this statement because in our original experiments we found that if the allograft transfer is done immediately, the papillary muscle may indeed survive for many years (36–40).

For the above reasons the transplanting surgeon must realize that the papillary anastomosis is a "delicate part of the procedure" (1) and "should be given special attention" (51). In their earlier paper, Acar et al. (1–5) recommended that the papillary muscle should be dipped in 0.6% glutaraldehyde solution for 45 min (2–4) to increase its resilience. They later abandoned this technique (1).

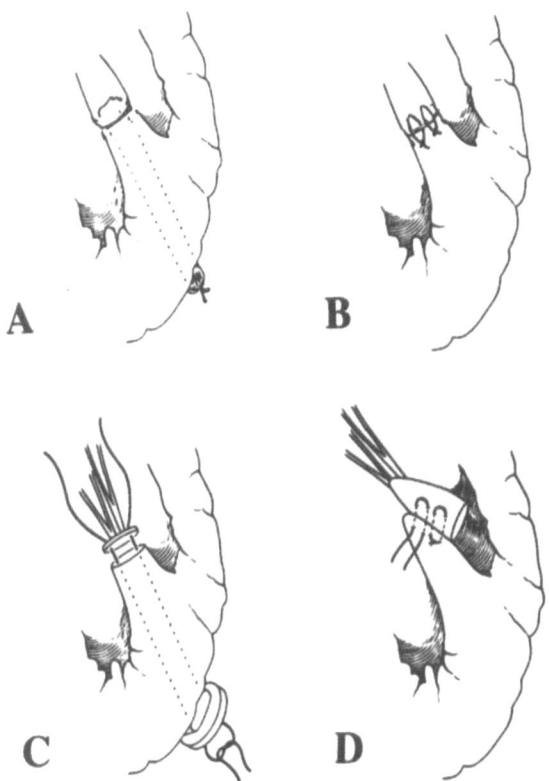

Fig. 9. Different methods of fixation of the papillary muscles.

The above problems have been addressed by different authors throughout the years. As far as the matter of papillary muscle attachment is concerned, we (36–40), as well as later others (19, 29, 42, 90), have recommended that the suture(s) anchoring the donor papillary muscle be driven through the stump of that of the host's and the entire width of the ventricular myocardium and tied on the epicardial surface over a buttress. Others suggested different alternatives such as simple end-to-end anastomosis of the papillary muscle (18) or side-to-side anastomosis between the appropriate papillary muscles using a double row of unpledgeted, interrupted, non-absorbable, monofilament 5-0 sutures, starting with the posterior papillary muscle (1). Based on the study of three clinical late failures, Yankah et al. (51) now agree that the attachment of papillary muscle site should be securely supported by transmural fixation (36) and that the chordae be reinforced (14, 46, 47, 52). To solve the "papillary muscle problem," Vetter et al. also recommended that a PTEE patch of 0.4 mm thickness should be placed over the truncated papillary muscle tip of the host to reinforce the attachment of the papillary muscle of the homograft (46, 47) (Fig. 10).

One may wonder that in favorable anatomical situations, consideration may be given to retain the host's papillary muscle and chordae tendineae together with a distal rim of the leaflet and limit the transplantation to the leaflets only attaching them to the annulus of the host on one side, and to the rim of the distal remnant of the host's mitral valve containing the edge of the leaflet with the host's chordae shortened on the other. This transfer of the line of transplantation from the base of the donor

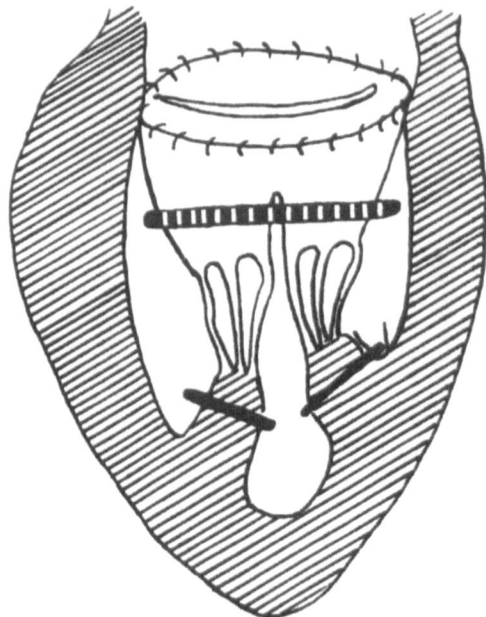

Fig. 10. The lower line of the graft-attachment if the entire valve (solid line) or only the leaflets are transplanted (dotted line).

papillary muscle to slightly above the leaflet-chordae junction may solve the problem of chordae and papillary muscle durability.

Indications

Because of the still existing uncertainty regarding the durability of atrioventricular unstented allografts, the indication for their usage is far from being firmly established. Some of their principal advantages such as low thrombogenicity are also shared with bioprostheses which have well-proven durability up to 6–8 years. The main advantage of allografts, i.e., a relatively high resistance to infections has been implied, but never proven conclusively.

Additional reasons mentioned by Acar et al. (1) for mitral allograft replacement include severe calcification of the host's mitral leaflets, extensive destruction of the valve apparatus in cases of acute bacterial endocarditis, especially with calcareous vegetations or with acute valvular abscess formation (1). In such patients the abnormal portion of the valve may be excised together with associated sub-valvular apparatus, and the defect repaired with suitable portion of the mitral homograft (1).

Chauvaud et al., also from the Carpentier group, most recently reported the case of a 17-year-old girl with severe mitral incompetence and hemodialisis due to renal insufficiency caused by systemic lupus erythematous. She was successfully treated with a cryopreserved mitral allograft. At 1 year after surgery echocardiographic study revealed mild leaflet-thickening, but good valve function (13).

Again, to give a more definite answer regarding indication in the future, we will have to first clear the matter of durability. Therefore, we believe that at the present time there is only one solid indication for the application of unstented fresh allograft in the atrio-ventricular position: that is to replace the destroyed tricuspid valve by septic endocarditis which fails to respond to conservative measures. Such a situation may exist especially in intravenous drug addicts who not only infect by maintaining their drug habit, but keep reinfecting their valve.

Treating such a situation with allograft implants is multifold: 1) The atrio-ventricular valve allograft, while statistically not proven, theoretically appears to be the valve substitute most resistant to severe infection; 2) If there is a residual dysfunction of the transplanted valve, moderate to medium regurgitation is usually well tolerated in the tricuspid position; 3) Even if there is acute massive failure of the allograft in the tricuspid position, it is usually not as disastrous as when it occurs in other valve orifices.

In the relatively short period of recent atrio-ventricular allograft "renaissance," we are still left with a number of controversial issues: 1) Gludaraldehyde fixation of the papillary muscle (1–5), 2) Routine use of annuloplasty ring (1–5), 3) Reinforcement of chordae tendineae with PTFA sutures (46, 47), 4) Extending the size of the allograft with an atrial skirt (19), 5) The usage of fresh, preserved by conventional ways and cryopreserved homografts (1–5, 10, 24–26, 46, 47), 6) The method of attachment of the papillary muscle to the myocardium (1–5, 33, 34, 36–40, 46, 47). Well conducted experiments such as by Vetter et al. (46, 47) are rare, and even those are limited to a relatively small number of animals and a relatively short follow-up observation.

We are definitely in need of further studies both experimental and clinical, and in that particular order. These studies should involve groups large enough in numbers as well as long-range hemodynamic and clinical monitoring and detailed post-operative results. Most data presently available encompass but a few months; thus, they should be regarded as relevant, but certainly not conclusive. The initial attempts at unstented allograft transplantations of the tricuspid and mitral valves in the 1950s and 1960s were characterized by the desperate search for a valve substitute to alleviate an otherwise hopeless situation. Now it is different. We have to compare the results of this method not to the conservatively treated disease process, but to the gold standards of mechanical and bioprosthetic valves. While modern technology gives us a much better chance of success than what the earlier investigators had, it also puts on our shoulder a much higher responsibility.

Until reliable late results can be obtained, initial clinical studies, as we stated, should be limited to a few centers. Even in these, strict protocol should be established as far as the indication is concerned, and if the study is done for clinical research purposes only, it should be assured that informed consent of the patients is obtained.

By providing an appropriate forum to investigators and assuring a virtually immediate exchange of ideas and results, some of our speciality journals played a major role of calling attention to this very important new field of cardiac surgery. These early reports were also wisely balanced by several cautious editorials by some of the most respected experts in the field of cardiac valve surgery (10, 15, 19).

Now, however, we have come to a stage where the "let's get on the band-wagon" attitude should be eliminated. While we indeed need to know events regarding unstented mitral and tricuspid homografts as soon as possible, this could be accomplished by holding frequent informal workshops. Reports claiming advantages of the method should be accepted only if they relate to: 1) Sufficient number of patients, 2) An observation period of appropriate length, and 3) Present proof of uniformity in the group, especially regarding the storage and handling the valve.

Summary

Allotransplantation of unstented fresh (or preserved "live") atrio-ventricular (especially mitral) valves in the tricuspid and mitral position appears to be a method with high biological and clinical potential with the promise of better flow characteristics, less thrombogenicity, and probably more resistance to infection than other devices used for valve replacement.

The disadvantages of the method include: 1) A taller "learning" curve, and in general more surgical experience that what is needed for implementation of mechanical or bioprosthetic valve, 2) More difficult availability.

The main reasons at the present why one may also advise against wider application of this promising method: 1) Most of the experimental work done on this subject is now historical and even then atrio-ventricular allografts showed a high failure rate in most of the animals; 2) There is a scarcity of newer experimental research work regarding durability; 3) The entire clinical material which is available for study is limited to a handful of patients; even in those, the storage method of the valves was not uniform and the follow-up period has been short.

The above questions, especially valve durability, cannot yet be clarified. The method of allotransplantation of unstented mitral and tricuspid valves should be confined to a few institutions, and their general introduction, as of today, does not appear to be justified with the exception of tricuspid endocarditis resistant to other methods of treatment.

Further long-range experimental and clinical research in this field is mandatory.

References

1. Acar C, Gaer J, Chauvaud S, Carpentier A (1995) Technique of homograft replacement of the mitral valve. J Heart Valve Dis 4: 31–4.
2. Acar C, Deloche A, Farge A, et al. (1994) Partial and total replacement of the mitral valve using a cryopreserved mitral homograft. Eur Heart J 15 (abstr suppl): 230.
3. Acar C, Deloche A, Farge A, et al. (1994) A new surgical approach in acute mitral valve endocarditis: partial or total replacement using a mitral homograft. Circulation 90: I–I310.
4. Acar C, Farge A, Ramsheyi A, et al. (1994) Mitral valve replacement using a cryopreserved mitral homograft. Ann Thor Surg 57: 746–8.
5. Acar C, Iung B, Cormier B, Grare P, Berrebi A, D'Attellis N, Acar J, Carpentier A (1994) Double mitral homograft for recurrent bacterial endocarditis of the mitral and tricuspid valves. J Heart Valve Dis 3: 470–2.
6. Al-Janabi N, Ross DN (1973) Viability of fresh mitral homograft valves. Thorax 28: 293–4.
7. Baird RJ, Williams WG, Spratt EH, Cohoon WJ (1969) Experimental homograft replacement of mitral valve. Canad J Surg 12: 144–54.
8. Berghuis J, Rastelli G, Van Vliet V, Titus JL, Swan HJC, Ellis FH (1964) Homotransplantation of the canine mitral valve. Circulation 29(Suppl I): 47–53.
9. Bernhard A, Ringdal R, Babotai I, Linder E, Kroyenbuhln HP, Senning A (1965) Zur Homotransplantation der mitrolklappe. Technik und postopertivoe and funktionelle resultate. Thoraxchirurgie 13: 89–95.
10. Bodnar E (1994) Editorial: Clinical use of homologous and heterologous mitral valves. J Heart Valve Dis 3: 468–469.
11. Burch GE, DePasquale NP (1965) Time-course of tension in papillary muscles of heart. JAMA 192: 117–20.
12. Cachera JP, Salvatore L, Hermant J, Herbinet B (1964) Reconstruction plastiques de l'appareil mitral chez le chien au moyen de valves mitrales homologues conservees. Ann Chir Thorac Cardiovase 3: 459–474.

13. Chauvaud S, Kolangos A, Berrebi AJ, Gaer JAR, Acar C, Carpentier AF (1966) Systemic lupus erythematosus valvulitis: Mitral valve replacement with homograft. Ann Thor Surg 60: 1803–5.
14. Cochran RP, Kunzelman KS (1991) Comparison of viscoelastic properties of suture versus porcine mitral valve chordae tendineae. J Card Surg 6: 508–13.
15. Cosgrove DM (1993) Editorial: Mitral homograft for tricuspid valve replacement. J Heart Valve Dis 2: 124.
16. Dalichau H, Timm D, Waertel G, Lübbing H (1974) Mitralklappen – Totalrekonstruktion mit freien Transplantaten. Experimentelle Untersuchungen. Thoraxchirurgie 22: 355–9.
17. Davis PKB, Kinmonth JB (1963) The movements of the annulus of the mitral valve. J Cardiovasc Surg (Torino) 4: 427.
18. Dossche K, Vanermen H, Wellens F (1994) Partial mitral valve replacement with a mitral homograft in subacute endocarditis. Thorac Cardiovasc Surg 42: 240–2.
19. Duran CMG (1995) Mitral valve allografts. An opportunity. Editorial, J Heart Valve Dis 4: 29–30.
20. Huber R, Rothlin M, Senning A (1975) Spatresultate nach Atrioventrikularklappenersats mit Mitralallotransplantat. Thoraxchirurgie 23: 33–8.
21. Hubka M (1965) Homotransplantation of cardiac valves. Folia Biol Praha 11(4): 324–7.
22. Hubka M, Siska K, Brozman M, et al. (1966) Replacement of mitral and tricuspid valves by mitral homograft. J Thorac Cardiovasc Surg 51: 195–204.
23. Hubka M, Siška K, Holec V (1967) Replacement of the mitral valve with an aortic valve homograft implanted into the left atrium. J Thorac Cardiovasc Surg 53: 260–7.
24. Kumar AS, Trehan H (1994) Homograft mitral valve replacement. A case report. J Heart Valve Dis 3: 473–5.
25. Kumar AS, Chander H, Trehan H (1995) Surgical technique of multiple valve replacement with biological valves: A new option. J Heart Valve Dis 4: EDITOR, UPDATE!.
26. Kumar N, Gallo R, Al-Halees Z, Al-Fadley F, Duran CMG (1995) Unstented semilunar homograft replacement of tricuspid valve in Ebstein's malformation. Ann Thorac Surg 59: 320–2.
27. Kunzelman KS, Cochran RP, Verrier ED, Eberhart RC (1994) Anatomical basis for mitral valve remodeling. J Heart Valve Dis 3: 491–6.
28. Morea M, de Paulis R, Galloni M, Gastaldi L, de Summa M (1994) Mitral valve replacement with the Biocor stentless mitral valve: Early results. J Heart Valve Dis 3: 476–82.
29. O'Brien MF, Gerbode F (1964) Homotransplantation of the mitral valve. Preliminary experimental report and review of the literature. Aust and New Zealand J of Surg 34: 81–8.
30. Ohta S (1973) Late results of valve replacement with biological grafts. Nippon Kyoto Geko 5: 499–509.
31. Pappas G, Titus JL, Berchuis J, McKenzie MB, Ellis FH Jr (1966) Dog mitral valve homografts and heterografts. Surg Forum 17: 175–6.
32. Pollock AV, Thomas V (1965) Replacement of tricuspid valve cusp by a homologous cusp in dogs. Surg Gyn Obst 103: 731–5.
33. Pomar JL, Mestres CA (1993) Tricuspid valve replacement using a mitral homograft. Surgical technique and initial results. J Heart Valve Dis 2: 125–8.
34. Pomar JL, Mestres CA, Pare C, Miro JM (1994) Management of persistent tricuspid endocarditis with transplantation of cryopreserved mitral homografts. J Thorac Cardiovasc Surg 107: 1460–3.
35. Revuelta JM, Cagigas JC, Bernal JM, Val F, Rabasa JM, Lequerica MA (1992) Partial replacement of the mitral valve by homografts: An experimental study. J Thorac Cardiovasc Surg 104: 1274–9.
36. Robicsek F (1953) Szivbillentyu-apultetes. Orvosi Hetilap 25: 1–8.
37. Robicsek F (1954) Cardiac Valve Transplantation. Acta Medica Hung. 1–2: 81–91.
38. Robicsek F, Sanger PS, Taylor FH, Robicsek L (1962) Transplantability of heart valves. Arch Surg 84: 141–8.
39. Robicsek F (1986) First experiments on orthotopic heart valve transplantation–in Biologic Bioprosthetic Valves. Endre Bodnar and Magdi Yacoub eds. Yorke Med Group. London.
40. Robicsek F (1994) The application of biological tissues in cardiac valve surgery. The history of the first two decades. J Heart Valve Dis 3: 613–26.
41. Ross DN (1967) Replacement of aortic and mitral valves with a pulmonary autograft. Láncet 2: 956–8.
42. Senning A, Largiader F (1967) Homologe Transplantation von Mitralklappen beim Menschen. Transplantatbeschaffung und erste Anwendungen. Med. Mitt. (Melsungen) 41: 79–84.

43. Sievers HH, Lange PE, Yankah AC, Wessel A, Bernhard A (1985) Allogeneous transplantation of the mitral valve. An open question. Thorac Cardiovasc Surgeon 33: 227–9.
44. Summa M di, Donegani E, Zatlera G, Pansini S, Morea M (1993) Successful orthotopic transplantation of fresh tricuspid valve homograft in a human. Ann Thor Surg 56: 1407–8.
45. Van Vliet PD, Titus JL, Berghuis J, Ellis RH Jr (1965) Morphologic features of homotransplanted canine mitral valves. J Thor and CV Surg 49: 504–10.
46. Vetter HO, Dagge A, Liao K, et al. (1995) Echocardiographic evaluation of a stentless allograft mitral valve with chordal support implanted in the sheep. J Heart Valve Dis 4: EDITOR, UPDATE.
47. Vetter HO, Dagge A, Liao K, Erhorn A, Chryssagis K, Strenkert C, Reichart B (1995) Mitral allograft with chordal support: Echocardiographic evaluation in sheep. J Heart Valve Dis 4: 35–9.
48. Victor S, Mayak V (1994) Transplantation of atrioventricular valves. (Letter to the editor.) Ann Thor Surg 58: 1212.
49. Vrandecic M, Gontijo BF, Fantini FA, et al. (1992) Anatomically complete heterograft mitral valve substitute: Surgical technique and immediate results. J Heart Valve Dis 1: 254–9.
50. Yankah AC, Hetzer R, Miller DC, Ross DN, Somerville J, Yacoub MH (Eds) (1988) Cardiac valve allografts 1962–1987: Current concepts on the use of aortic and pulmonary allografts for heart valve substitutes. Springer-Verlag, New York.
51. Yankah AC, Sievers HH, Lange PE, Bernhard A (1995) Clinical report on stentless mitral allograft. J Heart Valve Dis 4: 40–4.
52. Zussa C, Polesel E, Da Col U, Galloni M, Valfré C (1994) Seven-year experience with chordal replacement with expanded polytetrafluoroethylene in floppy mitral valve. J Thorac Cardiovasc Surg 108: 37–41.

Authors' address:
F. Robicsek, MD
Surgeon-in-Chief
The Sanger Clinic, PA
1001 Blythe Boulevard,
Site 300
Charlotte, NC 28203
U.S.A.

Concluding remarks and prospects

A. C. Yankah

German Heart Institute Berlin, Berlin, Germany

The use of aortic valve allograft dates back to the experimental work of Heimbecker and Murray in the 1950s. Orthotopic implantation, i.e., sub-coronary insertion of the aortic allograft was demonstrated to be feasible in the animal laboratory by Gunning and Duran in 1962. Subsequently, Ross and Barratt-Boyes independently and successfully used this operation technique clinically to replace diseased aortic valves in June and August of the same year respectively. Ever since, the aortic valve allograft and, since 1983, the pulmonary allograft have become the accepted biological valve substitutes for diseased aortic valves, especially for infective endocarditis with annular abscesses, small and congenitally distorted aortic root and obstructive right ventricular outflow tract. Aortic and pulmonary allograft valves have now become an important part of the cardiac surgeon's armamentarium.

For many years guidelines and standards for quality control of allografts were based on limited scientific studies, and clinical experience of cardiac surgeons, tissue bankers and researchers working in this field therefore were poorly defined and formulated. After the International Allograft meeting in Berlin in 1987, continuing efforts have been made to formulate and establish guidelines and standards for procurement, preservation and viability of allograft valves which were practically nonexistent. In 1990, several meetings were conducted to this effect in USA between the Federal Drug and Food Administration (FDA) and American Association of Tissue Banks (AATB), and in Europe between the Commission of the Europe Community and several allograft banks in Europe, in order to harmonize guidelines for quality control of donor valves and to ensure safety of allograft valve recipients and ethical standards. There are many European governments which have issued a section in their code on human tissue which is similar to the standard operating procedures issued by the European Association of Tissue Banks (EATB) and AATB. Some parts of the AATB standards are even legally required by FDA for tissue bank accreditation, whereas those of the EATB are not enforced by law yet, with the exception of Belgium and France. Parker in London has stressed the continuing efforts which have been made by Association of Tissue Banks in Europe and the USA to develop and implement guidelines and standards to protect the recipients of allograft valves.

With regard to the definition of viability and fate of allograft valves, extensive studies have been done by Armiger and Barratt-Boyes in Aukland, Dawson and Brockbank from CryoLife in Atlanta, Hopkins and co-workers in Washington, DC, Yankah in Kiel and Berlin, and Feng in Antwerp to define cold and warm ischemia and critical time and temperature for allograft harvesting to cryopreservation. Now, difficulties of harvesting and preservation have been largely overcome. Cryopreservation seems to represent a distinct advance in preservation, while viability still remains an issue without consensus.

It is now well recognized that the clinical results and durability of cryopreserved aortic allografts might not only depend on the viability and quality of the tissue alone, but also on age at implantation, specific implantation techniques (including valve selection and evaluation of appropriate size for patients) and immunologic factors.

In the 1990s a debate began regarding the optimum implantation technique to achieve the best allograft valve durability in aortic position. This controversial topic on freehand subcoronary aortic valve and root replacement was highlighted and discussed at the Vancouver meeting in 1994 between Barratt-Boyes, O'Brien and Ross and Angell.

The important factor has been spelled out in the recent editorial comments by Barratt-Boyes and Yankah in the Journal of Heart Valve Disease of 1994 and 1996, respectively, as well as by Ross and Yacoub elsewhere, that the success of a allograft implantation, especially the freehand subcoronary technique, is dependent on knowledge, skill, implantation technique and experience of the implanting surgeon.

The aortic root replacement and reimplantation of the coronary arteries was initially developed and clinically applied by Ross for reconstruction of a tunnel type left ventricular outflow tract obstruction. This technique is now used for treating a destroyed infected aortic root. Ross has indicated in the foreword of the book that, after many years of clinical experience, the freestanding aortic root appears to be the surgical technique of preference. His recommendation is being supported by Yacoub in London, Clarke in Denver and Yankah in Berlin. The advantage of this surgical technique is that an appropriate adult size allograft can be used to match the native root particularly in a child without creating an early gradient across the valve and ventricular impairment. The child can grow to an adolescent age for a definite second valve substitute. In this book Yacoub, Yankah and Clarke discussed the medium term results and experience. In the clinical analysis factors favoring and opposing the use of subcoronary aortic valve implant and root replacement have been spelled out.

The technique of subcoronary implantation and root replacement with cryopreserved and homovital aortic allografts in the recent series of O'Brien in Brisbane, Yankah in Berlin, and Yacoub in Harefield and London provided identical early and mid-term results. In the same series subcoronary implant in adult patients <40 years of age have shown excellent medium term durability and hemodynamic performance providing evidence that long-term outcome with a meticulous subcoronary implantation technique was comparable to that with the aortic root replacement technique. If one compares Barratt-Boyes' results using 4.0 °C stored homografts with the series of O'Brien and co-workers using cryopreserved valves, as well as data of Langley and co-workers over 21 years of observation, the rates of reoperation after freehand subcoronary implantation are identical. These results demonstrate that the controversial risk factor for postoperative valve incompetence with this implantation technique can be minimized with patient selection and surgical perfection.

With regard to operative treatment of acute endocarditis Haydock in Aukland, Petrou and Yacoub in Harefield and London, and Yankah in Berlin have analyzed their clinical experiences and concluded that the aortic allograft valve is the valve substitute of choice for replacing infected aortic valve and prosthesis with annular abscessess because it heals well in place and has a very low incidence of reinfection. Oswalt in Texas, and Joyce and Petersen in Denmark even prefer pulmonary autograft for replacing the infected aortic valve because it is a viable, nonantigenic tissue which has the potential to grow. Whether this surgical therapeutic concept holds for endocarditis remains yet to be evaluated in a multicenter study. Freestanding root replacement is a preferred technique for annular destruction with abscess formation because in comparison , to subcoronary implant technique the incidence of pseudoaneurysm formation is minimum and nonexistent in Yankah's series.

The limitations of these two implantation techniques are also identical; the subcoronary implanted valve and root do not have any potential to grow and possibly some immunologic reaction cannot be excluded with either. These shortcomings may be overcome with the use of pulmonary autografts in selected patients. The aortic valve and root replacements with pulmonary autografts were pioneered by Ross in 1967 in London, but became unpopular among many cardiac surgeons because of high rate of morbidity due to coronary artery septal injuries during harvesting of the pulmonary autograft. The operation has been recently revived after being discredited for many years and is currently an undisputable alternative valve substitute in children because it has a potential to grow. The acceptance of this operation technique is also due to the improvement of harvesting the pulmonary autograft and implantation techniques and distinct knowledge in the configurations and distributions of the network of the septal and the first diagonal coronary arteries. A chapter on pulmonary autograft as an alternative valve substitute to allograft valves by Sievers in Kiel and Lübeck, Daenen in Leuven, Oswalt in Austin, Petersen in Denmark, Melo in Lisabon, and Metras in Marseilles is included in this volume. The authors' experiences underscore the benefits of this alternative operation method thus the increasing popularity and acceptance of this operation technique among pediatric cardiac surgeons of today.

The determinant factors for long-term durability and performance of cryopreserved aortic and pulmonary allografts are viability, valve and conduit size, age at operation and histocompatibility. Yankah and co-authors, Clarke and co-authors, as well as Meissner from the German Heart Center in Munich, demonstrated in their recent analysis of cryopreserved aortic and pulmonary allografts in the pulmonary circulation in children lower rate of early wall calcification and valve dysfunction in pulmonary allografts ($p < 0.05$) as compared to aortic allografts. The findings were also congruent with those reported by Monro and co-workers in Southampton. The results have confirmed and proved the importance and effect of orthotopic implantation of viable and larger size allografts in the pulmonary circulation (as a priviledged site), hence the pulmonary allograft is the preferential valve for reconstruction of the RVOT in children.

During the Berlin meeting in 1987, allograft mitral valve replacement was neglected as a subject for the oral presentation, it was only mentioned in the panel discussion by Barratt-Boyes, Yacoub, and Dr. Angell. Robiscek has rightly querried the omission of this special topic, although the global interest was patchy, episodic and without consensus. The operation methods were not well defined and this has been confirmed by Duran in his recent editorial comments in the Journal of Heart Valve Diseases.

In 1966, Senning in Zürich undertook to use mitral allograft for the replacement of diseased mitral and tricuspid valves, while Ross (1969) preferred to use pulmonary autograft and Yacoub (1969) top hat aortic allograft to replace the mitral valve. The operation methods were terminated with the exception of the top-hat technique, until when at least six groups in the world, Bernhard in Kiel (1985, 1994), Revuelta in Santander (1992), Vrandecic in Belo Horizonte (mitral heterograft 1992), Pomer and Mestres in Barcelona (1993), Acar in Paris (1994) and Kumar and Duran in Riyadh (1994), redeveloped the surgical technique including valve sizing, determination of graft length, suturing technique of papillary muscle union site and echocardiographic assessment of chordae-papillary alignment.

Revival of the operation recently was encouraged by intensive laboratory experimental work and great clinical experience in mitral valve reconstructive surgery by Carpentier and Acar as well as Pomar and Mestres. The mitral valve allograft and its subvalvular apparatus is known to possess sophisticated structures with sophisticated functions and therefore has to be viable and has the potential to maintain its viability, thus long-term function. This subject is still debatable, nonetheless, Yankah has been developing information concerning the immunologic aspects and modes of failure and the use of immunosuppression to maintain viability. Yacoub and Angell as well as Barratt-Boyes still regard the allograft stented valves to be the best valve in the mitral position in children and have used them for that purpose. It does not calcify early and they have patients in whom the stented allograft valves have lasted for 10–15 years.

With regard to immunogenicity of allografts, Hoekstra in Rotterdam, Yacoub and Johnson in Harefield, Melo in Lisabon, Simon in Kiel, and Schütz in Munich have demonstrated and confirmed in their in vivo experimental studies in humans the previous animal experimental studies Yankah (1985) in Kiel and Lupinneti in Ann Arbor (1991) on humoral and cellular immune response after implantation of cardiac valve allografts. So far these findings have not been translated into clinical practice although there is some experimental evidence shown by Yankah that the use of a short-course immunosuppression in allograft valve implantation might achieve tolerance.

Lastly, the improved preservation technique of arterial allograft has now allowed and encouraged revival of the former surgical concept of allograft arterial reconstruction pioneered by Dubost in Paris in 1952, which was associated with aneurysmal dilatation and calcification. Vogt in Zürich, Mestres and Pomer, Kieffer in Paris and Hetzer and Yankah in Berlin have been pursuing this concept with cryopreserved arterial conduits for treating infected synthetic graft of both abdominal and thoracic aorta as well as mycotic aneurysms using a short-term antibiotic therapy after operation as opposed to long-term postoperative antibiotic therapy and inherent risk of reinfection with synthetic grafts.

In summary, this book has brought together the current important knowledge and information on clinical and scientific homograft valve surgery.

Guidelines and standards for allograft cardiac valves are now established for cardiac surgeons, homograft bankers. Cryopreservation represents a distinct advance in preservation of allograft valves and maintainance of structural integrity without viable cells.

If one anticipates growth of an allograft valve with viable cellular components this can be achieved under immunosuppression of the host or under conditions of tolerance. Structural and cellular viability of allografts with regard to harvesting time and temperature has not been properly defined and needs to be established. Time of harvesting to cryopreservation and presence of quantitative number viable of cellular components will determine the strength of postimplant immune response and fate of the allograft. Young recipient age, small size and short allografts, malperfusion of nutritive vessels and maldiffusion of allograft vascular wall have been recognized to be determinant and risk factors for early allograft failure. Irrespective of the latter risk factors the pulmonary allograft, by virtue of its anatomical structure, appears to be more durable than the aortic allograft in the pulmonary circulation.

Freehand subcoronary aortic valve implant has comparable medium term results compared to that of root replacement technique if it is properly inserted.

To this effect meticulous implantation technique is mandatory and therefore requires proper tutorial guidance involving selection and evaluation of appropriate allograft size for recipient's annulus during the learning curve.

The limitations of the two methods are identical, i.e. the subcoronary implanted valve and the root do not have any potential to grow and the possibility of some immune response cannot be excluded with either. Adult size homografts are to be used since they do not have the potential for growth. These shortcomings may be overcome with the use of pulmonary autografts in selected patients.

The mitral allograft with its sophisticated structure and function demand specific implantation techniques. The revival of its use in the mitral and tricuspid position is justified, however, it demands perfect implantation and immunological understanding, especially with regards to viability and growth when this operation is going to be done in children and adolescents.

Prospects

A standard protocol for allograft harvesting, i.e. retrieval time and temperature to cryopreservation needs to be defined in order to define different grades of viability.

Standard methods for processing have to be established in view of selective elimination of cellular components of allovital valves.

In situations where growth of allografts is required a standard protocol would be useful for the use of histocompatible allovital valves either under or without the application of immunosuppression.

Parallel to the prospective randomized multicenter study a second protocol will compare the durability of pulmonary autografts with homovital allografts in aortic position with and without immunosuppression. Schütz and co-workers in Munich have developed and established the Cytoimmunological Monitoring (CIM) method for detecting and monitoring clinically the immune response after allograft valve implantation. The CIM might be a useful investigative tool for such randomized multicenter studies on mitral, aortic and pulmonary allografts.

A prospective, randomized multicenter study might be the appropriate method to assess and compare the two implantation techniques, the freehand subcoronary valve implantation and root replacement.